SBA and MTF MCQs for the Final FRCA

SBA and MTF MCQs
for the Final FRCA

The FRCAQ.com Writers Group

The Severn Deanery

Dr James Nickells
North Bristol NHS Trust

Dr Ben Walton
North Bristol NHS Trust

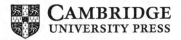

CAMBRIDGE
UNIVERSITY PRESS

University Printing House, Cambridge CB2 8BS, United Kingdom

Cambridge University Press is part of the University of Cambridge.

It furthers the University's mission by disseminating knowledge in the pursuit of education, learning and research at the highest international levels of excellence.

www.cambridge.org
Information on this title: www.cambridge.org/9781107620537

© Cambridge University Press 2012

First published 2012

A catalogue record for this publication is available from the British Library

Library of Congress Cataloguing in Publication data
Nickells, James.
SBA and MTF MCQS for the final FRCA / James Nickells, Benjamin Walton.
p.   ;   cm.
ISBN 978-1-107-62053-7 (pbk.)
I. Walton, Benjamin.   II. Title.
[DNLM: 1. Anesthesia – Examination Questions.   WO 218.2]
617.9´60076–dc23

2012032422

ISBN 978-1-107-62053-7 Paperback

. . . .

Contents

Contributors

The FRCAQ.com Writing Group for the Final FRCAQ.com site are:

DR ROBERT AXE MBChB, FRCA, Anaesthetic Trainee, Severn Deanery, Bristol, UK

DR EMMA BELLCHAMBERS MRCP, BMBS(Hons), BMedSci(Hons), Anaesthetic Trainee, Severn Deanery, Bristol, UK

DR JAMES BOWLER MA(OXON), MBBS, AICSM, Anaesthetic Trainee, Severn Deanery, Bristol, UK

DR TIM BOWLES BSc(Hons), MBBS, FRCA, Senior Registrar, Intensive Care Unit, Royal Perth Hospital, Western Australia

DR ALICE BRAGA MBChB(Hons), MRCP, FRCA, Anaesthetic Trainee, Severn Deanery, Bristol, UK

DR JULES BROWN BSc, MBChB, MRCP, FRCA, DICM, FICM, Consultant in Critical Care and Anaesthesia, North Bristol NHS Trust, Bristol, UK

DR HELEN CAIN BMBS, BMedSci, FRCA, Anaesthetic Trainee, Severn Deanery, Bristol, UK

DR AMY CREES BSc(Hons), MBChB, MRCP, Core Medical Trainee, Severn Deanery, Bristol, UK

DR ALIA DARWEISH MBChB, MSc, DRCOG, MRCS(Eng), FRCA, Anaesthetic Trainee, Severn Deanery, Bristol, UK

DR JAMES EVANS MBChB, MRCP, FRCA, Anaesthetic Trainee, Severn Deanery, Bristol, UK

DR TOBIAS EVERETT MBChB, FRCA, Consultant Anaesthetist, The Hospital for Sick Children, Toronto, Canada

DR ANDREW FOO BSc(Hons), MBBS, MRCS, FRCA, Anaesthetic Trainee, Severn Deanery, Bristol, UK

DR DAN FRESHWATER-TURNER MA, MBBChir, MRCP, FRCA, Consultant in Anaesthesia and Intensive Care, University Hospitals, Bristol NHS Foundation Trust, Bristol, UK

DR ANDY GEORGIOU MBChB, BSc(Hons), FRCA, DICM DIC, Consultant in Critical Care and Anaesthesia, Royal United Hospital, Bath, UK

DR JUAN GRATEROL Medico Cirujano, FRCA, Anaesthetic Trainee, Severn Deanery, Bristol, UK

DR BEN GREATOREX BMBS, BMedSci, FRCA, Anaesthetic Trainee, Severn Deanery, Bristol, UK

DR RUTH GREER BMBS, BMedSci, Anaesthetic Trainee, Severn Deanery, Bristol, UK

DR CLARE HOMMERS BMBS, MRCP, FRCA, DICM, Anaesthetic Trainee, Severn Deanery, Bristol, UK

DR TIM HOOPER MBBS, FRCA, EDIC, Anaesthetic Trainee, Severn Deanery and Defence Medical Services, Bristol, UK

DR TIM HOWES MBChB, FRCA, Anaesthetic Trainee, Severn Deanery, Bristol, UK

DR BEN HUNTLEY MBChB, FRCA, Consultant in Pain Medicine and Anaesthesia, Barking, Havering and Redbridge NHS Foundation Trust, UK

DR IZREEN IQBAL MBChB, FRCA, Anaesthetic Trainee, Severn Deanery, Bristol, UK

DR DOM JANSSEN BA, BSc(Med), MBBS, FRCA, Anaesthetic Trainee, Severn Deanery, Bristol, UK

DR IAN KERSLAKE BSc(Hons), FRCA, Anaesthetic Trainee, Severn Deanery, Bristol, UK

DR EMMA KING MBChB, FRCA, Anaesthetic Trainee, Severn Deanery, Bristol, UK

DR SIOBHAN KING FRCA, MRCP, MBBCh, BSc(Hons), Anaesthetic Trainee, Severn Deanery, Bristol, UK

DR SARAH LANCASTER MBChB, MRCS(Eng), Orthopaedic Trainee, Severn Deanery, Bristol, UK

DR ABBY LIND BSc, MBChB, MRCP, FRCA, Anaesthetic Trainee, Severn Deanery, Bristol, UK

DR CLINTON LOBO BSc, MBChB, MRCP, FRCA, Anaesthetic Trainee, Severn Deanery, Bristol, UK

DR HELEN MAKINS MBBS, FRCA, Anaesthetic Trainee, Severn Deanery, Bristol, UK

DR CHRIS MARSH MBChB, FRCA, PG Cert Adv HCP, Anaesthetic Trainee, Severn Deanery, Bristol, UK

DR ALEX MIDDLEDITCH MBChB, FRCA, Anaesthetic Trainee, Severn Deanery, Bristol, UK

DR HENRY MURDOCH BSc, MBBS, FRCA, Anaesthetic Trainee, Severn Deanery, Bristol, UK

DR CHRIS NEWELL BSc(Hons), MBChB, MRCP(UK), Anaesthetic Trainee, Severn Deanery, Bristol, UK

DR JAMES NICKELLS MBBS, FRCA, Consultant Anaesthetist, North Bristol NHS Trust, Bristol, UK

DR SONJA PAYNE MD, MSc, BSc(Hons), Anaesthetic Trainee, Severn Deanery, Bristol, UK

DR ANNABEL PEARSON BMedSci(Hons), BMBS, Anaesthetic Trainee, Severn Deanery, Bristol, UK

DR KIERON ROONEY MRCP, FRCA, DICM, EDIC, PGCMEd, Consultant in Anaesthesia and Intensive Care, University Hospitals, Bristol NHS Foundation Trust, Bristol, UK

DR SOPHIE SCUTT FRCA, MRCP, Anaesthetic Trainee, Severn Deanery, Bristol, UK

DR SIMON SLINN BSc(Hons), MBBCh, FRCA, Anaesthetic Trainee, Welsh Deanery, UK

DR JANINE TALBOT MBBS, BSc ,FRCA, PGCMEd, Anaesthetic Trainee, Severn Deanery, Bristol, UK

DR HELEN TURNHAM MBChB(Hons), FRCA, Anaesthetic Trainee, Severn Deanery, Bristol, UK

DR BENJAMIN WALTON MBChB, MRCP, FRCA, Consultant in Critical Care and Anaesthesia, North Bristol NHS Trust, Bristol, UK

DR SARAH WARWICKER BM, BCh, MA, FRCA, Anaesthetic Trainee, Severn Deanery, Bristol, UK

DR MARK WIGGINTON MBBS, FRCA, Anaesthetic Trainee, Severn Deanery, Bristol, UK

DR MARK YEATES BM, FRCA, MRCS, Anaesthetic Trainee, Severn Deanery, Bristol, UK

Preface

You are currently holding a book containing 180 MCQ questions designed to help you revise for the written component of the Final FRCA exam set by the Royal College of Anaesthetists. The book provides two papers, each consisting of 90 questions, with 60 multiple true false questions (MTF) followed by 30 single best answer questions (SBA). The split of question topic areas covers all those tested by the College. These topic areas are basic sciences, medicine and surgery, intensive care medicine, clinical anaesthesia and pain medicine. The papers in this book have the correct ratio of questions from all these five disciplines and the correct proportion of SBAs and MTFs across these disciplines. For example, each paper has five SBAs in pain and five MTFs in pain as per the real Final FRCA paper. After the question papers, the second section of the book provides answers and explanations for the questions. Each question has both a short explanation that should allow the user to determine, at a glance, why they may have selected an answer incorrectly and a long explanation which provides more in-depth information on the topic area. The questions have been prepared by anaesthetists or experts in areas of tested knowledge who have either recently sat the Final FRCA or have been involved in training candidates for the exam. This book represents 180 question files from the highly popular and successful FRCAQ.com website. This website has over 2600 question files available, covering all areas of the Final FRCA syllabus. Access to the website is available with a subscription at www.FRCAQ.com.

It is our experience that candidates are still more comfortable and familiar with answering MTF questions compared to the SBA questions. SBAs were introduced in to the Final exam in September 2010 with the idea that they test an area of understanding at a higher level than an MTF question. Traditionally, MTFs have been used to test points of knowledge. They often have the structure of making a statement about a specific area and asking you whether it is true or false. You have a fifty:fifty chance of getting the answer right or wrong if you knew nothing and had a wild guess. A typical pass mark for an MTF component of the Final FRCA MCQ paper is 75–80%. The SBA section usually involves a clinical scenario followed by the candidate being asked to select a best option. For example, this may be 'Select the best management plan' or 'What investigation should you perform next?' In SBAs, typically most of the available options are interrelated and plausible; it's just that one of the options is best. The pass mark for the SBA component of the exam is typically 50–55%. This should allow the mathematically astute candidate to realise that on average you are not being asked to select the best answer. You are being asked to whittle the list of five options down to two and then have a guess between the last two. Rather than Single Best Answer questions, they could be called 'Discount the Least Good Three Answers' questions. In training people for sitting these questions, this mindset has allowed us to teach people a very useful tactic for approaching these questions. The key is to discount the more ridiculous options and try to pare the options down to a small group (ideally a group of one, but two or occasionally three is not a disaster). Once a smaller group has been identified, an educated guess within that group will usually be sufficient to achieve an adequate score. When we first heard the news that SBAs were being launched for anaesthetic exams we thought that the answers would have to be based on emphatic knowledge and therefore guessed that questions would be drawn from areas of anaesthesia in which firm guidelines existed (such as resuscitation or the management of anaphylaxis). Subsequently it seems that this has not been the case, with the College content to examine areas in which controversy or differences of opinion occur. The criterion for determining the 'correct' answer is based on what the majority of a group of experienced anaesthetists would choose. The controversial nature of the SBA content and the fact that only 20% will be scored by wild guessing means that a user getting over 55% on this section of the paper is doing extremely well.

Each part of an MTF question counts for one mark in your final score. Sixty questions with five marks available for each contributes 300 marks to the final score. Four marks are given for each correct SBA question, so 30 questions contributes 120 marks to the final total of 420 available marks. If the pass mark for the SBA paper is around 50–55% and for the MTF section is 75–80%, the combined pass mark is usually around 70%.

Our general advice for using this book would be, in the first instance, to try to sit the two papers under as close to exam conditions as possible. Following an initial attempt at the questions, a review of the explanations will not only act as a revision aid, but also give some insight into how and why questions are set. If using this book has proved valuable, please come and visit us at www.FRCAQ.com, where we have nearly fifteen times the amount of content in this book for you to explore.

Good luck – and we look forward to seeing you at www.FRCAQ.com soon.

James Nickells and Ben Walton
Editors, FRCAQ.com

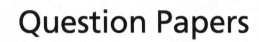

Question Papers

Paper 1

MTF Question 1

With regard to measurement of humidity, which of the following statements are correct?

a) Most instruments measure absolute humidity
b) Regnault's hygrometer has a silver tube containing ether
c) Absolute humidity can be measured by transducers
d) The hair hygrometer works on the principle that hair shortens as humidity increases
e) The wet and dry bulb hygrometer relies on the cooling effect by loss of latent heat of vaporisation for its function

MTF Question 2

Which of the following statements regarding ketamine are true?

a) Ketamine causes analgesia through its activity at opioid receptors
b) NMDA receptor antagonism is the main mechanism of ketamine effect
c) Ketamine blocks the release of glutamate in the CNS
d) Ketamine blocks activity at muscarinic receptors in the central nervous system
e) Like all general anaesthetic agents, ketamine has activity at the $GABA_A$ receptor

MTF Question 3

Causes of hypokalaemia include:

a) Pyloric stenosis
b) Villous adenoma of rectum
c) Conn's syndrome
d) Theophylline poisoning
e) Renal tubular acidosis

MTF Question 4

The physiological features of severe anorexia nervosa include:

a) Cardiomyopathy
b) Proteinuria
c) Bradycardia

d) Gastric dilation
e) Panhypopituitarism

MTF Question 5

Regarding the use of targeted temperature management after cardiac arrest:

a) The ideal target temperature is 30 °C
b) J waves are a common finding on the ECG of a patient at 31 °C
c) At the end of the cooling period, passive rewarming should be allowed
d) A heart rate of 38 beats per minute when the patient's temperature is 32 °C is an indication for rewarming
e) Shivering should preferentially be treated with a non-depolarising neuromuscular blocking drug (NMBD)

MTF Question 6

Regarding gabapentin, which of the following statements are true?

a) Gabapentin is an agonist at the γ-aminobutyric acid $(GABA)_A$ receptor
b) Gabapentin is metabolised by the CYP3A4 isoenzyme
c) Gabapentin is available in a transdermal drug delivery patch
d) Gabapentin can be used for the treatment of acute pain
e) Gabapentin enhances the action of morphine

MTF Question 7

Regarding the neuromuscular junction:

a) The synaptic cleft is 5 nanometres wide
b) There are 10 acetylcholine receptors for every molecule of acetylcholine released in a conducted impulse
c) Nerve fibres converge on the motor end-plate of the muscle fibre
d) The terminal portion of the motor neurone is unmyelinated
e) Prejunctional acetylcholine receptors have the same morphology as the postjunctional ones

MTF Question 8

Regarding the porphyrias:

a) They are rare acquired disorders of haem biosynthesis
b) They are rare genetic disorders of haem breakdown
c) Acute intermittent porphyria presents with neurovisceral crises and cutaneous manifestations
d) Urine porphobilinogens are not raised between attacks in acute intermittent porphyria
e) Treatment of an acute attack includes a low-carbohydrate diet

MTF Question 9

Regarding urinary tract infection:

a) Gram-negative organisms are usually involved
b) It rarely causes sepsis
c) More than 100 000 organisms/mm^3 on urinary microscopy is significant

d) Urinary catheterisation is rarely associated
e) Treatment should include urinary catheterisation

MTF Question 10

Which of the following statements regarding pharmacology in renal failure are true?

a) In acute kidney injury (AKI), the loading dose of a drug which undergoes excretion via the renal tract may need to be increased
b) The commonest reason for AKI caused by aminoglycosides is that they cause an interstitial nephritis
c) Imipramine is a cause of obstructive (post-renal) AKI
d) Acetazolamide is a cause of obstructive (post-renal) AKI
e) When using ketamine for analgesia, the dose should be reduced in patients with AKI

MTF Question 11

Regarding the role and location of central chemoreceptors in the control of breathing:

a) The central chemoreceptors are located near the dorsal surface of the pons
b) Central chemoreceptors respond rapidly to changes in carbon dioxide tension in the blood
c) Central chemoreceptors respond rapidly to changes in oxygen tension in the blood
d) The pH of cerebrospinal fluid is slightly acidic compared with plasma
e) Respiratory acidosis causes a greater increase in ventilation than metabolic acidosis

MTF Question 12

With regard to the cardiovascular complications associated with obesity, which of the following statements are correct?

a) Renal blood flow is increased in obesity
b) Cardiac arrhythmias can be caused by fatty infiltration of the conduction system
c) Obese individuals have an increased cardiac output predominantly due to an increased heart rate
d) Absolute blood volume is increased
e) Systemic hypertension is 2 times more prevalent than in the non-obese population

MTF Question 13

With regard to critical care outreach services (CCOS), which of the following are true?

a) There is no evidence that it reduces the number of patients who have received cardiopulmonary resuscitation (CPR) prior to ICU admission
b) There is strong (level 1A) evidence that it reduces ICU mortality
c) CCOS was introduced into the NHS without formal prospective evaluation processes
d) Early warning scores may form part of the track and trigger approach
e) Education of ward staff and junior doctors commonly forms part of its remit

MTF Question 14

Which of the following are true of hyperosmolar non-ketotic coma (HONK)?

a) It is the same as hyperosmolar hyperglycaemic state

b) It is more common in type 1 diabetes than in type 2 diabetes
c) It presents with a mild ketosis
d) It presents in the absence of coma
e) Severe hyperglycaemia causes a functional thrombocytopenia

MTF Question 15

Which of the following are recognised treatment options used in confirmed cyanide poisoning?

a) Dicobalt edetate
b) Hydroxocobalamin
c) Gastric lavage
d) Sodium nitroprusside
e) Sodium thiosulphate

MTF Question 16

Functional residual capacity (FRC):

a) Can be measured using Fowler's method
b) Is the sum of the residual volume and the expiratory capacity
c) Is a fixed volume
d) Exceeds the closing capacity in the elderly
e) May be reduced by restrictive lung disease

MTF Question 17

Which of the following statements are true regarding Turner syndrome?

a) Patients often suffer from menorrhagia
b) Common clinical features include short stature
c) It only affects females
d) Mental retardation is common
e) Coarctation of the aorta occurs in 10% of patients

MTF Question 18

Regarding psychological techniques in pain management:

a) There is no evidence to support psychological support in chronic pain patients
b) Psychological management is helpful to cure chronic pain conditions
c) Cognitive behavioural therapy challenges maladaptive thinking patterns
d) Encouraging patients to pace their activity facilitates coping with chronic pain
e) Psychological techniques encourage malingering behaviour

MTF Question 19

Which of the following statements regarding community-acquired pneumonia (CAP) are true?

a) A chest radiograph is necessary to make the diagnosis
b) Urea and electrolytes (U&E) offers important prognostic information

c) The white blood cell (WBC) count is an important prognostic determinant in non-immunosuppressed patients
d) *Staphylococcus aureus* is the most common causative organism
e) Macrolides should be discontinued in patients admitted to intensive care if the atypical pneumonia screen is negative

MTF Question 20

The following are true of the use of clonidine in critical care:

a) It is predominantly a postsynaptic α_2-adrenoreceptor agonist
b) It has an oral bioavailability approaching 100%
c) On starting the medication it may cause initial, short-lived, hypertension
d) It can be stopped abruptly without a reducing dosage regime
e) It is the first-line treatment for agitation in a recently extubated patient with traumatic brain injury and established acute alcohol withdrawal

MTF Question 21

Regarding current religious rulings and cultural attitudes to brainstem death in the UK, which of the following statements are true?

a) It is considered *haraam* (forbidden) for Muslims to become heart-beating organ donors
b) Orthodox Jewish law, *Halacha*, accepts brainstem death as comparable to cardiorespiratory death
c) *Shariah* (Islamic) law representatives in the UK consider brainstem death to be a true definition of death
d) Buddhist doctrine does not accept brainstem death to be a true definition of death
e) Brainstem death is still considered legal in the UK even if the patient's family reject the diagnosis on religious grounds

MTF Question 22

Concerning the pipeline medical gas supply to theatres:

a) Medical oxygen is supplied at a pressure of 4 bar via a white coloured hose
b) Air is supplied via a black and white hose at a pressure of either 4 or 7 bar
c) The pipeline gas distribution network upstream of the wall terminal outlets is made of reinforced PVC with an antistatic core
d) Each Schrader valve has a similar external diameter irrespective of the gas pipeline that ends at it
e) By law it must be possible to disconnect a hose from a Schrader valve using one hand only

MTF Question 23

Which of the following statements regarding local anaesthetics are true?

a) Ester and amide local anaesthetic agents have exactly the same mechanism of action
b) Local anaesthetic agents are weak acids
c) A local anaesthetic agent with a low pKa will have a fast onset of activity
d) Local anaesthetic agents only work after being 'trapped' inside nerve cells
e) Local anaesthetic agents preferentially bind to sodium channels in their open state

MTF Question 24

Which of the following statements about the intercostal nerves are correct?

a) The intercostal nerves contain sensory, motor and autonomic fibres
b) The intercostal nerves supply the skin over the sternum and over the spine
c) The intercostal nerves run between the internal intercostal muscle and the transversus thoracic muscle
d) Paravertebral block will provide adequate analgesia for a rib fracture
e) A chest drain should be inserted at the inferior aspect of the intercostal space

MTF Question 25

The following are features suggestive of carcinoid syndrome:

a) Diarrhoea
b) Hypertensive episodes
c) Facial flushing
d) Dementia
e) Wheeze

MTF Question 26

When performing an arterial blood gas, which of the following are true?

a) Excess heparin in the syringe will make the sample more acidic
b) Carbon dioxide levels are measured by changes in electrode pH
c) Air bubbles in the sample increase the carbon dioxide partial pressure
d) A pH of 7.4 is equivalent to 40 mmol/L of hydrogen ions
e) A sample kept at room temperature has a lower hydrogen ion concentration

MTF Question 27

Which of the following statements regarding the Glasgow Coma Scale (GCS) are true?

a) A decorticate response to stimulus will score 2 on the motor component
b) Moaning in pain will score 2 on the voice component
c) A sternal rub is an appropriate painful stimulus
d) With asymmetrical limb movement, the best limb should be scored for the motor component
e) The original Glasgow Coma Scale was scored out of 14

MTF Question 28

Which of the following cause a rise in end-tidal carbon dioxide?

a) Pulmonary embolism
b) Hypovolaemia
c) Hyperthermia
d) Sepsis
e) Flow rates of less than 150 mL/kg/min using a coaxial Mapleson D circuit during spontaneous ventilation

MTF Question 29

Regarding renin:

a) Renin is released from the macula densa in response to a decrease in circulating volume
b) Release is inhibited by angiotensin II
c) Sympathetic stimulation, via activation of α-adrenoreceptors, stimulates renin release
d) Release is stimulated by atrial natriuretic peptide
e) Renin directly stimulates the release of vasopressin

MTF Question 30

Regarding magnesium:

a) Magnesium is the second most abundant extracellular cation
b) Magnesium antagonises N-methyl-D-aspartic acid (NMDA) receptors in the central nervous system
c) The biggest stores of magnesium in the body are in the skeleton
d) Magnesium is a cofactor for Na^+/K^+-ATPase
e) Hypomagnesaemia may produce cardiac arrhythmias similar to those caused by hypokalaemia

MTF Question 31

With regard to the diagnosis and treatment of gestational hypertension:

a) Oral hydralazine should be commenced as first-line treatment
b) Gestational hypertension is defined as a sustained sitting blood pressure > 140/90 mmHg occurring after 20 weeks gestation
c) Gestational hypertension is defined as an increase in systolic blood pressure ≥ 30 mmHg or diastolic blood pressure ≥ 15 mmHg occurring after 20 weeks gestation
d) Oral labetalol at a dose of 50–100 mg twice daily is appropriate initial treatment unless there are contraindications
e) Amlodipine is an acceptable alternative to nifedipine to treat gestational hypertension

MTF Question 32

Regarding the cranial vault in a healthy adult:

a) The mass of a human brain is approximately 1000 g
b) Brain parenchyma occupies 85% of the cranial volume
c) Volume of cerebrospinal fluid in the cranial vault is 150 mL
d) Blood occupies 7% of cranial vault volume
e) Early compensation for raised intracranial pressure (ICP) includes reduced production of cerebrospinal fluid

MTF Question 33

Regarding pyloric stenosis:

a) It is more common in females
b) Metabolic acidosis is common
c) Surgery must be performed immediately upon diagnosis

d) It usually presents in the first week of life

e) Blood results typically show a hypokalaemic, hyperchloraemic metabolic alkalosis

MTF Question 34

Which of the following statements about desflurane are true?

a) Desflurane has a lower blood : gas partition coefficient than nitrous oxide

b) Desflurane increases the risk of haemorrhage during obstetric procedures

c) Desflurane increases respiratory secretions and may cause bronchospasm

d) Desflurane is likely to cause bradycardia if used at high concentrations

e) Desflurane requires a special vaporiser because it is unstable at room temperature

MTF Question 35

Regarding Duchenne muscular dystrophy (DMD):

a) DMD presents from early childhood and is progressive

b) DMD occurs equally in both sexes

c) Genetic counselling is recommended

d) Calf hypertrophy with lower motor neurone signs and restrictive lung function deficit are indicative of DMD

e) Diagnosis is confirmed by response to steroid therapy and plasmaphoresis or immunoglobulin infusion

MTF Question 36

Which of the following statements regarding the internal jugular vein are correct?

a) The internal jugular vein drains the sigmoid sinus

b) The internal jugular vein joins the subclavian vein posterior to the clavicle

c) The internal jugular vein begins at the foramen lacerum at the base of the skull

d) Horner's syndrome is a recognised complication of attempted cannulation of the internal jugular vein

e) The internal jugular vein is valveless

MTF Question 37

A 17-year-old girl is admitted to the emergency department with collapse following a 2-day history of vomiting. On examination she is slim, with patches of vitiligo. She is currently haemodynamically stable. Blood tests reveal sodium 129 mmol/L, potassium 6.9 mmol/L, urea 5.2 mmol/L, creatinine 89 µmol/L. ECG shows sinus rhythm with peaked T waves. Ideal initial management should include:

a) Intravenous hydrocortisone

b) Salbutamol nebuliser

c) Short adrenocorticotrophic hormone (ACTH) stimulation test

d) Calcium gluconate

e) Intravenous glucose and insulin infusion

MTF Question 38

Which of the following statements relating to an amniotic fluid embolism (AFE) are correct?

a) A maternal age of < 20 years makes the diagnosis of AFE more likely
b) A simple blood test can be performed to confirm the diagnosis of AFE
c) Pulmonary oedema leading to hypoxaemia is often seen in AFE
d) Coagulopathy is uncommon in AFE
e) The majority of cases occur in the immediate post-partum period

MTF Question 39

Regarding botulism, which of the following are true?

a) *Clostridium botulinum* is a Gram-negative anaerobic rod
b) Patients with botulism caused by wound infections should be treated with penicillin
c) Botulinum toxin blocks presynaptic release of acetylcholine
d) Patients present with flaccid paralysis and autonomic dysfunction
e) Botulinum antitoxin should be given to reverse the muscle weakness

MTF Question 40

Which of the following statements about the pharmacokinetics of drugs in patients following major trauma are correct?

a) Drugs administered via nasogastric tube have the same absorption kinetics as if they were taken orally
b) Hepatic enzyme activity is decreased following major trauma by the activity of pro- and anti-inflammatory cytokines
c) A patient anticoagulated with warfarin can expect to require a lower dose to maintain the same INR after major trauma
d) The volume of distribution of water-soluble drugs increases after major trauma
e) After head injury, brain levels of most drugs will increase

MTF Question 41

Regarding the impact of occupational, environmental and socioeconomic factors on critical illness:

a) Alcohol-related deaths are more frequent in males than in females
b) Patients from lower socioeconomic backgrounds have a higher incidence of obstructive sleep apnoea than the general population
c) Low socioeconomic status is associated with worse long-term survival after critical illness, after adjusting for effects of age, severity of illness and comorbidities
d) Patients with a history of drug dependence are at increased risk of delirium in intensive care
e) Where patients with alcohol dependence require supplemental enteral nutrition, protein restriction is recommended to reduce the risk of hepatic encephalopathy

MTF Question 42

Regarding human lymphatics, which of the following statements are true?

a) The adult flow of lymph is 2–4 L/h
b) Collecting lymphatics have smooth muscle in their walls and have valves

c) Entrainment promotes lymph flow
d) Radical mastectomy and axillary node clearance results in upper-limb lymphoedema in 50% of patients
e) In a test tube, pure lymph will clot

MTF Question 43

Regarding drug prophylaxis in migraine, which of the following are considered first-line treatment?

a) Atenolol
b) Propanolol
c) Bisoprolol
d) Amitriptyline
e) Nortripyline

MTF Question 44

Which of the following are true in relation to the use of ultrasound in clinical practice?

a) Increased frequency of ultrasound during B-mode scanning results in higher-resolution scans
b) There is no risk of damage to red blood cells with Doppler ultrasound scanning
c) The use of Doppler in conjunction with standard ultrasound imaging reduces the risk of damage to tissues by cavitation
d) Increased frequency of ultrasound results in greater depth of tissue penetration
e) The heating effect of ultrasound fields is more marked in bone compared to soft tissues

MTF Question 45

Which of the following are part of the definition of the systemic inflammatory response syndrome (SIRS)?

a) Heart rate > 100 beats/minute
b) Systolic blood pressure < 100 mmHg
c) Respiratory rate > 20 breaths/minute
d) Temperature < 36 °C
e) White blood cell count < 4000 cells/mm^3

MTF Question 46

Regarding sphincters:

a) The lower oesophageal sphincter maintains a tonic constriction producing intraluminal pressure of 30 mmHg
b) Pre-capillary sphincters are located at the junction of arterioles and metarterioles
c) The pyloric sphincter poses little resistance to the passage of fluids
d) The sphincter of Oddi is located at the junction between the cystic duct and the duodenum
e) The internal bladder sphincter is innervated by the pudendal nerve

MTF Question 47

In combined data from placebo versus drug trials, which of the following produced no significant risk reduction for postoperative nausea and/or vomiting (PONV)?

a) Magnesium
b) Glycopyrrolate
c) Metoclopramide
d) Ginger
e) Clonidine

MTF Question 48

Regarding inflammation:

a) Vasodilation is mediated by bradykinin
b) Increased vascular permeability inhibits the inflammatory response
c) Histamine increases vascular permeability
d) Chemotaxis is the process that limits the inflammatory response
e) Prostaglandin E_2 mediates vasodilation

MTF Question 49

Regarding hereditary angio-oedema:

a) It results from a disorder with complement
b) It has an autosomal dominant inheritance pattern
c) The majority of attacks occur spontaneously
d) Treatment options include administration of fresh frozen plasma
e) Upper airway obstruction is rarely a problem

MTF Question 50

A 48-year-old asthmatic patient is reviewed in preoperative assessment clinic prior to admission for cholecystectomy in 4 weeks. He has spirometry showing FEV_1 1.2L, FVC 2.5L (predicted 2.6/3.2). He has had nightly symptoms for a week, but on clinical examination he is not distressed. His medication includes fluticasone 250 g bd and salmeterol 50 g bd. The likely management needed prior to surgery includes:

a) Admission for intravenous hydrocortisone
b) Addition of a leukotriene receptor antagonist to his medication
c) Specialist review
d) Commencement of antibiotics
e) Increase in his inhaled steroid medication

MTF Question 51

Concerning open fractures:

a) Approximately 25% of tibial fractures are open fractures
b) Intravenous antibiotics should be commenced within 6 hours of the acute injury
c) All open fractures should be debrided within 6 hours of the injury
d) Up to 30% of patients with an open fracture will develop a significant infection following the injury

e) Definitive skeletal stabilisation of an open fracture should occur within 48 hours of the injury

MTF Question 52

The following are properties of bisoprolol in ischaemic heart disease:

a) Bisoprolol is a selective β_2-adrenoreceptor blocker
b) It reduces the activity of the heart muscle, reducing oxygen demand
c) It has a half-life of 12 hours and is therefore administered once daily
d) Bisoprolol has a higher cardioselectivity than atenolol
e) A dose of 20 mg should be started after a myocardial infarction as prophylaxis against recurrent infarction

MTF Question 53

The following drugs and doses are correctly stated parts of the algorithm for the routine ALS management of cardiac arrest:

a) Adrenaline, 1 mg
b) Atropine, 3 mg
c) Sodium bicarbonate, 50 mmol
d) Amiodarone, 300 mg
e) Magnesium, 2 g

MTF Question 54

A previously well 48-year-old female is admitted to the emergency department with acute onset of productive cough, fever to 39.8 °C, heart rate of 130 bpm (sinus tachycardia) and a blood pressure of 75/40 mmHg. Chest x-ray shows opacification of the right lung field with air-bronchogram. Which of the following statements about her initial management are correct?

a) Antibiotic administration should be delayed until after a sample of cerebrospinal fluid has been obtained for microscopy and culture
b) Antibiotic administration should be delayed until after blood samples have been collected for culture
c) Antibiotic administration should be delayed until after laboratory evidence of leucocytosis is available to confirm presence of infection
d) Fluid resuscitation should be delayed until central venous pressure monitoring is in situ in order to assess the haemodynamic response to fluid boluses
e) Noradrenaline is an appropriate initial vasopressor if the haemodynamic parameters fail to respond to fluid boluses

MTF Question 55

The following are recognised adverse effects of treatment with amiodarone:

a) Steatohepatitis
b) Perception of everything tasting bitter
c) Yellowing of axillary skin
d) Epiphora
e) Peripheral myopathy

MTF Question 56

Regarding the thalassaemias:

a) Red blood cell destruction occurs intravascularly
b) A complete absence of β-globin (β°/β°) is associated with intrauterine death (Bart's hydrops)
c) The same patient can have both α- and β-thalassaemia
d) Inadequate transfusion is known to result in frontal bossing
e) Splenomegaly is common in β-thalassaemia minor

MTF Question 57

Concerning patient-controlled analgesia (PCA):

a) Adding ketamine into a morphine PCA improves postoperative analgesia
b) Giving low-dose ketamine IV perioperatively will improve analgesia when PCA is used postoperatively
c) The main proven advantage of PCA is improved patient satisfaction
d) PCA decreases the total morphine dose the patient requires perioperatively when compared with conventional analgesia
e) PCA produces a clinically small but statistically significant improvement in perioperative analgesia compared with conventional analgesia

MTF Question 58

It is true to say of rocuronium that:

a) It is less potent than vecuronium
b) It is 10% protein-bound
c) The dose for modified rapid sequence induction is 0.5 mg/kg
d) Its effects can be reversed by administration of γ-cyclodextrin
e) It can be administered via the intramuscular route

MTF Question 59

During an adult cardiac arrest, which of the following drugs are recommended as being suitable to be administered down an endotracheal tube?

a) Amiodarone
b) Vasopressin
c) Calcium gluconate
d) Adrenaline
e) Sodium bicarbonate

MTF Question 60

Regarding aortic aneurysms:

a) Patients with an abdominal aortic aneurysm with a diameter > 55 mm should be offered surgical repair
b) In patients fit for either EVAR (endovascular aneurysm repair) or open aneurysm repair, EVAR has lower 30-day postoperative mortality than open repair
c) In patients unfit for open repair, EVAR demonstrates a lower long-term mortality than non-operative measures

d) The majority of abdominal aortic aneurysms are suprarenal
e) During dissection of an abdominal aneurysm, blood dissects between the tunica media and tunica adventitia

SBA Question 61

A patient is fitted with a VVI pacemaker. Which one of the following is INCORRECT regarding the functions of this pacemaker?

a) An intrinsic rhythm of a P wave transmitted to the ventricles will result in inhibition of pacing output
b) An ectopic of ventricular origin will result in inhibition of pacing output
c) A supraventricular tachycardia (SVT) transmitted to the ventricles will result in inhibition of pacing output
d) Polyfocal ectopics as a result of a wire introduced during insertion of a central venous catheter result in activation of pacing output
e) Administration of glycopyrronium bromide is more likely to increase than decrease the rate of pacing output

SBA Question 62

After a long day, you quickly stop in the hospital shop to grab a snack for the drive home. Whilst waiting to pay, your attention is drawn to a frantic woman calling for help for her choking child. She is kneeling over a 3-year-old girl who is conscious and appears to be coughing, but no noise is made. Which of the following is the single most appropriate immediate action?

a) Deliver five back blows
b) Continue to encourage coughing
c) Call for help and deliver up to five abdominal thrusts
d) Perform a finger sweep to dislodge the object
e) Place the child in the recovery position

SBA Question 63

Regarding POSSUM risk scoring, which of the following is the LEAST correct?

a) POSSUM provides an estimation of both morbidity and mortality, to guide appropriateness of surgery
b) The POSSUM equation was modified to the P-POSSUM equation, as the former was deemed to over-predict death in low-risk patients
c) The P-POSSUM risk scoring includes 12 preoperative physiological parameters
d) Peritoneal contamination is an operative parameter included in the P-POSSUM risk estimation
e) The white blood cell count is a physiological parameter included in the P-POSSUM risk estimation

SBA Question 64

Having performed a rapid sequence induction using 5 mg/kg thiopental and 1 mg/kg suxamethonium for an appendectomy, you attach a nerve stimulator to monitor degree of neuromuscular blockade. After 20 minutes there are no twitches seen in response to a supramaximal stimulus. Which of the following statements would NOT explain the observed phenomenon?

a) The patient is mildly hypermagnesaemic (plasma magnesium 2.8 mmol/L)
b) The patient is 30 weeks pregnant
c) The patient has chronic hepatic failure
d) The patient is taking regular cyclophosphamide
e) The patient is clinically malnourished

SBA Question 65

Which ONE of the following treatment modalities is best explained by the gate control theory of pain?

a) Capsaicin cream
b) Lidocaine patches
c) Transcutaneous electrical nerve stimulation
d) Guanethidine block
e) Gabapentin

SBA Question 66

A 74-year-old man is admitted to hospital with abdominal pain and distension. He gives a 3-month history of weight loss and diarrhoea. His past medical history is unremarkable except for recently diagnosed asthma. A CT scan shows an obstructive lesion at the rectosigmoid junction, with a single hepatic metastasis. He undergoes a Hartmann's procedure. During manipulation of the tumour he becomes slightly hypo-tensive and tachycardic, and develops marked facial erythema and a significant wheeze. Which one of the following is the best treatment in this situation?

a) Intravenous (IV) hydrocortisone and nebulised salbutamol
b) IV fluids and IV chlorpheniramine
c) IV fluids, IV magnesium sulphate, IV hydrocortisone
d) IV fluids and IV octreotide
e) IV adrenaline infusion

SBA Question 67

Which of these is the current International Association for the Study of Pain (IASP) definition of 'neuropathic pain'?

a) Pain caused by a lesion or disease of the somatosensory nervous system
b) Pain initiated or caused by a primary lesion or dysfunction in the nervous system
c) Pain caused by a lesion or disease of the central somatosensory nervous system
d) Pain caused by a lesion or disease of the peripheral somatosensory nervous system
e) Pain defined by a specific series of clinical parameters in the presence or absence of demonstrable damage to nerve tissue

SBA Question 68

You are called to see a postoperative patient in the recovery room, whom you find has developed a corneal abrasion. The most likely position the patient was in during the procedure is:

a) Lateral
b) Lithotomy with reverse Trendelenburg
c) Prone knees/chest

d) Prone jack-knife
e) Supine

SBA Question 69

A 4-week-old boy presents with projectile vomiting and weight loss. He is clinically dehydrated and a diagnosis of pyloric stenosis is confirmed by ultrasound scan. Blood chemistry taken at the time of presentation is likely to show:

a) Na^+ 129 mmol/L, K^+ 2.9 mmol/L, Cl^- 110 mmol/L, HCO_3^- 24 mmol/L, pH 7.38
b) Na^+ 145 mmol/L, K^+ 3.0 mmol/L, Cl^- 111 mmol/L, HCO_3^- 34 mmol/L, pH 7.32
c) Na^+ 140 mmol/L, K^+ 4.4 mmol/L, Cl^- 84 mmol/L, HCO_3^- 31 mmol/L, pH 7.49
d) Na^+ 127 mmol/L, K^+ 2.8 mmol/L, Cl^- 85 mmol/L, HCO_3^- 33 mmol/L, pH 7.54
e) Na^+ 128 mmol/L, K^+ 2.9 mmol/L, Cl^- 88 mmol/L, HCO_3^- 21 mmol/L, pH 7.52

SBA Question 70

A 79-year-old woman with a metastatic pelvic tumour complains of pain on her left hip and leg secondary to a pathological fracture. It is intense on movement but can be absent at rest. The prognosis is poor, and survival at 1 year is minimal. Because of other comorbidities it is not amenable to surgery. Which ONE intervention is most likely to produce long-lasting pain relief with minimal side effects?

a) Femoral nerve block
b) Sciatic nerve block
c) Guanithidine block
d) Percutaneous cordotomy
e) Systemic opioids

SBA Question 71

When considering your choice of anaesthetic for thoracic surgery, which ONE of the following operations is an absolute indication for using a double-lumen endotracheal tube?

a) Oesophagectomy
b) Right upper lobectomy
c) Open surgery on the left main bronchus
d) Left total pneumonectomy
e) Open thoracic aortic aneurysm repair

SBA Question 72

A patient presents to the pain clinic complaining of pain in the right suprascapular area. On examination a palpable taut band within the skeletal muscle is found. It has a hypersensitive spot that is able to reproduce referred pain when stimulated. Which of the following interventions is MOST likely to produce immediate pain relief?

a) Systemic opioids
b) Anticonvulsants
c) Antidepressants
d) TENS
e) Psychotherapy

SBA Question 73

Which of the following is the most appropriate indication for use of intra-aortic balloon pump (IABP) therapy in critical care?

a) A confused 76-year-old gentleman, 2 days post admission following an acute myocardial infarction who has developed cardiogenic shock and is oliguric
b) A 56-year-old lady who has developed hypotension and chest pain, 2 days after admission for a fractured humerus following a road traffic accident
c) A 66-year-old gentleman who had an acute myocardial infarction and developed cardiogenic shock 2 days post femoral–popliteal bypass for severe peripheral vascular disease
d) A 54-year-old hypotensive gentleman with a history of ischaemic heart disease, admitted under the surgeons with a suspected leaking abdominal aortic aneurysm, whom they want to stabilise preoperatively
e) A 23-year-old intravenous drug user in septic shock who has developed worsening shortness of breath and hypotension despite 2 weeks of intravenous antibiotics

SBA Question 74

An 80 kg 64-year-old man is scheduled for an elective laparoscopic right hemicolectomy to remove an adenocarcinoma. Following induction of anaesthesia, and neuromuscular blockade using 40 mg atracurium, you are unable to visualise the vocal cords via direct laryngoscopy, after four attempts using a variety of laryngoscope blades. You are also unable to pass a bougie but can still ventilate easily. Assistance is on the way but will take some time to arrive. Select the most suitable course of action from the following:

a) Continue oxygenation via facemask and inform the surgeon of the problem. Wake the patient up once four twitches are visible on train of four and plan an elective awake fibreoptic intubation
b) Insert a standard LMA and, if oxygenation is adequate, proceed with the case and ask the surgeon to limit the pressure of gas used for laparoscopy to 10 mmHg
c) Give a further 10 mg of atracurium, continue bag-mask oxygenation, ask the anaesthetic assistant to fetch the intubating bronchoscope and perform an asleep fibreoptic intubation
d) Insert a standard LMA and, if oxygenation is adequate, attempt to perform a fibreoptic intubation, proceeding with surgery if successful
e) Perform an emergency cricothyroidotomy using either an open or Seldinger technique and proceed with surgery

SBA Question 75

A 28-year-old male is brought into the emergency department (ED) unconscious. His partner tells you that as well as consuming alcohol and cocaine, he saw him drink from a bottle of amyl nitrate, having mistaken it for a 'shot'. He is deeply cyanosed and tachypnoeic. The pulse oximeter shows a haemoglobin saturation of 52%. An arterial blood sample is chocolate-brown in colour. His arterial blood gas analysis is as follows: pH 7.46; PaO_2 18 kPa; $PaCO_2$ 2.3 kPa; HCO_3 16.4 mmol/L; base excess −8 mmol/L; oxygen saturation 96%. What is the most appropriate treatment?

a) Preoxygenate the patient, intubate and transfer to ICU for ventilation and heamofiltration
b) Give high-flow oxygen and telephone the nearest centre providing hyperbaric oxygen therapy

c) Intubate the patient and give 10mL of 1% methylene blue solution
d) Intubate the patient and contact the nearest centre with the facility for ECMO (extracorporal membrane oxygenation).
e) Intubate the patient in the ED, send a toxicology screen and give N-acetyl cysteine

SBA Question 76

A previously fit 43-year-old is brought into the emergency department following a fall from a height of 15 metres. He was unconscious at scene with obvious facial injuries and bruising over his left flank and pelvis and an open fracture of his left femur. The paramedics inserted a laryngeal mask airway (LMA) at the scene and are ventilating him with increasing difficulty. He has an 18 gauge cannula in situ and has received 500 mL of crystalloid en route. He was initially cardiovascularly stable but the crew report that he has been getting progressively more hypotensive with a BP on arrival of 73/46 mmHg, although his pulse rate has dropped from 110 to 65 bpm and he is centrally cyanosed. On examination he has poor air entry, much worse on the left. Which of the following is the most urgent initial management strategy?

a) Obtain urgent chest, abdominal and pelvic x-rays in the emergency department
b) Remove the LMA, preoxygenate, then proceed to urgent rapid sequence intubation and ventilation
c) Arrange an urgent trauma series CT scan (head, CTL spine, chest, abdomen and pelvis)
d) Insert an intercostal drain
e) Insert two large-bore intravenous access, arrange urgent cross-match and commence cautious fluid resuscitation titrated against a palpable radial pulse and apply a pelvic binder

SBA Question 77

A 45-year-old insulin-dependent diabetic presents first on your list for an inguinal hernia repair. He tells you his glucose levels are well controlled with twice-daily injections of Novomix30 and that, as advised by the pre-assessment nurse, he has halved his morning dose. His HbA1c is 7.8% and capillary blood glucose this morning is 8.9 mmol/L. Which one of the following is the most suitable intraoperative fluid regimen for this person?

a) 0.45% sodium chloride with 5% glucose and 0.15% potassium chloride
b) 0.45% sodium chloride with 5% glucose and 0.3% potassium chloride
c) 0.9% sodium chloride with 5% glucose and 0.15% potassium chloride
d) 0.9% sodium chloride
e) Hartmann's solution

SBA Question 78

Regarding the use of intravenous anaesthetic agents in obese patients, all of the following statements are correct, EXCEPT which one?

a) Induction dose of propofol should be calculated using ideal body weight
b) Initial dose of midazolam should be calculated using total body weight
c) Remifentanil dose should be calculated using ideal body weight
d) Suxamethonium dose should be calculated using ideal body weight
e) Morphine dose should be calculated using ideal body weight

SBA Question 79

A 72-year-old male with a history of chronic obstructive pulmonary disease (COPD) is 7 days post emergency laparotomy. He remains intubated and ventilated on pressure-controlled ventilation with an inspired pressure of $26\,cm/H_2O$, a PEEP of $8\,cm/H_2O$ and an FiO_2 of 0.5. He has recently developed a secondary ventilator-associated pneumonia and has been restarted on antibiotics and noradrenaline infusion (0.1 g/kg/h) to maintain his mean arterial pressure (MAP). He is currently stable, lightly sedated but cooperative. A tracheostomy is planned after the weekend in view of his likely protracted clinical course. The physiotherapist comes to you, as the registrar on the unit, for advice about her management of this patient. Which ONE of the following describes the best approach to this patient's physiotherapy?

a) All physiotherapy should be delayed until after the tracheostomy
b) His vasopressors should be weaned off before any aggressive physiotherapy is undertaken
c) Chest physiotherapy alone should be undertaken regularly to improve secretion clearance and oxygenation
d) Passive mobilisation and positioning are more important than chest physiotherapy
e) A combination of regular chest physiotherapy and early passive and then active mobilisation (as tolerated) should be undertaken

SBA Question 80

A 68-year-old man with a past medical history of hypertension (treated with atenolol 50 mg daily and ramipril 10 mg daily) underwent an elective right hemicolectomy for colonic adenocarcinoma 5 days ago. He has suffered significant pain (treated with paracetemol, diclofenac and a morphine PCA), and has an ongoing ileus with abdominal distension. Over the last 24 hours, his creatinine has doubled from his baseline of 130 mmol/L to 270 mmol/L, accompanied by a reduced urine output. As the ICU registrar, you have been asked to see him regarding his acute kidney injury (AKI). Which of the following statements is LEAST correct?

a) Hypovolaemia is likely to be contributing significantly to his AKI
b) His past medical history is likely to be relevant
c) Medication administered for his pain is likely to have contributed to his AKI
d) He is likely to have raised intra-abdominal pressure contributing to his AKI
e) The single dose of gentamicin he received as routine prophylaxis interoperatively is likely to be contributing to his AKI

SBA Question 81

You have just extubated a 5-year-old girl following tonsillectomy. She has coughed once but you now cannot ventilate her. You think she is in complete laryngospasm. Which of the following best describes the afferent (sensory) and efferent (motor) pathways involved in this reflex arc?

a) Afferent: external branch of superior laryngeal nerve. Efferent: recurrent laryngeal nerve.
b) Afferent: recurrent laryngeal nerve. Efferent: internal branch of superior laryngeal nerve.
c) Afferent: internal branch of superior laryngeal nerve and recurrent laryngeal nerve. Efferent: external branch of superior laryngeal nerve and recurrent laryngeal nerve.
d) Afferent: internal branch of superior laryngeal nerve. Efferent: pharyngeal branches of vagus.

e) Afferent: external branch of superior laryngeal nerve. Efferent: pharyngeal branches of vagus.

SBA Question 82

Spinal anaesthesia is administered to a 52 kg 89-year-old undergoing hip hemiarthroplasty. Her only medical condition is well-controlled hypertension, for which she takes atenolol and ramipril. Following the block her blood pressure drops from 130/70 mmHg to 65/40 while her heart rate remains stable at 80 bpm. She has received 500 mL crystalloid in the past 30 minutes. What is the most appropriate action?

a) Position the patient slightly head down, raising her legs and give the remaining 500 mL of crystalloid, rechecking the blood pressure every 1–2 minutes
b) Give 3 mg incremental boluses of ephedrine
c) Give the remaining 500 mL of crystalloid and recheck the blood pressure every 1–2 minutes
d) Give 0.5 mg incremental boluses of metaraminol and recheck the blood pressure every 1–2 minutes
e) Give 250 mL colloid and 3mg incremental boluses of ephedrine, rechecking the blood pressure

SBA Question 83

Five patients in different wards within your hospital have developed watery diarrhoea. Stool samples are sent for detection of *Clostridium difficile* toxin. In which patient's sample is the toxin most likely to be present?

a) The 52-year old male with chronic renal failure, otherwise fit, who attends the hospital three times weekly for intermittent haemodialysis; on day 3 of a short course of trimethoprim for a urinary tract infection
b) The 82-year-old female, day 1 post primary total hip replacement, who has a penicillin allergy and was given 24 hours of perioperative clindamycin as prophylaxis against operative site infection
c) The 68-year-old male, on a general surgical ward, day 11 after anterior resection for colonic carcinoma, on day 5 of intravenous vancomycin for a methicillin-resistant *Staphylococcus aureus* (MRSA) wound infection
d) The 5-year-old male, admitted to a general paediatric ward 7 days previously with lobar pneumonia, on day 7 of co-amoxiclav
e) The 68-year-old male, day 8 in intensive care after sustaining thoracic injuries in a road traffic collision, intubated and ventilated; has received 6 days' ciprofloxacin therapy for a urinary tract infection; also receiving proton-pump inhibitor therapy

SBA Question 84

Which one of the following is LEAST appropriate in the management of pancreatic pain?

a) Eating low-fat meals
b) Radiofrequency ablation of the coeliac plexus
c) Opioids
d) Pancreatic enzyme supplementation
e) Splanchnic nerve block

SBA Question 85

You are asked to see a woman who is 34/40 weeks gestation in the antenatal clinic. She is a primigravida who is morbidly obese with a body mass index (BMI) of 52 (weight 126 kg, height 1.55 m). What would be the best piece of advice that you could give her in order to prepare for labour?

a) Advise her to avoid gaining weight in the last 4–6 weeks of pregnancy
b) Advise her that it may not be possible to deliver her baby safely within 30 minutes should a category 1 caesarean section be needed
c) Advise her to request an epidural early in labour so that operative procedures can be more easily dealt with under epidural top-up
d) Advise her that the incidence of failed or difficult intubation rises from 1 in 280 to approximately 1 in 3 in the obese obstetric population
e) Advise her to avoid an epidural if possible as she would have a four times greater risk of suffering a severe headache afterwards

SBA Question 86

You are called to review your patient in the recovery room who has developed a tachycardia with a regular rate of 145 beats per minute. Blood pressure is recorded as 75/40 mmHg. An ECG shows a QRS of duration 0.14 s. Preoperatively, you noted a left bundle branch block. Which is the single most appropriate immediate action?

a) Give amiodarone 300 mg intravenously followed by a 900 mg infusion
b) As known bundle branch block, give adenosine 6 mg as a rapid intravenous bolus
c) Control rate with β-blocker
d) DC cardioversion with 150 J biphasic shock
e) Synchronised DC cardioversion with 100 J monophasic shock

SBA Question 87

A 60-year-old man presents for hernia repair on your day-case general surgical list. He has a history of type 2 diabetes, asthma and hypertension. As you make your preoperative assessment you note that he is overweight with a potentially difficult airway. He volunteers that he has not taken his morning medication in order to be nil by mouth for the procedure. In which ONE of the following circumstances would this patient be unsuitable for discharge on the day of the procedure?

a) He has a history of obstructive sleep apnoea with nasal CPAP at home
b) Following the procedure he suffers postoperative nausea that is resistant to antiemetics
c) His preoperative blood pressure is 157/93 mmHg
d) He has a body mass index of 42 kg/m^2
e) He experiences an episode of laryngospasm in the recovery room

SBA Question 88

Regarding transcutaneous electrical nerve stimulation (TENS), which type of nerve fibres are said to be stimulated?

a) Aα
b) Aβ
c) Aδ

d) B
e) C

SBA Question 89

A 32-year-old man is undergoing open reduction and internal fixation of a distal forearm fracture. An arterial tourniquet is inflated at the mid-humeral level. The surgeons do not want to deflate the tourniquet. Which of the following provides the best reason for allowing the tourniquet to stay inflated?

a) The patient received ketamine preoperatively to reduce the hypertension caused by tourniquet use
b) Every 30 minutes of tourniquet inflation only increases the risk of nerve damage by 50%
c) The patient is at a lower risk of neurological injury as he is relatively young
d) The tourniquet will help to reduce anaesthetic requirements by reducing physiological sensory nerve conduction from the surgical site
e) The tourniquet had only been inflated for 2 hours

SBA Question 90

You are anaesthetising an obese 45-year-old man for an emergency laparotomy to investigate a suspected bleeding duodenal ulcer. He has a BMI of 40 and Hb of 9.5 g/dL. With regard to oxygenation in this patient, which one of the following statements is true?

a) Impending hypoxaemia will be detected by monitoring his arterial oxygen saturations
b) He will desaturate at the same rate as a patient matched for age and size who is not critically ill
c) Because he is anaemic, there will be a reduction in the time to critical hypoxia despite adequate preoxygenation
d) Preoxygenating obese patients in a head-up position reduces the time to critical hypoxaemia
e) As an adult, he will remain oxygenated longer during apnoea than an equivalently unwell 5-year-old child, principally due to his relatively larger functional residual capacity

Paper 2

MTF Question 1

Regarding advance decisions made by competent patients, which of the following are true?

a) They may be ignored by a healthcare worker as they are not legally binding in the UK
b) They can authorise doctors to carry out a specific form of treatment
c) They should only be applied to a specific set of circumstances and pathologies
d) They should be disregarded in patients with dementia
e) They allow patients to refuse any type of treatment

MTF Question 2

A 25-year-old woman is admitted to hospital with recurrent chest infections. She is also known to have cystic fibrosis (CF). Which of the following statements are true?

a) The most likely organism causing the chest infection is *Pseudomonas aeruginosa*
b) Nebulised antibiotics are used in chronic infections
c) Physiotherapy is contraindicated in this patient, as it can increase the risk of pneumothorax
d) Restricted dietary intake is important in this case, to reduce bronchial secretions
e) The patient is likely to have had functionally abnormal lungs since birth

MTF Question 3

Regarding electrical hazards, which of the following are true?

a) A current of 5 mA will cause ventricular fibrillation if applied directly to the myocardium
b) Direct current is less likely to cause ventricular fibrillation than alternating current
c) The muscles present the highest impedance to current flow when current is applied to the patient
d) As current frequency increases above 50 Hz the risk of ventricular fibrillation increases linearly
e) Microshock can occur when external ECG leads are applied to the chest

MTF Question 4

Regarding epidural steroid injections for low back pain of >6 months duration, which of the following statements are true?

a) In 2009 NICE recommended the use of epidural steroids in the treatment of nerve root pain
b) Fluoroscopy is mandatory in all epidural steroid injections for low back pain
c) Caudal injection of epidural steroids in adults has an increased risk of accidental dural puncture
d) Congestive cardiac failure is a relative contraindication to epidural steroid injection
e) Particulate steroid preparations risk anterior spinal artery syndrome

MTF Question 5

Regarding urinary electrolytes:

a) Electrolytes usually found in urine include sodium, glucose and potassium
b) Urinary sodium levels can indicate volume status
c) Urinary sodium levels increase in syndrome of inappropriate antidiuretic hormone secretion (SIADH)
d) Urinary potassium levels increase with increased aldosterone levels
e) Values vary according to diet

MTF Question 6

Regarding Paget's disease of bone:

a) Serum alkaline phosphatase levels are raised in 85% of patients with untreated Paget's disease
b) The disease presents with increased serum calcium and phosphate
c) The risk of sarcoma is around 1%
d) Pain is worse in the morning but improves during the day
e) Bisphosphonates are first-line treatment

MTF Question 7

Regarding the management of tachyarrhythmias:

a) It is generally easy to distinguish between supraventricular tachycardia (SVT) and ventricular tachycardia (VT) on the 12-lead ECG
b) Atrial fibrillation (AF) will normally cardiovert in response to an adequate dose of adenosine
c) New AF in critically ill patients is generally related to an underlying structural cardiac abnormality
d) Digoxin therapy is contraindicated in the treatment of AF in the presence of Wolff–Parkinson–White (WPW) syndrome
e) In the presence of an arterial blood pressure of 86/43 mmHg, VT should normally be treated with amiodarone in the first instance

MTF Question 8

Regarding the measurement of pH with the pH electrode, which of the following are true?

a) The active (measuring) electrode is silver/silver chloride
b) Calibration is not necessary
c) The potential difference created is in the order of 60 mV per unit of pH
d) The system must be maintained at 37 °C
e) A linear relationship exists between the potential difference and the pH

MTF Question 9

Regarding hepatitis C:

a) It is a DNA virus
b) Early infection is often asymptomatic
c) Approximately 85% of patients develop cirrhosis by 20 years
d) On blood testing, the AST : ALT ratio is > 1 : 1 in the absence of cirrhosis
e) Interferon-α if given in acute infection can decrease progression to chronicity

MTF Question 10

When considering intubation in the pre-hospital environment, which of the following statements are true?

a) All practitioners in the pre-hospital environment should be capable of tracheal intubation
b) Securing the airway should be the priority in the critically injured pre-hospital patient
c) Appropriately trained paramedics are permitted to use drugs to facilitate tracheal intubation and maintenance of anaesthesia
d) Standards governing a pre-hospital intubation are the same as those governing an in-hospital intubation
e) When outdoors, pre-hospital tracheal intubation is likely to be easier on a sunny day than at night

MTF Question 11

With regard to the transfer of the critically ill patient, which of the following are correct?

a) The use of dedicated transfer teams improves the outcome of critically ill patients between hospitals
b) Routine transfers for capacity reasons alone are acceptable
c) The minimum personnel for the transfer team includes at least one attendant whose sole responsibility is care of the patient
d) The decision to transfer must be made by both the referring and the receiving consultant
e) Fixed-wing aircraft should be considered for transfer distances greater than 240 km (150 miles)

MTF Question 12

An HIV-positive patient presents with sore throat, malaise with bloody diarrhoea, blurring of vision and pain around the eye. Fundoscopy shows a 'pizza pie' appearance and a presumptive diagnosis of cytomegalovirus (CMV) is made. Which of the following are true?

a) Were this the diagnosis, large intracytoplasmic/intracellular inclusions – 'owl's eye bodies' – would be expected on tissue biopsy examination
b) CMV is mostly asymptomatic in newborns if transmitted in utero, with few complications later
c) The preferred treatment for CMV is intravenous fluconazole
d) Pneumonitis is more common than retinitis in HIV patients with CMV
e) CMV can lead to acute viral hepatitis

MTF Question 13

Regarding bicarbonate:

a) It is the principal buffer in erythrocytes
b) It is the principal buffer in plasma
c) Of the bicarbonate filtered at the glomerulus, 95% is reabsorbed in the proximal convoluted tubule
d) Its concentration in cerebrospinal fluid is the same as that in plasma
e) It is the moiety responsible for the titratable acidity of urine

MTF Question 14

The following congenital heart defects may progress to Eisenmenger's syndrome if left untreated:

a) Atrial septal defect (ASD)
b) Ventricular septal defect (VSD)
c) Tetralogy of Fallot (TOF)
d) Ebstein's anomoly
e) Patent ductus arteriosus (PDA)

MTF Question 15

With reference to the prevention and management of pressure ulcers:

a) Damage can be caused by pressure, shearing, moisture and/or friction
b) Risk factors include anaemia and/or the use of noradrenaline infusions
c) A positive microbiology wound swab from a pressure sore will require antibiotics
d) A grade 1 pressure ulcer, using the European Pressure Ulcer Advisory Panel (EPUAP) scoring system, frequently requires surgical intervention
e) Sheepskins are useful in preventing pressure ulcers

MTF Question 16

Which of the following statements regarding mannitol are true?

a) Mannitol increases cerebral blood flow
b) Mannitol is freely filtered at the glomerulus
c) Mannitol reduces intraocular pressure
d) Mannitol must be used with caution in patients with heart failure
e) Mannitol cannot be given orally due to its osmotic action on the gut mucosa

MTF Question 17

Regarding the use of troponins in diagnosing acute myocardial infarction:

a) Troponin levels rise after 1–2 hours
b) They peak at 12 hours
c) They can be raised for 5–10 days
d) They may be elevated in chronic renal failure, cardiac trauma and pulmonary embolus
e) CK-MB is more sensitive and more specific than troponin enzymes for myocardial infarction

MTF Question 18

Regarding thirst:

a) The thirst centre is located in the thalamus
b) The thirst centre is sensitive to angiotensin II
c) Low-pressure sensors in the right atrium send afferents to the thirst centre
d) The thirst centre has osmoreceptors that are sensitive to extracellular tonicity
e) The sensation of thirst is sated once normal osmolality is restored

MTF Question 19

A 78-year-old man is admitted to the emergency department with central, crushing chest pain and sudden, increasing shortness of breath. ECG shows ST depression and T-wave inversion in the anterior chest leads. Troponin level is significantly elevated. On examination, he is distressed and agitated. There is a loud systolic murmur and bibasal crepitations on auscultation. He is extremely dyspnoeic, hypoxic and tachycardic. Which of the following statements are correct regarding the acute management of this patient?

a) Non-invasive ventilation (NIV) is indicated in refractory hypoxia
b) Ultrafiltration plays no role
c) Glyceryl trinitrate (GTN) reduces in-hospital mortality rate
d) Primary percutaneous coronary intervention (PCI) should be considered
e) Use of inotropes carries prognostic benefits

MTF Question 20

Regarding intestinal pseudo-obstruction:

a) Bowel sounds are usually absent
b) A caecum dilated to 8 cm suggests likely perforation
c) Colonoscopy is contraindicated
d) Hyperkalaemia is a common cause
e) Neostigmine is contraindicated because of the risk of perforation

MTF Question 21

Regarding consent from adults to medical treatment:

a) Adults who lack capacity to consent for a procedure cannot consent but are able to refuse treatment
b) A medical practitioner can perform a procedure in an unconscious adult patient if it is in that patient's best interests, but the next of kin has refused to consent for the procedure
c) Artificial nutrition and hydration is not deemed medical treatment

d) A patient who can consent for a procedure but cannot read or write is legally obliged to mark the consent form or find someone to sign on his/her behalf

e) If, during an operation, another procedure is found to be necessary but has not been discussed with the patient, and therefore has not been consented for, the surgeon may still go ahead with the procedure

MTF Question 22

With regard to grown-up congenital heart disease in pregnancy:

a) In women with right-to-left shunts the drop in systemic vascular resistance (SVR) caused by pregnancy improves the shunt and decreases hypoxia

b) Pregnant women with pre-existing aortic regurgitation should be started on β-blockers, and tachycardia in labour should be avoided

c) Asymptomatic patients with small septal defects can be managed at their local district general hospital in a 'normal' manner

d) Pregnant women with pulmonary hypertension have the highest mortality out of all the specific cardiac lesions

e) Pre-eclampsia can cause significant cardiovascular decompensation in women with aortic regurgitation

MTF Question 23

Which of the following statements regarding the ligaments of the vertebral column are correct?

a) The posterior longitudinal ligament is found within the vertebral foramen

b) The ligamentum flavum connects adjacent laminae

c) The interspinous ligaments are continuous from the cervical vertebrae to the lumbar vertebrae

d) The supraspinous ligament connects the tips of the spinous processes and is continuous from the lower cervical vertebrae to the sacrum

e) The supraspinous ligament may become ossified

MTF Question 24

Regarding Parkinson's disease:

a) It consists of a tremor most marked on movement and absent when at rest

b) The cause is due to reduced activity of dopamine-secreting cells in the substantia nigra

c) Lewy bodies are seen at postmortem examination

d) Fatigability associated with blepharoptosis is a hallmark feature, but reflexes are normal

e) Surgery involving electrical stimulation of the sub-thalamic nucleus, thalamus or globus pallidus can be undertaken in those who become resistant to medication

MTF Question 25

Regarding cephalosporins:

a) Ceftazidime is more active than cefuroxime against Gram-positive bacteria

b) Cephalosporins were so named because they were good at crossing the blood–brain barrier and stopping bacterial proliferation

c) Cephalosporins are classified into one of four generations according to international consensus

d) Cephalosporins, in combination with probenecid, are effective against *Clostridium difficile*

e) In the absence of acquired bacterial resistance, first-generation cephalosporins can be used to treat any infection that is sensitive to penicillins

MTF Question 26

Which of the following are true regarding the use of heat and moisture exchange (HME) filters in anaesthetic practice?

a) As well as bacterial and viral particles, HME filters also filter latex particles

b) An HME filter that has no bacterial or viral filtration properties should be green in colour

c) According to the manufacturer's instructions, insertion of an HME filter between a patient and a breathing circuit allows that breathing circuit to be used for more than one patient

d) In general, hydrophobic filters are better than electrostatic ones in the prevention of fluid contamination of anaesthetic breathing circuits

e) In general, hydrophobic filters are better than electrostatic ones in the prevention of particulate contamination of anaesthetic breathing circuits

MTF Question 27

Regarding the use of drugs as tocolytics:

a) The β-adrenoreceptor agonist ritodrine is a good first-line agent

b) Nifedipine produces more cardiovascular instability than terbutaline

c) Indomethacin is effective but may cause premature closure of the ductus arteriosus

d) Atosiban works as an oxytocin receptor antagonist

e) Atosiban is the agent of choice if comorbidities such as pre-eclampsia or placental abruption are present because of favourable cardiovascular stability

MTF Question 28

Which of the following statements regarding severe acute asthma in adults are correct?

a) Asthmatic patients should be fluid resuscitated prior to intubation

b) Ketamine should be avoided as it causes bronchospasm and bronchorrhoea

c) Nitric oxide has been shown to be beneficial as an adjunct in ventilation of near-fatal asthma

d) Heliox has been shown to be beneficial as an adjunct in ventilation of near-fatal asthma

e) Initial ventilator settings should use no PEEP, low respiratory rates and long expiratory times

MTF Question 29

A 10-year-old patient is admitted from the emergency department with palpitations. On examination his heart rate is 250 beats per minute. He is diagnosed with Wolff–Parkinson–White syndrome. Which of the following are features of this syndrome?

a) Delta wave on the ECG

b) Narrow QRS complex on the ECG
c) Prolonged PR interval on the ECG
d) Pre-excitation of the ventricles by the bundle of Kent
e) Most people remain asymptomatic throughout their lives

MTF Question 30

Regarding calcium channel antagonists:

a) They cause vasodilation of the arterioles and venous capacitance vessels
b) All produce clinically effective lowering of the blood pressure
c) Nimodipine improves outcome after subarachnoid haemorrhage
d) Sublingual nifedipine is commonly used as a first-line antihypertensive agent
e) The effects of calcium channel antagonists (CCAs) in overdose can be reversed by magnesium

MTF Question 31

Regarding cryoanalgesia:

a) Cryoanalgesia results in an area of sensory loss
b) The probe uses the Joule–Thomson effect
c) Cryoanalgesia has a higher incidence of neuroma formation than phenol ablation
d) Cryoanalgesia is painful and therefore often requires sedation
e) A larger lesion is created by continuous rather than pulsed cooling

MTF Question 32

With regard to anaesthesia and the elderly, which of the following are true?

a) In the face of normal renal function vecuronium is preferable to atracurium due to the more predictable offset of action of the former drug
b) Gas induction occurs more slowly as the cardiac output is reduced
c) Spinal anaesthesia lasts longer than in a 30-year-old
d) By the age of 80 years, MAC values have reduced by 30% from the value in a 30-year-old
e) Confused patients with pain receive one-quarter the amount of morphine compared to patients with a mini mental state score of 10/10

MTF Question 33

Regarding acute pulmonary thromboembolism (PTE):

a) Patients with proven pulmonary thromboembolism (PE) have a coexisting deep vein thrombosis in approximately 60% of cases
b) Acute PTE occurring within 6 weeks of surgery has a negligible recurrence rate
c) A patient suspected of having a massive PE should have urgent computed tomographic pulmonary angiography (CTPA) to confirm the diagnosis
d) The D-dimer assay is a useful diagnostic test in patients with a high probability of PE
e) Westermark's sign or Hampton's hump are signs on a chest radiograph suggestive of an acute PTE.

MTF Question 34

Regarding treatments for malaria:

a) ECG monitoring is essential for administration of quinine, but not for quinidine
b) Artemisinins should not be given to a woman in the second or third trimester of pregnancy
c) Chloroquine can be used alone as prophylaxis and gives full protection
d) Benign malarias should be treated with chloroquine
e) Mefloquine should be avoided if there is a past medical or family medical history of epilepsy

MTF Question 35

Regarding the technique of defibrillation during cardiac arrest:

a) No person should touch the patient once the defibrillator has started charging
b) Oxygen should be disconnected from the tracheal tube before the shock is delivered
c) If using the standard sterno-apical pad position, the apical pad should be placed in the V_6 position
d) After shock delivery, CPR should not resume until a pulse check has confirmed the absence of return of spontaneous circulation
e) The recommended initial biphasic shock energy is 150–200 J

MTF Question 36

The following features are typical of a patient presenting with hypocalcaemia:

a) Carpal spasm when inflating a blood pressure cuff
b) Torsades de pointes
c) QT shortening
d) Constipation
e) Recurrent infections and short fifth metacarpal

MTF Question 37

Regarding the clinical use of steroids:

a) Steroids reduce mortality in acute respiratory distress syndrome (ARDS) but only if administered in the fibroproliferative phase of the disease process
b) Steroids are useful in symptomatic treatment of brain cancer
c) Low-dose hydrocortisone may be of use in the management of septic shock
d) Topical steroids may prevent the rash of chicken pox developing into shingles in later life
e) High-dose steroids are contraindicated for reducing swelling of the brain following head injury

MTF Question 38

Which of the following statements regarding epiglottitis are true?

a) It is caused by Haemophilus infuenzae type B infection in approximately 25% of adult cases
b) It is most common in children aged 8–12 years
c) It has an insidious onset

d) A lateral neck x-ray will be unremarkable
e) Pulmonary oedema is a recognised complication

MTF Question 39

Regarding visceral pain:

a) Repetitive noxious stimulation of viscera increases spinal cord neurone excitability
b) Frequency-dependent changes in neuronal excitability cause the 'wind-up' phenomenon
c) Somatic and visceral afferents both induce 'wind-up' by the same mechanism
d) Postsynaptic neurotransmitter actions are central to the effect of 'wind-up'
e) Positive feedback loops acting on visceral neurones may result in autonomic symptoms

MTF Question 40

Regarding cholangitis and cholecystitis:

a) Charcot's triad is classically seen in acute cholecystitis
b) The most common causative pathogens in ascending cholangitis are *Enterococcus* species
c) Patients with primary sclerosing cholangitis have a 25% chance of developing cholangiocarcinoma
d) Acalculous cholecystitis has a higher mortality than cholecystitis secondary to gallstones
e) Overall mortality of ascending cholangitis in the UK is approximately 10%

MTF Question 41

With regard to pre-existing medical diseases complicating pregnancy:

a) Approximately 50% of women with asthma will experience worsened symptoms during pregnancy
b) Carboprost should be avoided in the management of post-partum haemorrhage (PPH) in an asthmatic woman
c) Misoprostolol should be avoided in the management of post-partum haemorrhage (PPH) in an asthmatic woman
d) Obstetric cholestasis is an indication for delivery by 37–39 weeks
e) Carbimazole is the preferred anti-thyroid drug in pregnancy

MTF Question 42

Regarding the use of the serum lactate concentration in critical illness:

a) Serum lactate concentration is a reliable indicator of tissue hypoxia
b) Elevated lactate is associated with worse outcomes in severe sepsis
c) In severe sepsis, lactate rise does not correlate well with blood pressure
d) Venous lactate will significantly overestimate arterial lactate concentration
e) The administration of exogenous lactate (e.g. by infusion of Hartmann's solution) significantly reduces the value of the serum lactate concentration as a measure of tissue oxygenation

MTF Question 43

Regarding the modified Glasgow score for pancreatitis:

a) The modification from the original Glasgow score results in a score out of 9
b) A point is scored for a serum amylase > 1000 units/L
c) The modified Glasgow score has been validated for pancreatitis caused by hyperlipidaemia
d) A point is scored if a criterion is met at any time during the 48 hours after onset of symptoms
e) An admission albumin concentration of 30 g/L would score a point

MTF Question 44

After amputation of a limb:

a) Virtually all amputees will experience phantom limb pain
b) Phantom sensations occur almost immediately after amputation
c) Phantom pain can be precipitated by spinal anaesthetic
d) Stump revision is a useful treatment for intractable phantom limb pain
e) Pre-emptive epidural analgesia will reduce the risk of phantom limb pain

MTF Question 45

A 34-year-old African businessman attends his general practitioner for an annual health check-up. He has been well over the past year but has been under some stress at work recently. He is a non-smoker, takes regular exercise and eats a healthy, balanced diet. His blood pressure was 165/89 mmHg. His cardiovascular risk is estimated at 10–20%. Regarding his management:

a) His blood pressure is an indication for immediate pharmacological intervention on this occasion
b) Amlodipine would be an appropriate first-choice antihypertensive
c) Ramipril would be an appropriate first-choice antihypertensive
d) Investigations should include plasma free metadrenaline and renal artery arteriogram
e) This gentleman has a healthy lifestyle, so lifestyle advice would not be indicated here

MTF Question 46

Administration of 100% oxygen must be used with caution in the following patients:

a) An 18-month-old baby presenting for removal of an inhaled foreign body
b) A 22-year-old male presenting for elective surgery who has received chemotherapy in the past for testicular cancer
c) A 60-year-old male presenting with an acute exacerbation of chronic obstructive pulmonary disease (COPD)
d) A 50-year-old female presenting with a pulmonary embolus
e) A 70-year-old male with ischaemic heart disease presenting with carbon monoxide poisoning

MTF Question 47

Which of the following statements regarding radiation sickness are correct?

a) The earliest symptoms of acute radiation sickness are nausea, vomiting and fever
b) Frequent exposure to low-dose radiation does not cause radiation sickness
c) The absorbed dose of radiation is measured in a unit called the gray
d) There is higher incidence of cancer amongst survivors of radiation sickness
e) Decontamination by removing clothes and washing the skin can remove up to 50% of radioactive particles

MTF Question 48

The clinical features of sickle cell anaemia include:

a) Pulmonary artery hypertension
b) Obstructive sleep apnoea
c) Cholesterol gallstones
d) Functional asplenism
e) Haemorrhagic stroke

MTF Question 49

Which of the following substances have degradation products with significant clinical pharmacological effects?

a) Paracetamol
b) Morphine
c) Atracurium
d) Rocuronium
e) Enalapril

MTF Question 50

Concerning the classification of lasers:

a) All lasers used in operative surgery are class 4
b) The blink reflex will fully protect the eye from potential damage caused by a class 3 laser
c) It is safe to view class 1 lasers with the naked eye
d) Class 3 lasers can set fire to materials upon which they are projected
e) For a laser to be classified as a class 2 laser it must be in the visible spectrum

MTF Question 51

A 78-year-old lady with a childhood history of rheumatic fever is being investigated for a murmur, found incidentally during a preoperative assessment visit. The murmur is ejection systolic in nature. There are no signs of right or left heart failure and the apex is not displaced. Which of the following are differential diagnoses for her murmur?

a) Aortic stenosis
b) Tricuspid regurgitation
c) Pulmonary regurgitation
d) Pulmonary stenosis
e) Mitral regurgitation

MTF Question 52

Which of the following associations with aortic valvular heart disease are correct?

a) Aortic regurgitation and Quincke's sign (nail-bed capillary pulsations)
b) Aortic regurgitation and early diastolic murmur
c) Aortic stenosis and narrow pulse pressure
d) Aortic stenosis and Austin Flint murmur
e) Aortic stenosis and large-volume, 'collapsing' pulse

MTF Question 53

Which of the following are components of Brown-Séquard syndrome?

a) Flaccid paralysis at the level of the lesion on the ipsilateral side
b) Ipsilateral loss of temperature sensation
c) Ipsilateral spinocerebellar tract involvement
d) Ipsilateral extensor plantar response
e) No plantar reflex on the ipsilateral side

MTF Question 54

Regarding traumatic splenic injury:

a) Vaccination against pneumococcus is recommended at 3 months post injury
b) Lifelong antibiotics are no longer recommended, because of the risk of multiresistance
c) The splenic artery supplies the stomach as well as the spleen
d) Fluid above the left kidney at ultrasound suggests a splenic injury
e) Hypotension at presentation is an indication for urgent laparotomy

MTF Question 55

Regarding the differences between the sexes in chronic pain conditions:

a) Women of reproductive age have higher opioid binding than men of a similar age
b) Men are at greater risk of chronic pain than women as they complain about pain less
c) Women have greater pain tolerance than men
d) Chronic pelvic pain is a female-specific pain syndrome
e) Amitriptyline has an increased volume of distribution in women compared to men

MTF Question 56

Regarding invasive blood-pressure monitoring, which of the following statements are true?

a) A smaller cannula will lead to increased resonance
b) The transducer must be zeroed at the site of the catheter
c) The presence of air bubbles in the system leads to a damping effect
d) A low dicrotic notch is seen in sepsis
e) A damping value of 0.8 will lead to an elevated diastolic blood pressure reading

MTF Question 57

Regarding the sacral plexus:

a) The sciatic nerve exits the pelvis via the greater sciatic notch
b) The superior gluteal nerve supplies gluteus maximus
c) The lateral cutaneous nerve of the thigh arises from the sacral plexus
d) The sciatic nerve only innervates muscles distal to the popliteal fossa
e) The inferior gluteal nerve supplies semitendinosus and semimembranosus

MTF Question 58

Regarding the lumbar plexus block:

a) The block provides good analgesia for a fractured neck of femur
b) To perform the block, the patient lies in the prone position
c) The needle insertion point is where Tuffier's line crosses a line drawn parallel to the spinous processes passing through the posterior superior iliac spine
d) The standard needle depth to the lumbar plexus is 8–12 cm
e) If the hamstring muscles are stimulated, the needle is too medial

MTF Question 59

Which of the following are true regarding the use of high air flow oxygen enrichment (HAFOE) devices to deliver a fixed fractional inspired concentration of oxygen (FiO$_2$)?

a) Air entrainment through mask side holes helps determine delivered FiO$_2$
b) Gas flow must exceed peak inspiratory flow rate
c) A predetermined oxygen flow rate is required to give the desired FiO$_2$
d) They have no contribution to dead space
e) Re-breathing does not occur

MTF Question 60

Which of the following statements concerning the use of hypnosis and imagery-based psychological interventions in pain management are correct?

a) These interventions are contraindicated in personality disorder and psychosis
b) There is no evidence for their use in chronic pain management
c) They are relaxation techniques only and not associated with adverse effects
d) They are useful in the management of acute postoperative pain
e) They are not helpful in pain associated with malignancy

SBA Question 61

With regard to the use of a nerve stimulator for monitoring neuromuscular function following administration of a non-depolarising muscle relaxant, the following statements are true, EXCEPT for which one?

Answers

a) Satisfactory recovery from neuromuscular block has not occurred until the train-of-four (TOF) ratio is > 0.9
b) The train-of-four count should be at least 3 before administering a neuromuscular antagonist

c) The use of a nerve stimulator is contraindicated in a patient with myotonic dystrophy

d) It is preferable for a nerve stimulator to deliver a constant current, rather than a constant voltage

e) Double-burst stimulation allows detection of small degrees of residual neuromuscular block

SBA Question 62

Which of the following doses of sugammadex should be used to reverse neuromuscular blockade in an 85 kg man who received 100 mg of rocuronium bromide 3 minutes ago?

a) 170 mg
b) 340 mg
c) 680 mg
d) 1360 mg
e) 2720 mg

SBA Question 63

A previously healthy 64-year-old has presented with pneumonia and septic shock. He is hypotensive, with a serum lactate level of 6 mmol/L. He appears dehydrated. Which of the following statements is LEAST CORRECT regarding his fluid therapy?

a) Correct fluid therapy will reduce his mortality
b) Early fluid therapy should be limited to 4L to reduce the risk of acute respiratory distress syndrome (ARDS) and pulmonary oedema
c) Central venous pressure (CVP) should be used to help guide fluid therapy
d) Serial lactate concentrations will help guide fluid therapy
e) There is a place for blood products during fluid resuscitation from septic shock

SBA Question 64

A 34-year-old man is admitted to the emergency department after being found trapped under a tractor for several hours. Both his legs have been crushed and are now very swollen. His urine is dark. Which one of the following is the most important step in his management?

a) He should have delayed fasciotomies to prevent the sudden release of myoglobin
b) He needs to have a bicarbonate infusion to alkalinise his urine and prevent myoglobin precipitation
c) He needs to have a mannitol infusion to induce a diuresis and prevent myoglobin deposition
d) He should have immediate angiography to determine which parts of his legs are viable
e) He should be given a 0.9% saline infusion sufficient to induce a diuresis

SBA Question 65

Regarding fasting for elective surgery, which of the following patients is most appropriately starved for theatre?

a) A patient who has just drunk 500 mL of water 2 hours before surgery

b) A patient who is chewing gum 4 hours before surgery
c) A patient who has eaten a hamburger 6 hours before surgery
d) A patient eating a boiled sweet 4 hours before surgery
e) A patient who has drunk 500 mL of lemonade 2 hours before surgery

SBA Question 66

A man presents for elective knee arthroscopy with a history of regular acid indigestion for which he uses over-the-counter antacid remedies. During your preoperative assessment he describes waterbrash on bending forward, and tells you that he sleeps propped up in bed due to reflux symptoms. What would be the most appropriate premedication to administer?

a) Metoclopramide 10 mg orally 2 hours prior to induction
b) Ranitidine 150 mg orally 2 hours prior to induction
c) Rabeprazole 20 mg orally 2 hours prior to induction
d) Sodium citrate 0.3 M 30 mL orally prior to induction
e) Omeprazole 20mg orally the night before and the morning of surgery

SBA Question 67

Which ONE of the following measures to improve gastrointestinal integrity in critically ill polytrauma patients has been shown to reduce both septic complications and mortality?

a) Early enteral nutrition with glutamine supplementation
b) Arginine
c) Oropharyngeal decontamination
d) Probiotics
e) Dopexamine

SBA Question 68

Which of the following is NOT an evidence-based transfusion trigger?

a) Hb 10 g/dL in a patient with active bleeding
b) Hb 7 g/dL in a haemodynamically stable resuscitated trauma patient
c) Hct > 30% in the early resuscitation phase of severe sepsis
d) Hb 12 g/dL in a patient with evidence of myocardial ischaemia
e) Hb 7 g/dL in a long-term ventilated patient with a history of stable cardiac disease

SBA Question 69

A 76-year-old is listed for endovascular aneurysm repair (EVAR) of an extensive infrarenal abdominal aortic aneurysm. The surgeon wishes to use a fenestrated trouser graft, as the neck below the renal arteries is short. Which of the following is the LEAST suitable method of providing anaesthesia?

a) Lumbar epidural with sedation
b) Combined spinal–epidural
c) Local anaesthesia with sedation
d) Spinal
e) General anaesthesia

SBA Question 70

A 45-year-old man was admitted to the ICU 5 days ago with a right-sided community-acquired pneumonia and acute respiratory distress syndrome (ARDS). He remains ventilated and has developed a right-sided pleural effusion. A pleural aspiration was performed this morning and 30 mL of sero-sanguinous fluid was aspirated and sent for analysis. You have been asked to review the results: pH 7.1, LDH 1200 IU/L, protein 35 g/L, no organisms on Gram staining. Which one of the following would constitute the most appropriate management plan?

a) No immediate action is required; observe the patient clinically and radiologically
b) Insertion of a large-bore chest drain
c) Urgent CT chest
d) Insertion of a small-bore chest drain under ultrasound guidance
e) Thoracocentesis under ultrasound guidance to drain the remaining fluid

SBA Question 71

Which of the following is INCORRECT regarding the preoperative preparation of a patient with phaeochromocytoma?

a) Labetolol provides optimal preoperative preparation, as it is both an α-adreno- and β-adrenoreceptor blocker
b) Phenoxybenzamine provides irreversible α-adrenoreceptor blockade but may contribute to postoperative hypotension
c) Selective α-adrenoreceptor blockade does not necessitate β-adrenoreceptor blockade
d) Preoperative blockade is not essential in patients with normotensive phaeochromocytoma
e) Echocardiography should be performed in patients with persistent hypertension

SBA Question 72

You are anaesthetising a patient who is having laser surgery to his upper airway. You have placed a specific laser endotracheal tube and are ventilating with 40% oxygen and 2% sevoflurane in air. Suddenly, the surgeon tells you there is a fire in the airway. What is the most appropriate course of action after switching off the laser and flooding the site with saline?

a) As you are using a laser-specific endotracheal tube, continue to ventilate the patient through the tube with 40% oxygen and 2% sevoflurane in air
b) As you are using a laser-specific endotracheal tube, continue to ventilate the patient through the tube but with 2% sevoflurane in air
c) Disconnect the anaesthetic circuit, remove the endotracheal tube and ventilate the patient on air using a bag-valve-mask circuit
d) Disconnect the anaesthetic circuit, remove the endotracheal tube and ventilate the patient on 50% oxygen using a bag-valve-mask circuit
e) Disconnect the anaesthetic circuit, remove the endotracheal tube and ventilate the patient on 100% oxygen using a bag-valve-mask circuit

SBA Question 73

Which ONE of these interventions is recommended in the management of complex regional pain syndrome (CRPS) of the lower limb?

a) Surgical lumbar sympathectomy

b) Spinal cord stimulation
c) Intravenous regional sympathetic blockade with guanethidine
d) Acupuncture
e) Amputation of the affected limb

SBA Question 74

Extra steps are often taken to obtund the hypertensive response to laryngoscopy. In which of the following situations are these extra steps LEAST likely to be required in order to avoid increased morbidity or mortality?

a) A 49-year-old female who is fit and well presenting for coiling of a berry aneurysm
b) A 79-year-old treated hypertensive with asymptomatic triple-vessel disease presenting for repair of an incarcerated inguinal hernia
c) A 29-year-old male with complete spinal cord transection at C6 who presents for appendicectomy
d) A 42-year-old pre-eclamptic woman presenting for a caesarean section under general anaesthesia
e) A 19-year-old fit scaffolder presenting for removal of a metal shard from his eye under general anaesthesia

SBA Question 75

You are anaesthetising a 67-year-old male for a transurethral resection of a bladder tumour under general anaesthetic. Midway through the operation, the surgeon complains that the patient's right leg is moving as he resects the right side of his bladder tumour. Which of the following blocks would have been most likely to prevent this occurring?

a) A spinal anaesthetic
b) A lumbar plexus block
c) A femoral nerve block
d) A sciatic nerve block
e) A caudal block

SBA Question 76

69-year-old lady undergoes an abdominoperineal (AP) resection for colonic cancer. She has a thoracic epidural sited for analgesia that works well. On postoperative day 3 she complains of left-sided weakness in her ankle joint and altered sensation on the outside of her left lower leg. You are asked to review her sensory loss. The most likely explanation to this neuropathy is:

a) Unilateral epidural blockade
b) Direct nerve injury during insertion of the epidural catheter
c) Spinal haematoma
d) Peripheral neuropraxia from leg supports
e) Residual paraesthesia from epidural infusion

SBA Question 77

You are asked to see a woman on the maternity ward who is considering an epidural for pain relief. She is concerned as she has heard stories about nerve damage and has heard that this is 'quite common'. During your discussion, you quote an incidence of

postdural puncture headache, transient nerve root damage and vertebral canal haematoma. The correct values for these, respectively, are:

a) 1 in 200, 1 in 15 000, 1 in 55 000
b) 1 in 1000, 1 in 50 000, 1 in 500 000
c) 1 in 100, 1 in 3000, 1 in 160 000
d) 1 in 10, 1 in 1000, 1 in 75 000
e) 1 in 20, 1 in 5000, 1 in 260 000

SBA Question 78

A 68-year-old is on your list for a paraumbilical hernia repair. He is a well-controlled
insulin-dependent diabetic and otherwise had a myocardial infarction 5 years ago.
Previous surgery includes a carpal tunnel release and a right aorto-femoral bypass
graft. The surgeon asks you whether anti-embolic stockings are suitable for this gentleman. What is the best treatment option?

a) Anti-embolic stockings are not suitable in this patient
b) Left side only knee-length anti-embolic stockings
c) Bilateral knee-length anti-embolic stockings
d) Left side only thigh-length anti-embolic stockings
e) Bilateral thigh-length anti-embolic stockings

SBA Question 79

A primigravida who has been induced for labour is 2–3 cm dilated and is requesting an
epidural. She is currently being treated for pre-eclamptic toxaemia (PET). Her blood
pressure was 170/110 mmHg, and after commencing a labetalol and magnesium sulphate infusion this decreased to 140/85 mmHg. She has proteinuria of 7 g/24 hours and
her most recent platelet count, taken 4 hours ago, was 100×10^9/L (6 hours before that it
was 150×10^9/L). What is the best management of this parturient's labour analgesia?

a) Insert epidural as usual
b) Send repeat full blood count and clotting screen and await results. Only insert
   epidural if platelet count is $> 80 \times 10^9$/L and clotting screen is within acceptable
   limits
c) Advise remifentanil PCA
d) Give 50 mg intramuscular pethidine and send repeat full blood count and clotting
   screen and await results. Only insert epidural if platelet count is $> 80 \times 10^9$/L and
   clotting screen is within acceptable limits
e) Send repeat full blood count and clotting screen and await results. Only insert
   epidural if platelet count is $> 60 \times 10^9$/L and clotting screen is within acceptable limits

SBA Question 80

An 80-year-old patient with severe chronic obstructive pulmonary disease (COPD) is
undergoing an elective total hip replacement under spinal anaesthesia and propofol
target-controlled infusion (TCI) sedation (1.0–1.5 g/mL). As the hip is reduced following joint insertion there is a fall in SpO_2 associated with significant hypotension. What
is the likely cause?

a) A combination of severe COPD, sedation and hypoventilation worsening
   pulmonary hypertension and cardiac output
b) Acute coronary syndrome

c) Reduced systemic vascular resistance secondary to spinal anaesthesia with associated reduced coronary perfusion and cardiac output

d) A 'high spinal' resulting in progressive loss of intercostal muscle function on the background of severe COPD, resulting in hypoxia and pulmonary hypertension

e) Bone cement implantation syndrome

SBA Question 81

You are asked to intubate a 2-year-old for a routine operative procedure. When considering this child's airway, which one of the following would you consider the LEAST likely to present a challenge?

a) This child is likely to have frequent upper respiratory tract infections, which can increase the risk of laryngospasm and other respiratory complications

b) The narrowest part of this child's airway is the cricoid ring. Your endotracheal tube may cause trauma at this level

c) The child may have loose teeth that can be dislodged and aspirated

d) The child will have a relatively large occiput compared to an adult patient, and excessive head extension may occlude the airway

e) The distance between cricoid and main bronchi is short, increasing the risk of endobronchial intubation

SBA Question 82

All of the following will potentially render the pulse oximeter reading inaccurate, EXCEPT which one?

a) A patient with cyanide poisoning

b) A patient with methaemoglobinaemia

c) A patient with methaemoglobinaemia treated with methylene blue

d) A patient with a LiMON global liver function monitor in use

e) A patient with carbon monoxide poisoning

SBA Question 83

A patient is scheduled to undergo an awake craniotomy. Which of the following would be most likely to prevent the surgery being done in this way?

a) The presence of a frontal lobe tumour

b) That the patient is registered blind

c) That the patient has a benign essential tremor

d) The presence of significant dural involvement of the tumour

e) That the patient is known to be epileptic

SBA Question 84

A child presents for cleft palate repair and is known to have an associated syndrome. That syndrome is most likely to be:

a) Treacher Collins syndrome

b) Pierre Robin syndrome

c) Klippel–Fiel syndrome

d) Down's syndrome

e) DiGeorge syndrome

SBA Question 85

A 65-year-old man presents to the emergency department. He has a history of prostate cancer and describes a 2-month history of worsening low back pain which is now severe and unresponsive to simple analgesia. Which one of the following symptoms/ signs points AGAINST a diagnosis of cauda equina syndrome?

a) Saddle anaesthesia
b) Hyperreflexia in the lower limbs
c) Difficulty urinating
d) Constipation
e) Unilateral radicular pain

SBA Question 86

When anaesthetising a patient for a laparotomy, which ONE of the following options is the most important implementation to reduce heat loss during surgery?

a) Using a heat and moisture exchange (HME) filter
b) Ensuring the patient is not in contact with any cold metallic objects
c) Avoiding the use of neuromuscular blocking agents, to allow thermogenesis via shivering
d) Use of total intravenous anaesthesia (TIVA), to prevent inactivation of the central thermoregulatory mechanisms
e) Use of a forced-air warming device

SBA Question 87

A patient with Parkinson's disease has undergone general anaesthesia for an upper limb orthopaedic procedure. Postoperatively he feels nauseated, but is not vomiting. He is due his next dose of oral dopaminergic agent shortly. Which one of the following is the best first-line antiemetic therapy in this case?

a) Metoclopramide intravenously
b) Domperidone orally
c) Prochlorperazine intramuscularly
d) Droperidol intravenously
e) Olanzapine orally

SBA Question 88

A 32-year-old woman complains of headaches associated with photophobia, phono-phobia and visual disturbances. It has a throbbing, pulsating quality with moderate to severe intensity, and lasts between 4 and 6 hours. Which of the following best describes this condition?

a) Migraine
b) Tension-type headache
c) Cluster headache
d) Trigeminal neuralgia
e) Post-herpetic neuralgia

SBA Question 89

A 79-year-old male presents for cataract surgery. He has a past medical history of hypertension which is well controlled with medication, a previous myocardial infarction (5 years ago), type 2 diabetes (tablet-controlled) and atrial fibrillation for which he takes warfarin. His current INR is 2.8. What is the most suitable course of action?

a) Advise the patient that the surgery will have to be cancelled as his INR is too high to safely carry out a regional anaesthetic technique today
b) Give 1 mg of vitamin K by slow intravenous injection, repeat his INR in 4 hours and proceed with surgery if it is < 2
c) Providing the surgeon is happy, proceed with surgery under general anaesthesia
d) Providing the surgeon is happy, proceed with surgery, performing a peribulbar block
e) Providing the surgeon is happy, proceed with surgery, performing a sub-Tenon's block

SBA Question 90

A category 1 caesarean section delivers an apnoeic, pale, floppy, 40-week-gestation baby covered in thin meconium. Which of these signs would be most likely to suggest that this baby is in primary rather than terminal apnoea?

a) Meconium stains the vocal cords and is suctioned from the lungs
b) Heart rate is approximately 70 beats per minute
c) Colour and tone improve with inflation breaths and chest compressions
d) The baby starts to display shuddering gasps
e) Approximately 5 minutes has passed since delivery

Answers

Paper 1

Answers

1)	b, c, e	31)	b, d	61)	e
2)	b, c, d	32)	b, d	62)	a
3)	a, b, c, d, e	33)	all false	63)	a
4)	a, b, c, d, e	34)	a, b, c	64)	a
5)	b	35)	a, c, d	65)	c
6)	d, e	36)	a, b, d	66)	d
7)	b, d	37)	a, d	67)	a
8)	all false	38)	c	68)	a
9)	a, c	39)	b, c, d	69)	d
10)	a, c, d	40)	b, c, d, e	70)	d
11)	b, d, e	41)	a, b, c, d	71)	c
12)	b, d	42)	b, c, e	72)	d
13)	c, d, e	43)	a, b, c, d, e	73)	a
14)	a, c, d	44)	a, e	74)	d
15)	a, b, c, e	45)	c, d, e	75)	c
16)	e	46)	a, c	76)	d
17)	b, c, e	47)	c	77)	e
18)	c, d	48)	a, c, e	78)	d
19)	b	49)	a, d	79)	e
20)	b, c	50)	c, e	80)	e
21)	c	51)	a, d	81)	c
22)	a, b, d, e	52)	b, c, d	82)	d
23)	a, c, d, e	53)	a, d	83)	e
24)	a, d, e	54)	b, e	84)	b
25)	a, c, d, e	55)	a, b, e	85)	c
26)	a, b	56)	c, d	86)	d
27)	b, d, e	57)	b, c, e	87)	b
28)	c, d, e	58)	a, d, e	88)	b
29)	b	59)	all false	89)	a
30)	b, c, d, e	60)	a, b	90)	c

Paper 2

Answers

1) c, e	31) a, b	61) c
2) a, b	32) d, e	62) d
3) a, b	33) b, e	63) b
4) d, e	34) d, e	64) e
5) b, c, d, e	35) c, e	65) a
6) a, d, e	36) a, b, e	66) b
7) a, d	37) a, b, c, e	67) a
8) a, c, d, e	38) a, e	68) d
9) b, e	39) a, b, e	69) d
10) d	40) d, e	70) d
11) a, d, e	41) b, d	71) a
12) a, e	42) b, c	72) c
13) b, d	43) d, e	73) b
14) a, b, e	44) b, c	74) c
15) a, b	45) b, d	75) b
16) a, b, c, d	46) b, c	76) d
17) b, c, d	47) a, b, c, d	77) c
18) b, c, d	48) a, b, d, e	78) a
19) a, c, d	49) a, b, e	79) b
20) all false	50) a, c, e	80) e
21) b, e	51) a, d	81) c
22) c, d, e	52) a, b, c	82) a
23) a, b, d, e	53) a, c, d	83) d
24) b, c, e	54) c, d	84) b
25) all false	55) a, e	85) b
26) a, d, e	56) c, d, e	86) e
27) c, d	57) a	87) b
28) a, e	58) a, c, d, e	88) a
29) a, b, d, e	59) b, c, d, e	89) e
30) c	60) a, d	90) d

Explanations

Paper 1

MTF Question 1: Measurement of humidity

With regard to measurement of humidity, which of the following statements are correct?

a) Most instruments measure absolute humidity
b) Regnault's hygrometer has a silver tube containing ether
c) Absolute humidity can be measured by transducers
d) The hair hygrometer works on the principle that hair shortens as humidity increases
e) The wet and dry bulb hygrometer relies on the cooling effect by loss of latent heat of vaporisation for its function

Answer: b, c, e

Short Explanation
Most instruments measuring humidity measure relative humidity. The hair hygrometer works on the principle that hair lengthens as humidity increases.

Long Explanation
Humidity can be expressed in two ways: relative and absolute. Absolute humidity is the mass of water vapour present in a given volume of air; it is usually expressed as mg/L or g/m^3. Relative humidity is the ratio of the mass of water vapour in a given volume of air to the mass required to saturate that given volume of air at the same temperature; it is usually expressed as a percentage. It is important to consider the difference between these two terms when looking at the measurement of humidity.

Most hygrometers measure relative humidity. Examples of hygrometers include the hair hygrometer, wet and dry bulb hygrometer, Regnault's hygrometer, humidity transducers, the mass spectrometer and ultraviolet light absorption hygrometers.

The hair hygrometer gives a direct reading of relative humidity. It consists of a pointer attached to a human hair whose length changes with differing humidity; as the humidity increases, the hair lengthens. It is simple but inaccurate. Animal tissue or paper has also been used in this instrument.

The wet and dry hygrometer gives another measure of relative humidity. As the name suggests, it consists of two bulb thermometers, one dry and the other wrapped in a wet wick. The dry bulb is in contact with its surroundings and reads the true ambient temperature. The wet bulb reads at a lower temperature owing to the cooling effect from the evaporation of water from the wick surrounding the bulb and the consequent loss of latent heat of vaporisation. The difference between the temperatures of the two bulbs is related to the rate of evaporation, which in turn depends on the ambient humidity. It is then possible to determine relative humidity from a set of tables. Accuracy of this system depends on adequate air movement around the bulbs.

Regnault's hygrometer consists of a silver tube containing ether which is cooled by blowing air through it with a rubber bulb. When condensation appears on the outside, the air is saturated with water at that temperature (the dew point). From a graph of saturated air against temperature, water content at dew point at that temperature can be determined. This gives a measurement of absolute humidity, from which relative humidity can be calculated.

Absolute humidity can also be measured by humidity transducers, the mass spectrometer and ultraviolet light absorption hygrometers.

Davis PD, Kenny GNC. *Basic Physics and Measurement in Anaesthesia*, 5th edn. Oxford: Butterworth–Heinemann, 2003; pp. 128–30.

Yentis S, Hirsch N, Smith G. *Anaesthesia and Intensive Care A–Z: an Encyclopaedia of Principles and Practice*, 3rd edn. Edinburgh: Butterworth-Heinemann, 2004; pp. 252–3.

MTF Question 2: Ketamine

Which of the following statements regarding ketamine are true?

a) Ketamine causes analgesia through its activity at opioid receptors
b) NMDA receptor antagonism is the main mechanism of ketamine effect
c) Ketamine blocks the release of glutamate in the CNS
d) Ketamine blocks activity at muscarinic receptors in the central nervous system
e) Like all general anaesthetic agents, ketamine has activity at the $GABA_A$ receptor

Answers: b, c, d

Short Explanation

Ketamine's main action is non-competitive antagonism at NMDA glutamate receptors. It also blocks glutamate release and antagonises other receptors, including muscarinic receptors. Although ketamine has complex actions at opioid receptors its analgesic activity is not blocked by naloxone. Unlike other anaesthetic agents it has no affinity for GABA receptors.

Long Explanation

Ketamine is a synthetic derivative of phencyclidine. Its main action appears to be non-competitive antagonism at the NMDA glutamate receptor. This complex receptor is responsible for opening a sodium/calcium channel and has been implicated in synaptic plasticity. Glutamate is the principal excitatory neurotransmitter of the CNS, and ketamine also reduces the amount of glutamate released from the presynaptic terminal. Ketamine also has complex interactions with opioid receptors (antagonist at MOP receptors and agonist at DOP and KOP receptors), although these interactions are much weaker than its affinity for NMDA receptors. Naloxone does not reverse the analgesic effects of ketamine, suggesting that they are modulated through other neuronal pathways.

Ketamine also antagonises monoaminergic, muscarinic and nicotinic receptors, and at high doses has a local anaesthetic activity due to a direct effect on voltage-gated sodium channels. Unlike other anaesthetic agents, it does not seem to have any affinity for GABA receptors.

Anaesthesia produced by ketamine is dissociative, with relative preservation of respiratory tone and reflexes; excessive salivation can be problematic. The overall cardiovascular effects are stimulatory, with tachycardia and hypertension usually seen, but these are caused by an increased sympathetic tone, and ketamine itself has a negatively inotropic direct effect on the heart.

Pai A, Heining M. Ketamine. *Contin Educ Anaesth Crit Care Pain* 2007; **7**: 59–63. Available online at ceaccp.oxfordjournals.org/content/7/2/59 (accessed 30 June 2012).

MTF Question 3: Hypokalaemia

Causes of hypokalaemia include:

a) Pyloric stenosis
b) Villous adenoma of rectum
c) Conn's syndrome
d) Theophylline poisoning
e) Renal tubular acidosis

Answer: a, b, c, d, e

Short Explanation
All these are associated with hypokalaemia. Causes of deficit of any ion may be considered in terms of inadequate intake, intercompartmental shift or failure of retention/excessive loss.

Long Explanation
Inadequate intake of potassium may result in hypokalaemia, but a dietary deficiency must be severe before this alone would cause a potassium deficit. There are several factors that may promote potassium shift into cells. Insulin and β-adrenoreceptor agonists (e.g. salbutamol, terbutaline) will do so. An alkalosis will produce hypokalaemia, not just by renal excretion, but by inducing shift into cells. Acute myocardial infarction will, via β-adrenergic stimulation, cause redistribution of potassium intracellularly.

Excessive loss may be renal or gastrointestinal. Considering renal losses, this is commonly induced iatrogenically by thiazide or loop diuretics or agents with mineralocorticoid activity (e.g. steroids). Increased aldosterone production occurs in Conn's and Cushing's syndromes but is also seen in liver failure, heart failure and adrenocorticotrophic hormone (ACTH)-secreting tumours. Intrinsic renal disease such as renal tubular acidosis (types 1 and 2) or gentamicin-induced nephrotoxicity may also result in hypokalaemia. Gastrointestinal losses are intuitive – potassium-rich juices or secretions are lost or drained in vomiting, diarrhoea, villous adenoma, ileostomy, fistulae or via third spacing in intestinal obstruction.

Theophylline acts with endogenous catecholamines to agonise β-adrenoreceptors, with consequent hypokalaemia if the drug is taken in overdose.

MTF Question 4: Anorexia

The physiological features of severe anorexia nervosa include:

a) Cardiomyopathy
b) Proteinuria
c) Bradycardia
d) Gastric dilation
e) Panhypopituitarism

Answer: a, b, c, d, e

Short Explanation

Myocardial damage may be induced by starvation or secondary to drug toxicity. Bradycardia is an adaptation to prolonged starvation and a reduction in basal metabolic rate. Over 50% of anorexic patients have proteinuria, while gastric dilation is seen in patients who binge eat and purge. Panhypopituitarism is seen rarely.

Long Explanation

Whist primarily a psychiatric diagnosis, anorexia nervosa may lead to profound physiological compromise. There are generally two types of anorexia nervosa described, the restricting type, where the patient limits nutritional intake and often exercises excessively, and the binge-eating/purging type, which is associated with self-induced vomiting, use of emetics, slimming pills and laxatives. The latter type generally has the greater mortality and is associated with the greatest electrolyte disturbances.

Myocardial damage may be induced directly by starvation, or it may be secondary to drug toxicity. Ipecac syrup (an emetic) induces inflammatory change and myofibril degeneration, and some antipsychotics are also associated with cardiomyopathy. Cardiomyopathy also increases the likelihood of arrhythmias, which are also seen independently in severe anorexia. Common ECG changes include atrioventricular conduction blocks, ST depression, T-wave inversion and QT prolongation.

Proteinuria is found in more than 50% of patients with anorexia, and impaired renal function and electrolyte disturbances are common. Vomiting leads to hyponatraemia, hypokalaemia, hypochloraemia, hypomagnesaemia and a metabolic alkalosis. Dehydration activates the renin–angiotensin–aldosterone system and further exacerbates the potassium loss, as does the abuse of diuretics or laxatives.

Gastric dilation is seen most often in patients who binge eat and purge, although gastric emptying times are also prolonged in starvation. There is also the direct corrosive effect of gastric acid and mechanical damage from repeated vomiting. Respiratory changes include pneumothoraces and aspiration pneumonia from vomiting, and reduced lung compliance from starvation.

The most common endocrine abnormality is amenorrhoea from reduced luteinising hormone, follicle-stimulating hormone and gonadotrophin-releasing hormone, but hypothalamic function is generally reduced from carbohydrate deprivation and hypoglycaemia. Features of panhypopituitarism are therefore seen in a minority of patients. Thyroid metabolic function is decreased, although thyrotropin-releasing hormone levels are usually normal. Immune function may be impaired when patients have lost 50% of their normal body weight.

Structural neurological changes include grey and white matter loss, while coma and seizures tend to be the result of electrolyte disturbances or hypoglycaemia. Electrolyte disturbances also cause myalgia and occasionally myopathy. Severe anorexia nervosa is also associated with osteoporosis and consequently an increased risk of fractures.

Denner AM, Townley SA. Anorexia nervosa: perioperative implications. *Contin Educ Anaesth Crit Care Pain* 2009; **9**: 61–4. Available online at ceaccp.oxfordjournals.org/content/9/2/61 (accessed 30 June 2012).

MTF Question 5: Post-arrest management

Regarding the use of targeted temperature management after cardiac arrest:

a) The ideal target temperature is 30 °C
b) J waves are a common finding on the ECG of a patient at 31 °C
c) At the end of the cooling period, passive rewarming should be allowed
d) A heart rate of 38 beats per minute when the patient's temperature is 32 °C is an indication for rewarming

e) Shivering should preferentially be treated with a non-depolarising neuromuscular blocking drug (NMBD)

Answers: b

Short Explanation

The core body temperature target should be 32–34 °C. Active, controlled rewarming is required. Sinus bradycardia is expected at this temperature. NMBDs may be required to control shivering, but can often be avoided.

Long Explanation

Targeted temperature management is the preferred term for therapeutic hypothermia after cardiac arrest. This has been shown to improve the odds of survival to hospital discharge after out-of-hospital VF or VT cardiac arrest, and has now widely been extended to all patients who remain comatose after return of spontaneous circulation (ROSC).

The patient's core temperature should be reduced as rapidly as possible after ROSC. The patient will require intubation and deep sedation, and may require vasopressor support to tolerate this. The temperature should be brought to the target of 32–34 °C over an ideal maximum of 4 hours. This temperature should be maintained for 12–24 hours, although the ideal time is not known, and many sources recommend at least 24 hours.

At the end of the period of hypothermia, controlled rewarming is required. Rapid restoration of normal temperature is deleterious, as is overshoot to pyrexia. Rewarming should occur at a maximum rate of 0.5 °C per hour. Passive rewarming does not consistently allow this slow rewarming, and therefore the patient should be rewarmed by slowly increasing the target temperature on the active cooling device.

Targeted temperature management poses several particular problems, including cardiovascular management. J waves are expected at temperatures around 32 °C (delta waves are associated with pre-excitation syndromes). Sinus bradycardia is almost ubiquitous, and is not an indication for rewarming the patient. Intense vasoconstriction may occur, raising the systemic vascular resistance. This is normally well tolerated, but in the presence of left ventricular dysfunction may precipitate heart failure.

Shivering is common during the active cooling phase. Neuromuscular blocking drug (NMBD) administration may be required to treat this. However, metabolism of NMBDs is unreliable during hypothermia, and ideally they should be avoided. Alternatives that may help include placing the hands in warm water, magnesium administration and pethidine administration.

During the period of hypothermia, usually intensive care management is required. Hypo- or hyperglycaemia should not be tolerated. Patients treated with targeted temperature management are at increased risk of infection, so ventilator care and central line insertion bundles should be followed meticulously. Although an ileus may complicate hypothermia, enteral feeding should be attempted.

Resuscitation Council UK. Adult advanced life support. Resuscitation Guidelines 2010. Available online at www.resus.org.uk/pages/als.pdf (accessed 30 June 2012).

MTF Question 6: Other analgesic agents

Regarding gabapentin, which of the following statements are true?

a) Gabapentin is an agonist at the γ-aminobutyric acid $(GABA)_A$ receptor
b) Gabapentin is metabolised by the CYP3A4 isoenzyme
c) Gabapentin is available in a transdermal drug delivery patch

d) Gabapentin can be used for the treatment of acute pain
e) Gabapentin enhances the action of morphine

Answer: d, e

Short Explanation

Gabapentin is a structural analogue of γ-aminobutyric acid but is not an agonist at the receptor. Gabapentin is not metabolised and is not available as a transdermal patch.

Long Explanation

Gabapentin is a structural analogue of γ-aminobutyric acid (GABA) but is not an agonist at the receptor. The mechanism of action is unclear but includes binding to voltage-dependent calcium channels in the central nervous system, in particular the 2δ subunit; this is upregulated in chronic pain syndromes. Binding to the calcium channel prevents calcium influx and reduces the release of neurotransmitters. Gabapentin also has action at the NMDA receptor. Gabapentin is not metabolised in humans and is excreted in urine. Gabapentin is only available as an oral formulation.

Gabapentin is licensed for chronic pain syndromes such as post-herpetic neuralgia but has also been used to good effect in the acute postoperative setting, reducing opioid and epidural requirements. It also enhances the action of morphine when coadministered.

Sasada M, Smith S. *Drugs in Anaesthesia and Intensive Care*, 3rd edn. Oxford: Oxford University Press, 2003; p. 168.

MTF Question 7: Neuromuscular junction structure

Regarding the neuromuscular junction:

a) The synaptic cleft is 5 nanometres wide
b) There are 10 acetylcholine receptors for every molecule of acetylcholine released in a conducted impulse
c) Nerve fibres converge on the motor end-plate of the muscle fibre
d) The terminal portion of the motor neurone is unmyelinated
e) Prejunctional acetylcholine receptors have the same morphology as the postjunctional ones

Answer: b, d

Short Explanation

The neuromuscular junction (NMJ) is a specialised termination of a motor neurone where an arriving impulse is potentially propagated across the synapse to elicit a contraction in the designated muscle. It is 50 nanometres wide. The motor end-plate receives input from only one nerve – nerves do not converge on a muscle. Pre- and postjunctional acetylcholine receptors have different antagonists and different morphologies.

Long Explanation

A single muscle fibre is innervated by a single branch of a motor neurone – together they are termed a motor unit. Although a single motor neurone may send branches to a number of muscle fibres, each muscle fibre receives input from only one nerve.

Where the nerve comes into immediate proximity with the muscle to make synaptic but not physical contact, both the nerve and the muscle are physically adapted to the purpose of signal transmission. This is termed the motor end-plate. The terminal portion of the motor neurone is unmyelinated as it reaches its destination muscle. An arriving action potential precipitates a number of intracellular events that culminate in release of vesicles of preformed acetylcholine. These diffuse the 50 nanometres across the cleft to bind the subunits of the acetylcholine receptors on the crests of the junctional folds, affecting a conformational change in the receptors that opens its ion pore, allowing the flux of principally (but not exclusively) sodium ions.

Each vesicle will produce a small end-plate potential. If enough of these potentials are summed together, this may be sufficient to reach the threshold firing potential of the muscle fibre, causing an action potential that will be propagated across the muscle, resulting in its contraction. It is an amplification cascade whereby a single nerve action potential arriving brings about the action potential of the whole (larger) muscle cell.

Presynaptic acetylcholine receptors are responsible for mediating a positive feedback loop in the nerve terminal button that mobilises further stores of acetylcholine if the stimulation is sustained. Curiously, although both receptors are activated by acetylcholine they are not antagonised by the same molecules, implying different morphology pre- and postsynaptically. There is a great excess of acetylcholine receptors for every molecule of acetylcholine released when a nerve action potential prompts its release. This 'spare receptor' phenomenon explains why such a large receptor occupancy by non-depolarising muscle relaxants is needed before any noticeable muscle weakness is produced.

MTF Question 8: Porphyria

Regarding the porphyrias:

a) They are rare acquired disorders of haem biosynthesis
b) They are rare genetic disorders of haem breakdown
c) Acute intermittent porphyria presents with neurovisceral crises and cutaneous manifestations
d) Urine porphobilinogens are not raised between attacks in acute intermittent porphyria
e) Treatment of an acute attack includes a low-carbohydrate diet

Answer: all false

Short Explanation
The acute porphyrias are rare genetic disorders of haem biosynthesis. Acute intermittent porphyria (AIP) is the commonest, characterised by gastrointestinal and neurological symptoms presenting in acute attacks. There are no cutaneous manifestations. Urine porphobilinogens are raised between attacks in 50% of patients. Treatment of attacks includes a high-carbohydrate diet.

Long Explanation
The porphyrias are classified into acute and non-acute. The acute porphyrias are autosomal dominant (variable pentrance) disorders of haem biosynthesis resulting in the toxic accumulation of porphobilinogen and δ-aminolaevulinic acid (porphyrin precursors). Acute intermittent porphyria (AIP) is the commonest acute porphyria and is characterised by acute neurovisceral crises but no cutaneous symptoms. Urine porphobilinogens are raised during attacks, and between attacks in 50% of patients.

Variegate porphyria and hereditary coproporphyria are characterised by photosensitive blistering skin rashes and/or acute attacks. Porphobilinogens are only raised during attacks in these variants.

Clinical features of acute attacks may mimic an acute abdomen with severe colicky abdominal pain, vomiting, fever and a raised white cell count. The patient may be hypotensive or shocked, with hyponatraemia or hypokalaemia. Neurological symptoms include psychosis, peripheral neuritis, paralysis or seizures. Drugs that may precipitate an acute attack include alcohol, barbiturates, halothane, some antibiotics (e.g. tetracyclines), oral hypoglycaemic agents and the oral contraceptive pill. Treatment is mainly supportive with symptom control but also includes a high carbohydrate diet and intravenous haematin.

The non-acute porphyrias are porphyria cutanea tarda, erythropoietic protoporphyria and congenital erythropoietic porphyria. They only exhibit cutaneous symptoms, and the defect results in porphyrin overproduction only, not porphyrin precursors.

Longmore JM, Wilkinson IB, Rajagopalan S. *Oxford Handbook of Clinical Medicine*, 6th edn. Oxford: Oxford University Press, 2004; p. 708.

MTF Question 9: Urinary tract infection

Regarding urinary tract infection:

a) Gram-negative organisms are usually involved
b) It rarely causes sepsis
c) More than 100 000 organisms/mm^3 on urinary microscopy is significant
d) Urinary catheterisation is rarely associated
e) Treatment should include urinary catheterisation

Answer: a, c

Short Explanation
Gram-negative organisms are usually involved in causing urinary tract infections. Greater than 100 000 organisms/mm^3 on urine microscopy is diagnostic of a urinary tract infection. Urinary catheterisation markedly increases the infection risk, and catheters should be removed as soon as possible to prevent infections. Urinary tract infections are a common cause of sepsis.

Long Explanation
A urinary tract infection occurs when bacteria in the urine cause inflammation to the genitourinary system. The kidney (pyelonephritis), bladder (cystitis), prostate (prostatitis) or urethra (urethritis) can all be affected. Women are more likely to have infections, because of the shorter urethra. Other risk factors include diabetes, pregnancy, impaired voiding and instrumentation of the urethra. Prophylactic antibiotics are usually given when instrumenting the urinary tract.

Gram-negative organisms are usually involved in causing urinary tract infections. *E. coli* and *Pseudomonas* species are commonly associated. The presence of white blood cells and > 100 000 organisms/mm^3 on urine microscopy are diagnostic of a urinary tract infection. Cultured organisms are tested for their sensitivity to different antibiotics.

Urinary catheterisation increases the infection risk markedly. Organisms gain entry to the bladder via the catheter lumen or along its outer surface. Urinary catheterisation should only be performed when necessary, and great care should be taken in placing urinary catheters with an aseptic technique. The risk of urinary tract infection increases the longer the catheters are left in situ, and hence catheters should be removed as soon as possible to prevent infections.

Urinary tract infections are a common cause of sepsis. Treatment involves antibiotics according to the sensitivity of the organism.

Longmore JM, Wilkinson IB, Rajagopalan S. *Oxford Handbook of Clinical Medicine*, 6th edn. Oxford: Oxford University Press, 2004; pp. 262–3.
Yentis S, Hirsch N, Smith G. *Anaesthesia and Intensive Care A-Z: an Encyclopaedia of Principles and Practice*, 3rd edn. Edinburgh: Butterworth-Heinemann, 2004; p. 526.

MTF Question 10: Pharmacology in renal failure

Which of the following statements regarding pharmacology in renal failure are true?

a) In acute kidney injury (AKI), the loading dose of a drug which undergoes excretion via the renal tract may need to be increased
b) The commonest reason for AKI caused by aminoglycosides is that they cause an interstitial nephritis
c) Imipramine is a cause of obstructive (post-renal) AKI
d) Acetazolamide is a cause of obstructive (post-renal) AKI
e) When using ketamine for analgesia, the dose should be reduced in patients with AKI

Answer: a, c, d

Short Explanation

Aminoglycosides cause acute tubular necrosis, not interstitial nephritis. Ketamine is metabolised in the liver, via norketamine, to inactive metabolites, which are renally excreted.

Long Explanation

The loading dose of a drug required to produce a desired plasma concentration is dependent on the volume of distribution (V_D). Since fluid retention is often seen in acute kidney injury (AKI), V_D increases, and an increase in dose may be required. However, the subsequent dosing will need to be altered if the drug is renally excreted, with dose reduction or increased dose interval.

Drugs may bring about kidney injury via pre-renal, post-renal or intra-renal damage. Pre-renal damage may be effected by non-steroidal anti-inflammatory drugs (NSAIDs) (which impair renal perfusion), ACE inhibitors (particularly in the context of renal artery stenosis), or indeed by any drug which causes volume depletion. Post-renal injury may occur in the context of crystalluria (leading to obstruction), which is a possible side effect of acetazolamide. Tricyclic antidepressants (e.g. imipramine) have anticholinergic side effects; prolonged urinary retention will give rise to a post-renal nephropathy. Intra-renal damage usually takes the form of a hypersensitivity reaction leading to either interstitial nephritis (e.g. NSAIDs, thiazides, penicillins) or glomerulonephritis (e.g. penicillamine, gold); other drugs have a direct toxic effect on the tubules (e.g. aminoglycosides).

Ketamine undergoes hepatic metabolism, via norketamine, to inactive metabolites which are renally excreted; its kinetics are therefore unaffected by renal impairment.

MTF Question 11: Central chemoreceptors

Regarding the role and location of central chemoreceptors in the control of breathing:

a) The central chemoreceptors are located near the dorsal surface of the pons
b) Central chemoreceptors respond rapidly to changes in carbon dioxide tension in the blood
c) Central chemoreceptors respond rapidly to changes in oxygen tension in the blood
d) The pH of cerebrospinal fluid is slightly acidic compared with plasma
e) Respiratory acidosis causes a greater increase in ventilation than metabolic acidosis

Answer: b, d, e

Short Explanation

The central chemoreceptors are located near the ventral surface of the medulla. These chemoreceptors have an important role in responding to changes in the arterial tension of CO_2, but not oxygen as would be expected.

Long Explanation

Control of breathing is complex and involves a number of receptors (chemoreceptors and lung receptors), central controllers (brainstem and cortex) and effectors to do the work (diaphragm and accessory muscles).

Chemoreceptors are extremely important in sensing changes in acid–base status, which are then communicated to the central controllers to mediate their desired respiratory changes via the effectors. The central chemoreceptors are located near the ventral surface of the medulla by the exit of the ninth and tenth nerves. They are surrounded by extracellular fluid of the brain, which is in contact with the cerebrospinal fluid (CSF).

The pH of cerebrospinal fluid is slightly acidic compared with plasma because it contains fewer proteins and hence a lesser ability to buffer pH changes. It is the changes in H^+ ions that actually mediate changes in respiration. Changes in the concentration of H^+ are caused by the easy diffusion of CO_2 across the blood–brain barrier into the extracellular fluid. The barrier is relatively impermeable to charged particles, and therefore H^+ and bicarbonate do not easily diffuse across. The increased CO_2 causes a shift in the equilibrium of the Henderson–Hasselbalch equation, which promotes the formation of H^+ and decreases the pH. It is this change in pH that mediates the appropriate increase in ventilation.

The changes in pH in the CSF caused by the increased CO_2 are exaggerated when compared with plasma, because of its limited buffering capacity. Respiratory acidosis causes a greater increase in ventilation than metabolic acidosis simply because the blood–brain barrier is permeable to CO_2. Patients who are chronic CO_2 retainers have a compensated near-normal CSF pH, so ventilation is comparatively low for the level of CO_2. These patients rely on their hypoxic drive (and hence the peripheral chemoreceptors) for ventilation.

West JB. *Respiratory Physiology*, 7th edn. Philadelphia, PA: Lippincott Williams & Wilkins, 2005; pp. 122–9.

A brief article on the control of breathing is available online at www.nda.ox.ac.uk/wfsa/html/u02/u02_011.htm (accessed 30 June 2012).

A pdf file on the control of breathing is available online at www.physiol.ox.ac.uk/~par/teaching/bm1_1ect/lecture6.pdf (accessed 30 June 2012).

MTF Question 12: Obesity

With regard to the cardiovascular complications associated with obesity, which of the following statements are correct?

a) Renal blood flow is increased in obesity
b) Cardiac arrhythmias can be caused by fatty infiltration of the conduction system
c) Obese individuals have an increased cardiac output predominantly due to an increased heart rate
d) Absolute blood volume is increased
e) Systemic hypertension is 2 times more prevalent than in the non-obese population

Answers: b, d

Short Explanation

Renal blood flow remains relatively unchanged in obesity. Obese individuals have an increased cardiac output predominantly due to an increased stroke volume. Systemic hypertension is 10 times more prevalent than in the non-obese population.

Long Explanation

Cardiovascular disease is a major cause of morbidity and mortality in obese individuals. Ischaemic heart disease is more common in the obese population. Underlying causes include hypercholesterolaemia, hypertension, diabetes, low high-density lipoprotein levels and physical inactivity. The increased metabolic demand of the adipose tissue causes an increase in total blood volume, cardiac output, oxygen consumption and arterial pressure. Absolute blood volume is increased mainly due to a combination of secondary polycythaemia and increased activity in the renin–angiotensin–aldosterone system. The actual blood volume is low relative to body mass and can be as small as 45 mL/kg.

The increased blood flow is directed mainly to tissue beds with increased fat deposition. Blood flow to the renal and cerebral systems remains relatively constant. Initially, with an increase in blood volume there is an increase in left ventricular filling and hence stroke volume and cardiac output.

Systemic hypertension is 10 times more common in the obese population. An expansion of the extracellular volume leading to hypervolaemia, and an increased cardiac output, are characteristic of obesity-induced hypertension. Left ventricular dilation results in an increased left ventricular wall stress and hypertrophy, which leads to reduced compliance of the ventricular wall. Diastolic dysfunction occurs, with impaired ventricular filling and an elevated left ventricular end-diastolic pressure. This combination leads to heart failure, and 'obesity cardiomyopathy' occurs when wall hypertrophy fails to keep pace with dilation. Left ventricular failure and pulmonary vasoconstriction result in pulmonary hypertension and eventually right heart dilation and failure. There is an increased risk of arrhythmias for many reasons; these include myocardial hypertrophy, coronary artery disease, increased circulating catecholamines, electrolyte disturbances related to diuretic therapy and fatty infiltration of the conducting and pacing systems.

Adams JP, Murphy PG. Obesity in anaesthesia and intensive care. *Br J Anaesth* 2000; **85**: 91–108.

Lotia S, Bellamy MC. Anaesthesia and morbid obesity. *Contin Educ Anaesth Crit Care Pain* 2008; **8**: 151–6. Available online at ceaccp.oxfordjournals.org/content/8/5/151 (accessed 30 June 2012).

Yentis S, Hirsch N, Smith G. *Anaesthesia and Intensive Care A–Z: an Encyclopaedia of Principles and Practice*, 4th edn. Edinburgh: Butterworth-Heinemann, 2009.

MTF Question 13: Critical care outreach

With regard to critical care outreach services (CCOS), which of the following are true?

a) There is no evidence that it reduces the number of patients who have received cardiopulmonary resuscitation (CPR) prior to ICU admission
b) There is strong (level 1A) evidence that it reduces ICU mortality
c) CCOS was introduced into the NHS without formal prospective evaluation processes
d) Early warning scores may form part of the track and trigger approach
e) Education of ward staff and junior doctors commonly forms part of its remit

Answers: c, d, e

Short Explanation

There is some evidence that CCOS is associated with significant decreases in the proportion of ICU admissions receiving CPR prior to admission. While there is evidence that it may reduce hospital mortality, there is little evidence, if any, that it reduces ICU mortality. One of the major problems in assessing its effectiveness is that there was no formal prospective evaluation implemented when CCOS was introduced.

Long Explanation

With the publication of *Comprehensive Critical Care* in 2000, CCOS was introduced widely into the NHS as an important component of the vision for the future of critical care services. However, without a structured model for its implementation it has taken on many forms across the NHS. It was also introduced without any formal prospective evaluation, making assessment of effectiveness and outcome particularly difficult.

There is insufficient robust research to fully assess the impact of CCOS on patient or service outcomes. Most studies were uncontrolled before-and-after studies and many were of poor methodological quality. Only one study has provided level 1 evidence for the UK, and this demonstrated that CCOS significantly reduced hospital mortality. In addition, two observational studies, which scored higher in terms of study quality, also demonstrated significant reductions in hospital mortality. However, the multicentre cluster RCT conducted by the MERIT team in Australia found no significant differences in any of the outcomes measured.

The three essential objectives of CCOS are to avert admissions, to enable discharges and to share critical care skills with staff on general hospital wards. This has been interpreted in many different ways, and CCOS activities are therefore diverse. They include training and education of general ward staff, track and trigger systems, telephone hotlines, post-critical-care follow-up and direct bedside support.

Track and trigger systems use periodic observation of vital signs (the 'tracking') with predetermined criteria (the 'trigger') for requesting the attendance of more experienced staff. Vital signs typically include heart rate, systolic blood pressure, respiratory rate, temperature, conscious level and urine output. There are different types of systems, ranging from a single-parameter system, where vital signs are compared against a simple set of criteria with predetermined thresholds, to aggregate weighted scoring systems, where vital signs are weighted according to importance.

Department of Health. *Comprehensive Critical Care: a Review of Adult Critical Care Services*. London: Department of Health, 2000. Available online at www.dh.gov.uk/en/Publicationsandstatistics/Publications/PublicationsPolicyAndGuidance/DH_40065 85 (accessed 30 June 2012).

MERIT Study Investigators. Introduction of the medical emergency team (MET) system: a cluster-randomised controlled trial. *Lancet* 2005; **365**: 2091–7.

Rowan K. Evaluation of outreach services in critical care. National Institute for Health Research Service Delivery and Organisation programme. Project SDO/74/2004. Available online at www.sdo.nihr.ac.uk/files/project/74-final-report.pdf (accessed 30 June 2012).

MTF Question 14: Hyperosmolar non-ketotic coma (HONK)

Which of the following are true of hyperosmolar non-ketotic coma (HONK)?

a) It is the same as hyperosmolar hyperglycaemic state
b) It is more common in type 1 diabetes than in type 2 diabetes
c) It presents with a mild ketosis
d) It presents in the absence of coma
e) Severe hyperglycaemia causes a functional thrombocytopenia

Answer: a, c, d

Short Explanation

HONK is more formally known as hyperosmolar hyperglycaemic state (HHS). It can occur in all age groups, but is most commonly seen in older patients with type 2 diabetes mellitus. There may be a mild ketosis, and true coma is uncommon. Patients are primarily at risk of thrombotic events.

Long Explanation

Hyperosmolar hyperglycemic state (HHS) is a life-threatening emergency manifested by marked elevation of blood glucose, hyperosmolarity, and little or no ketosis. HHS has replaced the term hyperosmolar non-ketotic coma (HONK) to acknowledge that the hyperosmolar hyperglycaemic state may involve a mild to moderate degree of clinical ketosis, and changes in consciousness may present without coma. Less than 20% of patients are comatose, and these patients represent the most severe end of the disease spectrum. Significant acidosis is rare, because of the low levels of ketones. HONK terminology is still used in clinical practice.

There are multiple precipitants, but infection is the most common. These patients are profoundly dehydrated and require aggressive fluid resuscitation (average of 9 L over 48 hours) and insulin infusions. They will also require careful monitoring of electrolytes and are likely to require electrolyte replacement. The hyperosmolar state adversely affects blood rheology, and hyperglycaemia itself potentiates collagen-induced platelet activation, leading to an increased risk of vascular occlusive events (e.g. mesenteric artery thrombosis and myocardial infarction). These patients should be on prophylactic low-molecular-weight heparin (LMWH) at a minimum, and consideration should be given to formal anticoagulation until they are adequately rehydrated.

Disseminated intravascular coagulation (DIC) has also been reported. Dextrans are fluids consisting of complex branched polysaccharides that increase blood glucose measurement; they are used as anti-platelet agents through reduction in platelet adhesiveness and their effect on von Willebrand factor.

Kitabchi AE, Umpierrez GE, Miles JM, Fisher JN. Hyperglycemic crises in adult patients with diabetes. *Diabetes Care* 2009; **32**: 1335–43.
Stoner GD. Hyperosmolar hyperglycemic state. *Am Fam Physician* 2004; **71**: 1723–30.

MTF Question 15: Cyanide: management of poisoning

Which of the following are recognised treatment options used in confirmed cyanide poisoning?

a) Dicobalt edetate
b) Hydroxocobalamin
c) Gastric lavage
d) Sodium nitroprusside
e) Sodium thiosulphate

Answer: a, b, c, e

Short Explanation

Dicobalt edetate, hydroxocobalamin and sodium thiosulphate are all recognised antidotes used in cyanide poisoning, although dicobalt edetate is reserved for cases of confirmed severe poisoning. Gastric lavage is suggested for patients presenting within 1 hour of ingestion with features of moderate or severe toxicity. Sodium nitroprusside can cause cyanide poisoning.

Long Explanation

Cyanide is a mitochondrial toxin that is among the most rapidly lethal poisons known to man. It can cause death within minutes to hours of exposure. Though significant cyanide poisoning is uncommon, it must be recognised rapidly to ensure prompt administration of life-saving treatment.

The most common source of cyanide poisoning in the UK is from fires and the combustion of household materials. Cyanide is used in a number of industrial processes, so there is also an occupational risk. Cyanide toxicity can also develop from the use of certain medications – commonly sodium nitroprusside, which is used in the treatment of hypertensive emergencies. There is also a potential risk of cyanide poisoning from the ingestion of certain food groups. Cyanide toxicity secondary to sodium nitroprusside is due to the release of cyanide groups during metabolism of the nitroprusside molecule.

Cyanide acts at a mitochondrial level by inhibiting electron transport and blocking ATP production, leading to reduced cellular oxygen utilisation. This causes anaerobic metabolism and a lactic acidosis. Symptoms of cyanide toxicity depend on the level of exposure, and can range from nausea, vomiting, drowsiness and anxiety to coma, seizures and cardiovascular collapse.

Initial management includes an ABC approach and administering high-flow oxygen. Blood cyanide levels can be measured, but only in a few laboratories, and the results may take some time, so it is recommended not to withhold treatment in cases of suspected moderate or severe cyanide toxicity. A lactate > 7 mmol/L, an elevated anion gap acidosis and a reduced arteriovenous oxygen gradient are all features that may suggest cyanide poisoning.

There are specific treatments available for cyanide poisoning, including hydroxocobalamin, sodium thiosulphate and dicobalt edetate (which should only be used in confirmed severe poisoning). Hydroxocobalamin combines with cyanide to form cyanocobalamin (vitamin B_{12}), which is renally cleared. Sodium thiosulphate enhances the conversion of cyanide to thiocyanate, which is renally excreted. Dicobalt edetate acts as a chelating agent by forming a stable complex with cyanide ions. Because this is a relatively rare form of poisoning seen in hospitals, it is sensible to seek help from your local poisons unit if cyanide poisoning is suspected.

Cummings TF. The treatment of cyanide poisoning. *Occup Med (Lond)* 2004; **54**: 82–5. Available online at occmed.oxfordjournals.org/content/54/2/82.full.pdf (accessed 30 June 2012).

MTF Question 16: Functional residual capacity

Functional residual capacity (FRC):

a) Can be measured using Fowler's method
b) Is the sum of the residual volume and the expiratory capacity
c) Is a fixed volume
d) Exceeds the closing capacity in the elderly
e) May be reduced by restrictive lung disease

Answer: e

Short Explanation
The functional residual capacity (FRC) is not a fixed volume but varies with respiration and postural changes. It is the sum of the residual volume and the expiratory reserve volume. In the elderly, the FRC is reduced and the closing capacity is increased. Therefore, FRC = closing capacity (CC) in the upright position at 65 years. Fowler's method is used to measure anatomical dead space and closing capacity.

Long Explanation
The functional residual capacity (FRC) is the volume of gas present in the lungs at the end of normal expiration. It is the sum of the residual volume and the expiratory

reserve volume and measures approximately 2.5–3.0 litres in an average adult male. (Remember, lung volumes are measured directly while lung capacities are the sum of two or more volumes). The FRC cannot be measured using simple spirometry, as it includes the residual volume. It can be measured using helium dilution, nitrogen washout or body plethysmography. Physiologically, the FRC is important, as it acts as an oxygen reservoir and helps minimise large variations in the arterial partial pressure of oxygen (PaO_2) during respiration. In addition, the relationship between the FRC and closing capacity (CC) predicts airway closure during expiration.

CC is the volume at which airway closure occurs during expiration, mainly in the dependent regions of the lung. In a normal, young adult, FRC exceeds CC, thereby holding the airways open. If the FRC is reduced, hypoxaemia may occur, due to either of the aforementioned principles. The FRC is reduced by the supine position (by 20–25%), obesity, pregnancy, extremes of age, restrictive lung disease (pulmonary fibrosis) and anaesthesia (although the mechanism is unknown). The FRC is increased by positive intrathoracic pressure, emphysema and asthma.

Fowler's method is a single-breath nitrogen washout used to measure anatomical dead space and closing capacity. This test differs from the nitrogen washout test used to determine FRC as the latter examines the total volume of expired gas over several minutes, not a single breath.

Smith T, Pinnock C, Lin T. *Fundamentals of Anaesthesia*, 3rd edn. Cambridge: Cambridge University Press, 2009; pp. 360–2.
Yentis S, Hirsch N, Smith G. *Anaesthesia and Intensive Care A–Z: an Encyclopaedia of Principles and Practice*, 3rd edn. Edinburgh: Butterworth-Heinemann, 2004; pp. 122–3.

MTF Question 17: Turner syndrome

Which of the following statements are true regarding Turner syndrome?

a) Patients often suffer from menorrhagia
b) Common clinical features include short stature
c) It only affects females
d) Mental retardation is common
e) Coarctation of the aorta occurs in 10% of patients

Answer: b, c, e

Short Explanation

Turner syndrome is a chromosomal abnormality where all or part of the X chromosome is absent, resulting in an XO genotype. Patients can have learning difficulties, but they do not have mental retardation. Turner syndrome patients are amenorrheic and infertile.

Long Explanation

Turner syndrome (TS) is a chromosome abnormality caused by complete or partial deletion of the X chromosome. The incidence is approximately 1 in 2000 live female births. Turner syndrome can be divided into 'classic Turner syndrome', in which an X chromosome is completely missing, and 'mosaic Turner syndrome', in which a complete X chromosome is only missing from some cells. Confirmation of a diagnosis is by karyotype. Prenatal diagnosis can be made by chorionic villous sampling, amniocentesis or ultrasound. Diagnosis should be considered in a neonate found to have coarctation of the aorta or oedema of the hands and feet. However, most girls are diagnosed in childhood by the absence of a pubertal growth spurt, when the lack of development of secondary sexual characteristics becomes apparent.

Other clinical features include lymphoedema of the hands and feet, broad chest with widely spaced nipples, droopy eyelids, low hairline, low-set ears, web neck, high arch palate, hearing problems, myopia, pigmented naevi, spoon-shaped nails.

Life expectancy in Turner syndrome is reduced by approximately 10 years. Treatment aims to reduce complications. During regular check-ups blood pressure treatment may be necessary, as well as tests of thyroid function, glucose levels and bone mineral density, along with hormone treatments and psychological support. Growth-hormone treatment for short stature and in-vitro fertilisation (IVF) for infertility are optional treatments.

Davenport ML. Approach to the patient with Turner syndrome. *J Clin Endocrinol Metab* 2010; **95**: 1487–95. Available online at jcem.endojournals.org/content/95/4/1487 (accessed 30 June 2012).

Hjerrild BE, Mortensen KH, Gravholt CH. Turner syndrome and clinical treatment. *Br Med Bull* 2008; **86**: 77–93.

MTF Question 18: Psychological techniques in pain management

Regarding psychological techniques in pain management:

a) There is no evidence to support psychological support in chronic pain patients
b) Psychological management is helpful to cure chronic pain conditions
c) Cognitive behavioural therapy challenges maladaptive thinking patterns
d) Encouraging patients to pace their activity facilitates coping with chronic pain
e) Psychological techniques encourage malingering behaviour

Answer: c, d

Short Explanation

A growing body of evidence attests to the value of cognitive behavioural therapy and recognising pain as a biopsychosocial problem, requiring multidisciplinary management. Psychological techniques promote acceptance of pain conditions, but do not offer a cure. There is no evidence to suggest that malingering behaviour is encouraged.

Long Explanation

Until Melzack and Wall's gate control theory of pain was published in 1965, the experience of pain was considered to be a biomedical issue, with pain expected to be proportional to the extent of tissue damage observed. Psychological dimensions to the pain experience were thought to be due to patient hysteria, and the pain was described as 'functional' if it was thought that the responses were disproportionate to the trauma observed.

After 1965 thinking shifted towards psychological factors as being intrinsic to the pain experience, including acute pain. Melzack and Wall suggested that cognitive activity (thoughts and inward interpretations of the pain experience) are also relevant to opening and closing the pain gate, or enhancing or diminishing the impact of pain.

Psychological management of chronic pain begins with accepting the patient's problem: pain is what the individual says it is, irrespective of the physical observations. A growing body of evidence attests to the value of developing behavioural modification programmes, based on the clinicians accepting that the patient has pain, the patient accepting his or her pain condition and challenging fear-avoidance behaviour in anticipation of causing 'damage' by engaging in activity. Systematic modification of activity, encouraging pacing, and steady build-up of activity is more likely to produce better functional results than prolonged periods of inactivity, which lead to muscle deconditioning, inevitable weight gain and feelings of frustration. Pacing involves spreading activity evenly throughout the day with a view to getting the most out of one's daily energy. This may then allow a steady build up of activity over time. Sudden periods of over-activity can lead to flare-ups of pain, leading the patient into a self-defeating cycle.

Cognitive behavioural therapy (CBT) techniques have been developed to challenge the defeatist thoughts patients have around their chronic pain problem. While a 'cure' may not be offered, acceptance by the patient, with the pain decentralised from his or her life, is more likely to move him or her forward and result in a return to function. Catastrophising about symptoms (for example 'I will end up in a wheelchair because of my bad back; nothing can be done to help me') can trigger unhelpful emotional and behavioural responses which ultimately lead to chromic disability. CBT therefore aims to help identify negative thinking patterns and challenge such thoughts, to construct more useful appraisals of a patient's situation.

British Pain Society. *Recommended Guidelines for Pain Management Programmes for Adults.* London: BPS, 2007. Available online at www.britishpainsociety.org/book_pmp_main.pdf (accessed 30 June 2012).
Melzack R, Wall PD. Pain mechanisms: a new theory. *Science* 1965; **150**: 971–9.

MTF Question 19: Pathophysiology, diagnosis and management of pneumonia

Which of the following statements regarding community-acquired pneumonia (CAP) are true?

a) A chest radiograph is necessary to make the diagnosis
b) Urea and electrolytes offers important prognostic information
c) The white blood cell count is an important prognostic determinant in non-immunosuppressed patients
d) *Staphylococcus aureus* is the most common causative organism
e) Macrolides should be discontinued in patients admitted to intensive care if the atypical pneumonia screen is negative

Answer: b

Short Explanation
There is no convincing evidence to show that WBC count on presentation affects outcome other than in previously immunosuppressed patients. *Streptococcus pneumoniae*, *Haemophilus influenzae* and *Moraxella catarrhalis* are the most frequent pathogens. Combination antibiotic therapy which includes macrolides has been shown to reduce mortality in intensive care.

Long Explanation
A chest radiograph is not mandatory in the community, and patients can be treated for suspected community-acquired pneumonia (CAP) on clinical criteria, but hospitalised patients should have an x-ray performed. The components of the CURB-65 score are confusion, elevated urea (>7 mmol/L), respiratory rate (>30 breaths/min), blood pressure (systolic < 90 mmHg or diastolic <60 mmHg) and age > 65 years. One point is scored for each of these five components that meets these criteria. The cumulative total predicts 30-day mortality.

CURB-65 total	30-day mortality
0	0.6%
1	3.2%
2	13.0%
3	17.0%
4	41.5%
5	57.0%

Streptococcus pneumoniae, Haemophilus influenzae and *Moraxella catarrhalis* account for approximately 85% of community-acquired pneumonia pathogens. The spectrum of pathogens encountered in CAP is different to those found in patients with pneumonia on intensive care. Often the patients on intensive care have more severe illness or are from populations more likely to require extra support (e.g. *Staphylococcus aureus* following viral infections and *Klebsiella* in relative immunosuppression such as alcohol excess). Macrolides as part of combination antibiotic therapy have been shown to reduce mortality in ICU patients with severe sepsis.

Lim WS, Baudouin SV, George RC, *et al*. BTS guidelines for the management of community acquired pneumonia in adults: update 2009. *Thorax* 2009; **64** (Suppl 3): iii1–55.

Tejerina E, Frutos-Vivar F, Restrepo MI, *et al.*; International Mechanical Ventilation Study Group. Prognosis factors and outcome of community-acquired pneumonia needing mechanical ventilation. *J Crit Care* 2005; **20**: 230–8.

Waterer GW. Are macrolides now obligatory in severe community-acquired pneumonia? *Intensive Care Med* 2010; **36**: 562–4.

MTF Question 20: Clonidine use in critical care

The following are true of the use of clonidine in critical care:

a) It is predominantly a postsynaptic α_2-adrenoreceptor agonist
b) It has an oral bioavailability approaching 100%
c) On starting the medication it may cause initial, short-lived, hypertension
d) It can be stopped abruptly without a reducing dosage regime
e) It is the first-line treatment for agitation in a recently extubated patient with traumatic brain injury and established acute alcohol withdrawal

Answer: b, c

Short Explanation

Clonidine acts by stimulating the presynaptic α_2-adrenoreceptors. Rapid withdrawal can lead to life-threatening rebound hypertension and tachycardia. Although commonly used for agitation associated with traumatic brain injury and alcohol withdrawal, it is not a first-line treatment.

Long Explanation

Clonidine is an imidazoline compound with α-adrenoreceptor agonist properties and an α_2 : α_1 ratio of approximately 20 : 1, making it predominately an α_2-agonist. Licensed for the treatment of hypertension, migraine and menopausal flushing, it also has analgesic, sedative and anxiolytic properties, making it a useful agent in anaesthesia and intensive care.

It acts by stimulating the presynaptic α_2-adrenoreceptors, thereby decreasing noradrenaline release from both central and peripheral sympathetic nerve terminals. By acting on the locus coeruleus, in the floor of the fourth ventricle, and depressing thalamic transmission to the cerebral cortex, it provides both sedation and analgesia. Hypotension is caused by its action on the dorsal nucleus of the vagus nerve.

Clonidine is rapidly and well absorbed orally, with a bioavailability of 100%. It can also be given intravenously either as a bolus dose or as an infusion. It causes an initial, shortlived, increase in blood pressure and systemic vascular resistance due to activation of vascular postsynaptic α_2-adrenoreceptors. A decrease in heart rate and blood pressure follows through a centrally mediated reduction in sympathetic tone and vagal stimulation. Rapid withdrawal can lead to a life-threatening rebound hypertension and bradycardia.

Clonidine is used as both an analgesic and a sedative in the intensive care setting, and it has been used successfully in both ventilated and spontaneously breathing patients. It can be used in a variety of conditions including the control of autonomic and psychological symptoms of alcohol and drug withdrawal and agitation secondary to traumatic brain injury. However, clonidine is not a first-line treatment for these conditions, and evidence for its use in intensive care, although promising, is still lacking.

Dexmeditomidine is a newer α_2-adrenoreceptor agonist with similar properties to clonidine. Recent trial evidence concerning its use as a sedative on intensive care is promising.

Jamadarkhana S, Gopal S. Clonidine in adults as a sedative agent in the intensive care unit. *J Anaesthesiol Clin Pharmacol* 2010; **26**: 439–45.

MTF Question 21: Cultural and religious factors influencing attitudes to brainstem death

Regarding current religious rulings and cultural attitudes to brainstem death in the UK, which of the following statements are true?

a) It is considered *haraam* (forbidden) for Muslims to become heart-beating organ donors
b) Orthodox Jewish law, *Halacha*, accepts brainstem death as comparable to cardiorespiratory death
c) *Shariah* (Islamic) law representatives in the UK consider brainstem death to be a true definition of death
d) Buddhist doctrine does not accept brainstem death to be a true definition of death
e) Brainstem death is still considered legal in the UK even if the patient's family reject the diagnosis on religious grounds

Answer: c

Short Explanation

There is no specific legislation for a medical declaration of death to be rejected in UK law. Brainstem death is controversial in Jewish law and is not currently accepted by Orthodox Jews in the UK. Buddhism accepts brainstem death as cessation of vitality that will lead to 'heart death'. The UK Muslim Law Council accepted brainstem death as a true definition of death in 1996, and decreed that Muslims could become heart-beating organ donors.

Long Explanation

Brainstem death occurs after neurological injury when the brainstem has been irreversibly damaged but the heart is still beating and the body is kept alive by a ventilator. International variations in brainstem death criteria, together with traditional and religious influences, evoke opposing and controversial views on how 'acceptable' brainstem death is within different cultures. Altruism is highly regarded in Judaism, Islam and Buddhism, and organ donation is considered to be a final selfless act, but opinions are divided within these communities as to whether it is acceptable to donate body parts after death, howsoever it is deemed to occur medically.

In some Islamic societies, organ donation is not acceptable: violation of the human body, either living or dead, is forbidden (*haraam*). Islamic governing law, *Shariah*, in the UK currently accepts brainstem death as an acceptable definition of cessation of life: the UK Muslim Council in 1996 agreed that 'current medical knowledge considers brainstem death to be a proper definition of death … constituting the end of life for the purpose of organ transplantation.' It legitimised UK Muslims to carry donor cards, and to become heart-beating organ donors should they so wish.

Orthodox Jews internationally are currently intensely debating the validity of brainstem death. The collective body of Jewish law, *Halacha*, in the UK has rejected the definition of brainstem death, it not being compatible with cardiorespiratory death, which constitutes a traditional *halachic* death (January 2011).

Buddhist scripture implies that death only occurs when vitality, heart and consciousness have all left the body. By embracing the concept that brainstem death will inevitably lead to the cessation of all bodily functions, together with the importance of consciousness for moral standing, Buddhists have accepted brainstem death. Organ donation, however, is less widely accepted. Tampering with a corpse in the critical days after death is believed by some to interfere with the rebirth of the soul. However, other Buddhist scholars suggest that organ donation is a final compassionate act as a means to acquire merit for a better rebirth.

In the state of New Jersey, USA, there is a specific provision for religious objection to insist on asystole before death has occurred. No such legislation exists in UK law.

Keown D. *Buddhism and Bioethics*, new edn. London: Palgrave Macmillan, 2001.
Religion, organ transplantation, and the definition of death [editorial]. *Lancet* 2011; **377**: 271.
UK's Muslim Law Council approves organ transplant. *J Med Ethics* 1996; **22**: 99. Available online at www.ncbi.nlm.nih.gov/pmc/articles/PMC1376922 (accessed 30 June 2012).

MTF Question 22: Pipeline and suction systems

Concerning the pipeline medical gas supply to theatres:

a) Medical oxygen is supplied at a pressure of 4 bar via a white coloured hose
b) Air is supplied via a black and white hose at a pressure of either 4 or 7 bar
c) The pipeline gas distribution network upstream of the wall terminal outlets is made of reinforced PVC with an antistatic core
d) Each Schrader valve has a similar external diameter irrespective of the gas pipeline that ends at it
e) By law it must be possible to disconnect a hose from a Schrader valve using one hand only

Answer: a, b, d, e

Short Explanation
The pipeline distribution network upstream from the Schrader valve is made from phosphorus-containing, deoxidised, non-arsenical copper.

Long Explanation
Oxygen, nitrous oxide, medical air and Entonox are distributed throughout a hospital using a colour-coded pipeline network. The pipes are labelled at regular intervals and

are made from phosphorus-containing, deoxidised, non-arsenical copper. They are heat-treated to withstand high pressure and all joins are made using a specific brazing alloy made from silver.

All of the above are delivered at an end pipeline pressure of 4 bar with the exception of medical air, which in theatres is delivered to an anaesthetic machine at 4 bar but with a separate 7 bar air supply allowing use of air-powered theatre equipment, e.g. drills for orthopaedic surgery. This pipeline network terminates at colour-coded, labelled, self-sealing, gas-specific sockets known as Schrader valves. These valves are made non-interchangeable via a collar indexing system that is unique to each gas. Although the external diameter of each valve is similar, each valve has a collar indexing system that will only allow connection with a gas-specific hose ending in a Schrader probe. It is a legal requirement that this probe should be able to be both removed and inserted quickly using one hand only.

The anaesthetic responsibility for checking this gas supply is downstream from the Schrader valve only. The hoses connecting the individual Schrader valves to the anaesthetic machine are colour-coded (white for oxygen, blue for nitrous oxide, black and white for medical air, and blue and white for Entonox), have an internal diameter of 6.5 mm and are manufactured from reinforced PVC with an antistatic core.

MTF Question 23: Local anaesthetics

Which of the following statements regarding local anaesthetics are true?

a) Ester and amide local anaesthetic agents have exactly the same mechanism of action
b) Local anaesthetic agents are weak acids
c) A local anaesthetic agent with a low pKa will have a fast onset of activity
d) Local anaesthetic agents only work after being 'trapped' inside nerve cells
e) Local anaesthetic agents preferentially bind to sodium channels in their open state

Answer: a, c, d, e

Short Explanation
Amides and esters work in the same way: un-ionised drug enters the cell where it is 'trapped' in the ionised, active form and binds sodium channels in their open state. Local anaesthetics are weak bases, and hence a lower pKa means a higher percentage in the un-ionised state at pH 7.4.

Long Explanation
Local anaesthetic (LA) agents are widely used in anaesthesia. There are two classes of LA drugs based on their chemical structure: esters and amides. However, the mechanisms of action are the same for both.

LAs work by selectively binding voltage-gated sodium channels in their active state. These channels are present in neural tissue, opening when the membrane potential becomes sufficiently depolarised and triggers the propagation of an action potential. After opening for a short period they become inactivated and refractory for a few milliseconds, before being reset by the repolarisation of the membrane. This prevents retrograde transmission of nerve impulses and tonic activity of the nerve. LAs bind open sodium channels on the intracellular side, and hence they need to cross the cell membrane and enter the cell to have their effect.

All LAs are weak bases, meaning that they are largely ionised at neutral pH, and only the un-ionised form of the drug can cross the cell membrane. The pKa value (the pH at which a substance is 50% ionised) of the LA determines its speed of onset, since a basic drug with a lower pKa will have a greater proportion present in the un-ionised state at pH 7.4 than one with a higher pKa (e.g. lidocaine pKa 7.9, bupivacaine pKa 8.1). Once inside the cell, the pH is lower, causing the drug to become ionised again. Only the ionised form interacts with the sodium channel, and this means that the active form of the drug is 'trapped' in the cell where it is required. This explains the lack of efficacy of LAs in acidic environments (such as infected tissue): less drug is present in the un-ionised form and hence less enters the cell.

Other important characteristics of LAs include their degree of protein binding (correlated to duration of action), lipid solubility (weakly correlated to potency) and intrinsic vasodilator activity (which affects both potency and duration).

Peck T, Hill S, Williams M. *Pharmacology for Anaesthesia and Intensive Care*, 3rd edn. Cambridge: Cambridge University Press, 2008.

Yentis S, Hirsch N, Smith G. *Anaesthesia and Intensive Care A-Z: an Encyclopaedia of Principles and Practice*, 4th edn. Edinburgh: Butterworth-Heinemann, 2009.

MTF Question 24: Intercostal nerves

Which of the following statements about the intercostal nerves are correct?

a) The intercostal nerves contain sensory, motor and autonomic fibres
b) The intercostal nerves supply the skin over the sternum and over the spine
c) The intercostal nerves run between the internal intercostal muscle and the transversus thoracic muscle
d) Paravertebral block will provide adequate analgesia for a rib fracture
e) A chest drain should be inserted at the inferior aspect of the intercostal space

Answer: a, d, e

Short Explanation

The intercostal nerves are formed from the ventral primary rami of the spinal nerves of T1–T11. The dorsal primary rami supply the skin over the spine. Both rami contain sensory, motor and autonomic fibres and can be anaesthetised by a paravertebral block. The intercostal nerves run between the internal and the innermost intercostal muscles at the superior end of the intercostal space.

Long Explanation

The spinal nerves are mixed motor, sensory and autonomic nerves. They emerge from the intervertebral foramina before dividing into dorsal and ventral primary rami. The dorsal primary rami pass posteriorly to innervate the muscles, bones, joints and skin of the back. The ventral primary rami of T1–T12 then pass anteriorly, T1–T11 as pairs of intercostal nerves and T12 as a pair of subcostal nerves.

As with the spinal nerve from which they originated, these nerves contain motor, sensory and autonomic fibres. A well-placed thoracic paravertebral block will anaesthetise the ventral primary ramus, providing analgesia from fractured ribs.

The intercostal nerves initially run in the middle of the intercostal space, but by the time they reach the angle of the rib they are sheltered by the costal groove of the rib at the superior aspect of the intercostal space. The nerves are the most inferior component of the neurovascular bundle in the costal groove (the vein is superior and the artery lies in the middle). Because of the position of the neurovascular bundle, chest drains should be inserted at the inferior aspect of the space, just above a rib. At this point the intercostal nerves lie between the internal and innermost intercostal muscles. The transversus thoracis muscles are slips of muscle running between the xiphoid process and the inferior costal cartilages (they are continuous inferiorly with the transversus abdominis muscle).

The intercostal nerves give off the following branches as they course around the chest wall:

• Collateral branches, which supply the intercostal muscles.

- Lateral cutaneous branches, which pierce the external intercostal muscle to provide sensation over the lateral chest wall.
- Anterior cutaneous branches, which supply the skin of the anterior thorax and upper abdomen.

Moore KL. The intercostal spaces. In: *Clinically Orientated Anatomy*, 3rd edn. Baltimore, MD: Williams & Wilkins, 1992; pp. 51–60.

MTF Question 25: Carcinoid syndrome

The following are features suggestive of carcinoid syndrome:

a) Diarrhoea
b) Hypertensive episodes
c) Facial flushing
d) Dementia
e) Wheeze

Answer: a, c, d, e

Short Explanation

Patients with carcinoid syndrome commonly exhibit symptoms of severe diarrhoea, flushing, wheeze and asthma attacks, and they may be hypotensive during these episodes. Dementia, along with dermatitis and diarrhoea, may result from niacin deficiency (pellagra) due to high serotonin levels.

Long Explanation

Carcinoid tumours originate from the neuroendocrine cells and are slow-growing. The majority of cases are located in the gastrointestinal tract, in particular the appendix and the ileum, but they may also be located in the respiratory tract, or very rarely in other intra-abdominal organs. They are highly vascularised, and most of these tumours produce 5-hydroxytryptamine (serotonin), which is taken up and stored in the platelets. If serotonin is present in excess, it is inactivated in the liver and lung and transformed into 5-hydroxyindoleacetic acid (5-HIAA).

Malignant carcinoid syndrome is the constellation of symptoms exhibited by patients with a metastatic carcinoid tumour which has spread to the liver, or in patients with a pulmonary carcinoid tumour. In these cases, serotonin is not degraded by the liver. Only 10% of patients with a carcinoid tumour will suffer from carcinoid syndrome, and the characteristic features are hot, red flushing of the face, severe diarrhoea and asthma attacks. The flushing results from increased secretion of kallikrein, which stimulates the productions of bradykinin, a powerful vasodilator. If there is cardiac involvement, murmurs may be audible on auscultation, and if there are liver metastases, there may be hepatomegaly. Peripheral oedema is also a feature. High levels of serotonin can cause a depletion of tryptophan leading to niacin deficiency, also known as pellagra, causing dermatitis, dementia and diarrhoea. After spreading to the liver, carcinoids can metastasise to the lungs, bone, skin, or almost any organ.

Serotonin causes vasodilation and can increase the risk of thrombosis by stimulating platelet aggregation, which may result in disseminated intravascular coagulation (DIC). However, serotonin is converted to 5-HIAA in the body. Carcinoids may also produce many other different polypeptides and amines.

The biochemical diagnosis of carcinoid tumours is based on the measurement of the serotonin metabolite 5-HIAA in a 24-hour urine collection. Urinary 5-HIAA excretion of 25 mg/day is diagnostic of carcinoid.

Bendelow J, Apps E, Jones LE, Poston GJ. 2008. Carcinoid syndrome. *Eur J Surg Oncol* 2008; **34**: 289–96.

Maroun J, Kocha W, Kvols L, *et al.* Guidelines for the diagnosis and management of carcinoid tumors. Part 1: the gastrointestinal tract. A statement from a Canadian National Carcinoid Expert Group. *Curr Oncol* 2006; **13**: 67–76

MTF Question 26: Blood gas samples

When performing an arterial blood gas, which of the following are true?

a) Excess heparin in the syringe will make the sample more acidic
b) Carbon dioxide levels are measured by changes in electrode pH
c) Air bubbles in the sample increase the carbon dioxide partial pressure
d) A pH of 7.4 is equivalent to 40 mmol/L of hydrogen ions
e) A sample kept at room temperature has a lower hydrogen ion concentration

Answer: a, b

Short Explanation
Air bubbles in the arterial blood gas sample increase the oxygen partial pressure and decrease the carbon dioxide partial pressure. A pH of 7.4 is equivalent to 40 nmol/L of hydrogen ions. At room temperature cellular metabolism continues, causing a reduction in oxygen partial pressure, and high carbon dioxide partial pressure and hydrogen ion concentration.

Long Explanation
An analyser requires a fresh arterial blood gas, which is heparinised and anaerobic. Heparin should only form a thin film on the interior of the syringe and fill the dead space. Excess heparin causes a lowering of the pH because it is acidic. If air bubbles are present in the sample, the partial pressure of oxygen increases and the partial pressure of carbon dioxide decreases. If a sample is left at room temperature, cellular metabolism persists. This causes a reduction in the partial pressure of oxygen as it is utilised and an increase in carbon dioxide partial pressure and hydrogen ion concentration. The sample should be kept on ice if there is a delay in analysis.

   The measured parameters on an arterial blood gas analyser are arterial blood oxygen partial pressure, carbon dioxide partial pressure and the pH. From these measurements other parameters are calculated, e.g. bicarbonate, base excess, oxygen saturation. Oxygen partial pressure and pH are measured by changes in their concentration. Carbon dioxide partial pressure is measured by measuring the changes in pH of an electrolyte solution using a modified pH electrode. The carbon dioxide diffuses across a membrane and reacts with water to produce hydrogen ions, changing the pH. A pH of 7.4 corresponds to 40 nmol/L, not 40 mmol/L.

Al-Shaikh B, Stacey S. *Essentials of Anaesthetic Equipment*, 2nd edn. London: Churchill Livingstone, 2002; pp. 164, 172.

MTF Question 27: Glasgow Coma Scale

Which of the following statements regarding the Glasgow Coma Scale (GCS) are true?

a) A decorticate response to stimulus will score 2 on the motor component
b) Moaning in pain will score 2 on the voice component
c) A sternal rub is an appropriate painful stimulus

d) With asymmetrical limb movement, the best limb should be scored for the motor component
e) The original Glasgow Coma Scale was scored out of 14

Answer: b, d, e

Short Explanation
Decorticate posturing is abnormal flexion (M3); decerebrate posturing is extension (M2). A sternal rub will provide an appropriate stimulus to assess eye opening, but may not allow differentiation between normal flexion (M4) and localisation to pain (M5).

Long Explanation
The original Glasgow Coma Scale described by Teasdale and Jennett in 1974 was scored out of 14 and omitted abnormal flexion. The scale in common usage is properly described as the Modified Glasgow Coma Scale.

Best motor response: M1 = none; M2 = decerebrate posturing, characterised by extension to pain (abduction of the arm, internal rotation at the shoulder, forearm pronation and wrist extension); M3 = decorticate posturing, i.e. abnormal flexion to pain (adduction of the arm, internal rotation of the shoulder, forearm pronation and wrist flexion); M4 = flexion/withdrawal to pain (elbow flexion, forearm supination, wrist flexion or pulling away from painful stimulus); M5 = localise to pain (purposeful movements towards painful stimulus, hand should rise above clavicle when supraorbital ridge pressure is applied); M6 = obeys simple commands.

Best voice response: V1 = none; V2 = incomprehensible sounds; V3 = inappropriate words; V4 = confused; V5 = orientated.

Best eye opening: E1 = none; E2 = opens eyes to painful stimulus; E3 = opens eyes to voice; E4 = eyes open spontaneously.

Teasdale G, Jennett B. Assessment of coma and impaired consciousness: a practical scale. *Lancet* 1974; **2** (7872): 81–4.

MTF Question 28: Capnography

Which of the following cause a rise in end-tidal carbon dioxide?

a) Pulmonary embolism
b) Hypovolaemia
c) Hyperthermia
d) Sepsis
e) Flow rates of less than 150 mL/kg/min using a coaxial Mapleson D circuit during spontaneous ventilation

Answer: c, d, e

Short Explanation
Any increase in metabolism and re-breathing will increase end-tidal carbon dioxide. Pulmonary embolism and hypovolaemia cause hypoperfusion and will reduce end-tidal carbon dioxide levels.

Long Explanation
Any increase in metabolic activity will increase the production of carbon dioxide and hence end-tidal carbon dioxide. Causes may include sepsis, malignant hyperthermia, hyperthermia, hypermetabolism and skeletal muscle activity. Other causes of a raised end-tidal carbon dioxide include hypoventilation and re-breathing. A coaxial map D circuit is efficient for controlled ventilation but inefficient for

spontaneous ventilation. At flow rates less than 150 mL/kg/min during spontaneous ventilation, re-breathing would occur.

Conversely, causes of a decreased end-tidal carbon dioxide level include hypothermia, hypometabolism and hyperventilation. Any cause of hypoperfusion will also cause a decrease in end-tidal carbon dioxide, such as hypotension, hypovolaemia and pulmonary embolus. Absence of end-tidal carbon dioxide can be useful for detecting disconnection, oesophageal intubation or loss of cardiac output!

Al-Shaikh B, Stacey S. *Essentials of Anaesthetic Equipment*, 2nd edn. London: Churchill Livingstone, 2002; pp. 117–20.

MTF Question 29: Renin

Regarding renin:

a) Renin is released from the macula densa in response to a decrease in circulating volume
b) Release is inhibited by angiotensin II
c) Sympathetic stimulation, via activation of α-adrenoreceptors, stimulates renin release
d) Release is stimulated by atrial natriuretic peptide
e) Renin directly stimulates the release of vasopressin

Answer: b

Short Explanation

Renin is released from the granular cells of the juxtaglomerular apparatus, not the macula densa. Vasopressin (antidiuretic hormone, ADH) release is activated indirectly by renin through the formation of angiotensin II. Stimulation of β_1-adrenoreceptors can also lead to renin release. Atrial natriuretic peptide is released from cardiac atrial cells in response to atrial stretch. This hormone causes a reduction in renin release.

Long Explanation

Renin is a proteolytic enzyme that is synthesised and stored by the juxtaglomerular apparatus. The juxtaglomerular apparatus is a microscopic structure within the kidney that regulates renal blood flow and the glomerular filtration rate (GFR). It consists of intrarenal baroreceptors and granular cells (containing renin) in the wall of the afferent arteriole and the macula densa within the walls of the early distal tubules.

The release of renin can be stimulated in three ways: (1) decreased sodium content in the distal tubules of the kidney, (2) sympathetic nervous system activation, (3) renal artery hypotension. A decrease in the sodium content of the tubular fluid is sensed by the specialised macula densa, leading to renin release. The granular cells are innervated by sympathetic nerve fibres. In response to a decrease in effective circulating volume (ECV), sympathetic activity increases to compensate for the fall in systemic blood pressure and cardiac output. The stimulation of β_1-receptors leads to renin release to ultimately help restore a normal circulating volume. Renal sympathetic stimulation also results in renal vasoconstriction upstream of the granular cells. Because of an increase in vascular resistance, arteriolar wall tension is decreased, which is sensed by baroreceptors present in the afferent arteriole. This further stimulates renin release. A decrease in circulating volume will have the same effect, also working via the afferent arteriolar baroreceptor reflex.

Once released from the granular cells, renin cleaves angiotensinogen into angiotensin I. Angiotensin-converting enzyme, present on the surface of endothelial cells in the lungs, further cleaves angiotensin I to form the active hormone, angiotensin II. Renin is the rate-limiting step in this process.

Smith T, Pinnock C, Lin T. *Fundamentals of Anaesthesia*, 3rd edn. Cambridge: Cambridge University Press, 2009; p. 346.

MTF Question 30: Magnesium

Regarding magnesium:

a) Magnesium is the second most abundant extracellular cation
b) Magnesium antagonises N-methyl-D-aspartic acid (NMDA) receptors in the central nervous system
c) The biggest stores of magnesium in the body are in the skeleton
d) Magnesium is a cofactor for Na^+/K^+-ATPase
e) Hypomagnesaemia may produce cardiac arrhythmias similar to those caused by hypokalaemia

Answer: b, c, d, e

Short Explanation
Magnesium is the fourth most abundant extracellular cation and the second most abundant intracellular cation.

Long Explanation
Magnesium is used as a cofactor in over 100 reactions in the body and also acts as a membrane stabiliser. It has a role in both protein and DNA production and nerve conduction. Hypomagnesaemia produces similar effects on the heart as those found with hypokalaemia. Magnesium is required for the effective functioning of Na^+/K^+-ATPase, and low magnesium levels may therefore lead to a reduction in the ability of cells to maintain an ionic concentration gradient.

Magnesium competes with calcium for transport systems across cell membranes. Low magnesium levels leave calcium to enter damaged cardiac cells more readily and accelerates the subsequent process of cell death. Magnesium antagonises NMDA receptors in the central nervous system and has been shown to act as an adjuvant to analgesics if administered intraoperatively.

Magnesium is the second most common intracellular cation and the fourth most common extracellular cation after sodium, potassium and calcium. 30% of the body's magnesium is within skeletal and cardiac muscle, but the majority of body magnesium is held within the skeleton.

Calvey N, Williams N. *Pharmacology for Anaesthetists*, 5th edn. Oxford: Blackwell, 2008; p. 300.

MTF Question 31: Pregnancy-induced hypertension

With regard to the diagnosis and treatment of gestational hypertension:

a) Oral hydralazine should be commenced as first-line treatment
b) Gestational hypertension is defined as a sustained sitting blood pressure > 140/90 mmHg occurring after 20 weeks gestation
c) Gestational hypertension is defined as an increase in systolic blood pressure ≥ 30 mmHg or diastolic blood pressure ≥ 15 mmHg occurring after 20 weeks gestation
d) Oral labetalol at a dose of 50–100 mg twice daily is appropriate initial treatment unless there are contraindications
e) Amlodipine is an acceptable alternative to nifedipine to treat gestational hypertension

Answer: b, d

Short Explanation

Oral hydralazine is not recommended as first-line treatment, and amlodopine has no established safety profile for pregnant women. The favoured current definition of gestational hypertension is new-onset hypertension with sustained sitting blood pressure > 140/90 mmHg occurring after 20 weeks gestation.

Long Explanation

Pregnancy-induced hypertension by definition occurs after 20 weeks gestation, and it is often used as an umbrella term to describe all hypertensive diseases that are caused by pregnancy. The definitions and terminology have changed over a number of years, but the National Institute for Health and Clinical Excellence (NICE) guidance issued in 2010 used the term 'gestational hypertension' to describe new onset of hypertension occurring after 20 weeks gestation without significant proteinuria. Hypertension is defined as mild, moderate, or severe:

	Diastolic BP (mmHg)	Systolic BP (mmHg)
Mild	90–99	140–149
Moderate	100–109	150–159
Severe	110	160

NICE recommends that women who are diagnosed with gestational hypertension have frequent measurements of urinary protein or urinary protein-to-creatinine ratio at antenatal visits. It is recommended that women have their blood pressure measured once-weekly for mild hypertension, and if the patient is deemed at high risk for developing pre-eclampsia then this should be more frequent. For moderate hypertension, blood pressure should be measured twice-weekly with blood tests to check full blood count, renal and liver profile.

Treatment for gestational hypertension should only be started if moderate or severe hypertension is diagnosed. It is recommended that women with severe hypertension are admitted until their blood pressure is under 159/109 mmHg. First-line treatment with oral labetalol is recommended, and alternatives include methyldopa and nifedipine if there are contraindications to labetalol. Fetal monitoring is recommended to check fetal growth, amniotic fluid volume and umbilical artery Doppler velocimetry. Generally delivery is planned for after 37 weeks.

Dalgleish DJ. Pre-eclampsia. *AnaesthesiaUK* 2006. Available online at www.anaesthesia uk.com/article.aspx?articleid=100463 (accessed 30 June 2012).

National Institute for Health and Clinical Excellence. *Hypertension in Pregnancy: the Management of Hypertensive Disorders During Pregnancy.* NICE Clinical Guideline **107**, August 2010. Available online at www.nice.org.uk/CG107 (accessed 30 June 2012).

MTF Question 32: Intracranial contents

Regarding the cranial vault in a healthy adult:

a) The mass of a human brain is approximately 1000 g
b) Brain parenchyma occupies 85% of the cranial volume
c) Volume of cerebrospinal fluid in the cranial vault is 150 mL
d) Blood occupies 7% of cranial vault volume
e) Early compensation for raised intracranial pressure (ICP) includes reduced production of cerebrospinal fluid

Answer: b, d

Short Explanation
The mass of the human brain is 1400 g. The volume of CSF within the cranial vault (as opposed to total CSF volume) is c. 75 mL. Early compensation mechanisms for rising ICP include displacement and reabsorption of CSF, but not reduced production.

Long Explanation
The fixed volume of the cranial vault contains brain parenchyma, arterial and venous blood and cerebrospinal fluid (CSF). An increase in the volume of any one of the components must be accompanied by a compensatory decrease in another to avoid raising intracranial pressure (Monro–Kellie doctrine).

The mass of the human brain is 1400 g. Its volume is around 1500 mL (as fat is less dense than water). A remarkable property of the brain being bathed in cerebrospinal fluid (CSF), on which it 'floats', is that the brain effective weight in vivo is 50 g. Some candidates may be perturbed when working though calculations regarding intracranial contents that the cranial vault appears to be of inadequate size to accommodate the brain. Remember, however, that not all of the brain resides in the cranial vault, yet it still contributes to its mass.

There is considerable variety in the quoted volumes and percentages of cranial contents depending on source, but the following is a reasonable aggregate. Total volume of CSF is 150 mL but 75 mL is in the spinal intrathecal space so only 75 mL is in the cranial vault (although this is sometime quoted as high as 100 mL intracranial). This represents 7–10% of the intracranial volume. Between 5% and 8% is the cerebral blood volume, leaving 85% of the intracranial volume occupied by brain parenchyma.

As intracranial pressure rises (by whatever mechanism), production of CSF by the choroid plexus remains remarkably consistent (at 0.35 mL/min or 500 mL/day) unless the intracranial pressure rises high enough to reduce cerebral perfusion pressure to less than 70 mmHg, whereupon CSF production decreases. Early compensation mechanisms for rising intracranial pressure are displacement of CSF into the spinal space, reduction in cerebral venous volume and increase in CSF reabsorption by the arachnoid villi. Resistance to reabsorption remains constant (thus absorption flow is proportional to pressure gradient) until the intracranial pressure reaches 30 cmH$_2$O, when the resistance to reabsorption falls.

MTF Question 33: Pyloric stenosis

Regarding pyloric stenosis:

a) It is more common in females
b) Metabolic acidosis is common
c) Surgery must be performed immediately upon diagnosis
d) It usually presents in the first week of life
e) Blood results typically show a hypokalaemic, hyperchloraemic metabolic alkalosis

Answer: all false

Short Explanation
Pyloric stenosis is more common in males. It presents between 4 and 6 weeks of age with projectile vomiting. Severe dehydration can occur. Blood results typically show a hypokalaemic, hypochloraemic metabolic alkalosis. It is important to correct the dehydration and metabolic abnormalities prior to surgical intervention.

Long Explanation

Pyloric stenosis is a common surgical problem, occurring in approximately 1 in 350 live births. Firstborn males are more commonly affected. The condition is caused by hypertrophy of the pyloric muscle, which then causes gastric outflow obstruction. The aetiology of pyloric stenosis is unknown.

Pyloric stenosis presents between 4 and 6 weeks of age with persistent vomiting (which can be projectile), dehydration, failure to thrive and a hypochloraemic, hypokalaemic metabolic alkalosis. Occasionally a mass can be palpated in the right upper quadrant or epigastrium. Diagnosis can be confirmed by ultrasound scan.

Prior to surgery it is important to correct any metabolic abnormality. For this reason, surgical correction is never an emergency. A nasogastric tube on free drainage should be sited. Prior to induction of anaesthesia the nasogastric tube should be aspirated in all four quadrants. This is done by moving the baby into right lateral, left lateral, supine and prone positions and aspirating the nasogastric tube in all positions. Induction of anaesthesia is most commonly performed by a rapid sequence induction, because of the increased risk of aspiration.

MTF Question 34: Desflurane

Which of the following statements about desflurane are true?

a) Desflurane has a lower blood : gas partition coefficient than nitrous oxide
b) Desflurane increases the risk of haemorrhage during obstetric procedures
c) Desflurane increases respiratory secretions and may cause bronchospasm
d) Desflurane is likely to cause bradycardia if used at high concentrations
e) Desflurane requires a special vaporiser because it is unstable at room temperature

Answer: a, b, c

Short Explanation

Blood : gas partition coefficients: desflurane 0.42; nitrous oxide 0.47. Like all volatiles, desflurane reduces uterine muscle tone. Desflurane is very irritating to the airways. If the inspired fraction is rapidly increased sympathetic stimulation causes tachycardia and hypertension. The special vaporiser is required because its boiling point is near room temperature.

Long Explanation

The most notable thing about desflurane is that it has a boiling point close to room temperature (22.8 °C) and a saturated vapour pressure close to atmospheric pressure. This makes it impossible to use in a standard plenum vaporiser, and instead a microprocessor-controlled vaporiser heats the agent to above its boiling point and then injects it directly into the fresh gas stream. This makes the desflurane vaporiser very accurate, although it is dependent on a power supply and will not work until the unit has reached operating temperature.

Desflurane has a lower blood : gas partition coefficient than nitrous oxide (0.42 vs. 0.47) but its equilibration rate is slower (probably because nitrous oxide is less lipid-soluble and is distributed differently to the peripheral compartments). However, it still has a very rapid onset and offset of action, and it is much more potent than nitrous oxide, with a MAC of 5–6%. It has little cardiovascular effect, producing a limited fall in SVR above 2 MAC and causing very little myocardial depression. It does not sensitise the heart to catecholamines.

It is pungent and irritating to the airways, making it unsuitable for inhalational induction, and indeed it causes increased bronchial secretions and may provoke bronchospasm in susceptible individuals. If the inspired fraction is increased rapidly at the onset of anaesthesia desflurane causes a sympathetic surge leading to transient tachycardia and hypertension, possibly as a result of airway irritation. Tidal volume falls and respiratory rate rises in patients breathing desflurane spontaneously, and there is a rise in $PaCO_2$. Cerebral metabolic requirements for oxygen fall under desflurane anaesthesia (as they do with all volatile agents) but it can cause a rise in cerebral blood flow and hence intracranial pressure; however, this is not significant below 1 MAC. It decreases skeletal and uterine muscle tone and potentiates neuromuscular blockade. It is excreted from the lungs largely unchanged, and only 0.02% undergoes hepatic metabolism.

Moppett I. lnhalational anaesthetics. *Anaesth lntens Care Med* 2008; **9**: 567–72.

Smith T, Pinnock C, Lin T. *Fundamentals of Anaesthesia*, 3rd edn. Cambridge: Cambridge University Press, 2009.

MTF Question 35: Muscular dystrophy

Regarding Duchenne muscular dystrophy (DMD):

a) DMD presents from early childhood and is progressive
b) DMD occurs equally in both sexes
c) Genetic counselling is recommended
d) Calf hypertrophy with lower motor neurone signs and restrictive lung function deficit are indicative of DMD
e) Diagnosis is confirmed by response to steroid therapy and plasmaphoresis or immunoglobulin infusion

Answer: a, c, d

Short Explanation
Duchenne muscular dystrophy is X-linked recessive, and occurs almost exclusively in males. Diagnosis is confirmed by a combination of history (including family history), clinical examination, muscle biopsy, DNA analysis, EMG (electromyography), ECG and blood tests. There are no specific treatment options.

Long Explanation
Myopathies can present in the form of muscular dystrophies, a group of genetically inherited diseases presenting with progressive weakness and degeneration of groups of muscles. The myopathy classically involves proximal, symmetrical development of muscle weakness – e.g. difficulty combing hair or climbing stairs, neck flexion being weaker than extension – with preservation of tendon reflexes. Other disease states need to be ruled out: for example, excess fatigability on exercise is more characteristic of myasthenia; fasciculations imply anterior horn or root disease; strangely firm muscles imply a pseudohypertrophic muscular dystrophy. Muscular tumours are rare.

Relevant tests for muscular dystrophies, aside from EMG studies and DNA analysis, include a number of blood tests – e.g. ESR, creatine phosphokinase (CPK), lactate dehydrogenase and aspartate transaminase (AST).

The Duchenne and Becker dystrophies are dystrophinopathies – diseases due to genetic mutations causing defective production of the large membrane-associated protein dystrophin. The Duchenne gene is located on the short arm of the X chromosome, and it is this gene that is responsible for both Duchenne and Becker dystrophy

As with other recessive genetic conditions associated with chromosomal abnormalities on the X chromosome, DMD and Becker dystrophy rarely present in females.

In order for a female to be affected both X chromosomes would need to be abnormal, whereas in males the Y chromosome offers no protection against an X-linked abnormality. Duchenne gives complete functional protein loss and leads to severe disease presentation, generally at about the age of 4 years. Ambulation is typically lost by the teenage years and death secondary to cardiorespiratory failure occurs between the ages of 20 and 30. There is no specific cure.

Becker dystrophy gives rise to a truncated form of the dystrophin protein but allows for partial protein functionality. Date of onset in Becker dystrophy can range from infancy to older adult age, and it has a better prognosis than Duchenne.

Hypertrophy of calf muscles with lower motor neurone signs and restrictive lung function deficit (particularly on lying flat) can aid diagnosis, along with history. Response to steroid therapy and plasmaphoresis or immunoglobulin infusion confirms the diagnosis of an entirely different condition (which happens also to present with weakness and restrictive lung function) – Guillain–Barré syndrome. Here the weakness is ascending and there are autonomic disturbances following recent infection.

MTF Question 36: Large veins and anterior triangle of neck

Which of the following statements regarding the internal jugular vein are correct?

a) The internal jugular vein drains the sigmoid sinus
b) The internal jugular vein joins the subclavian vein posterior to the clavicle
c) The internal jugular vein begins at the foramen lacerum at the base of the skull
d) Horner's syndrome is a recognised complication of attempted cannulation of the internal jugular vein
e) The internal jugular vein is valveless

Answer: a, b, d

Short Explanation

The internal jugular vein begins at the jugular foramen as the continuation of the sigmoid sinus. It passes anterior to the sympathetic chain (which may be damaged by attempted cannulation) and ends behind the sternal part of the clavicle by uniting with the subclavian vein. A bicuspid valve is found near its termination in the inferior bulb of the vein.

Long Explanation

The internal jugular vein is the largest vein in the neck and represents the continuation of the sigmoid sinus at the jugular foramen. It drains the brain and superficial areas of the head and neck. At its origin, a superior bulb is identified. From here, the vein courses inferiorly in the carotid sheath in the anterior triangle of the neck, lateral to the internal carotid and, more inferiorly, the common carotid artery. The vagus nerve lies between the vein and the artery within the carotid sheath.

Of note is that the cervical sympathetic chain lies immediately posterior to the carotid sheath, and so it is not impossible that recurrent failed attempts at cannulation of the internal jugular vein may injure the chain, producing a Horner's syndrome. This is caused by a lack of sympathetic supply to the head.

The vein exits the anterior triangle of the neck by passing inferior to the sternocleidomastoid muscle, passing deep to the gap between the sternal and clavicular head of this muscle, where it may be accessed for cannulation via a 'low' approach. Behind the sternal end of the clavicle the vein unites with the subclavian vein to form the brachiocephalic vein. Near its termination, the inferior bulb of the internal jugular vein is noted, and this contains a bicuspid valve.

Moore KL. The neck. In: *Clinically Orientated Anatomy*, 3rd edn. Baltimore, MD: Williams & Wilkins, 1992; pp. 802–16.

MTF Question 37: Hyperkalaemia

A 17-year-old girl is admitted to the emergency department with collapse following a 2-day history of vomiting. On examination she is slim, with patches of vitiligo. She is currently haemodynamically stable. Blood tests reveal sodium 129 mmol/L, potassium 6.9 mmol/L, urea 5.2 mmol/L, creatinine 89 μmol/L. ECG shows sinus rhythm with peaked T waves. Ideal initial management should include:

a) Intravenous hydrocortisone
b) Salbutamol nebuliser
c) Short adrenocorticotrophic hormone (ACTH) stimulation test
d) Calcium gluconate
e) Intravenous glucose and insulin infusion

Answer: a, d

Short Explanation

This patient with Addison's disease presents with adrenal crisis. Immediate management is parenteral hydrocortisone, which should not be delayed pending investigation. Calcium gluconate is cardio-protective in hyperkalaemia with ECG changes. Measures to reduce her potassium levels, including salbutamol and insulin infusion, are not indicated immediately, as treating the adrenal crisis may result in normalisation of potassium levels.

Long Explanation

Addison's disease is a cause of primary adrenal insufficiency with a functioning pituitary gland, raised adrenocorticotrophic hormone (ACTH), and glucocorticoid and mineralocorticoid deficiencies. Commonest causes include autoimmune disease (as suggested here, along with vitiligo), tuberculosis (commonest cause worldwide), bilateral adrenalectomy, HIV/AIDS and metastatic carcinoma.

Patients present with either chronic features or, as in this case, adrenal crisis. Patients presenting in crisis have nausea, vomiting, diarrhoea, muscle cramps and fever, and are often in circulatory shock. Blood tests reveal hyperkalaemia and hyponatraemia, and they may also have hypercalcaemia and hypoglycaemia.

In patients suspected of presenting in adrenal crisis, treatment should not be delayed pending results or further investigation. Immediate treatment is with parenteral glucocorticoid replacement, plus replacement of sodium if depleted. The patient may also need mineralocorticoid replacement.

Once the patient is stabilised, further investigation including the short ACTH stimulation test is indicated. This test is used to diagnose primary or secondary adrenal insufficiency and to assess the hypothalamic–pituitary–adrenal axis in patients taking suppressive glucocorticoid therapy, and it relies on ACTH-dependent adrenal atrophy in secondary adrenal insufficiency, so it may not detect acute insufficiency. Plasma cortisol is measured before and 30 minutes after Synacthen (ACTH) intramuscular injection. ACTH levels are also measured before Synacthen administration. Cortisol levels in Addison's disease fail to increase in response to Synacthen in primary or secondary adrenal insufficiency (levels < 460 nmol/L pre- and 30 minutes post-Synacthen). ACTH is low in secondary adrenocortical insufficiency and high in Addison's disease.

It is also important to treat the sequelae of electrolyte abnormalities. In this case the patient has profound hyperkalaemia, with ECG changes suggestive of cardiac strain as a result. ECG changes associated with hyperkalaemia include flattened P waves and widened QRS complexes due to inactivation of sodium channels and slow conduction of electrical impulses through the heart, and peaked T waves due to rapid repolarisation of the cardiac action potential. ECG changes, however, correlate poorly with the degree of hyperkalaemia.

The immediate management is with calcium gluconate, which is a cardio-protective agent, reducing the excitability of the cardiomyocytes by increasing the threshold potential and restoring the gradient between threshold and resting membrane potentials. Potassium-lowering treatments including salbutamol and insulin/glucose infusions are indicated in patients where potassium levels are not normalised with prompt treatment of the Addison's crisis.

Aslam S, Friedman EA, Ifudu O. Electrocardiography is unreliable in detecting potentially lethal hyperkalaemia in haemodialysis patients. *Nephrol Dial Transplant* 2002; **17**: 1639–42.

Ten S, New M, Maclaren N. Clinical review 130: Addison's disease 2001. *J Clin Endocrinol Metab* 2001; **86**: 2909–22.

MTF Question 38: Care of the pregnant woman in critical care: amniotic fluid embolism

Which of the following statements relating to amniotic fluid embolism (AFE) are correct?

a) A maternal age of < 20 years makes the diagnosis of AFE more likely
b) A simple blood test can be performed to confirm the diagnosis of AFE
c) Pulmonary oedema leading to hypoxaemia is often seen in AFE
d) Coagulopathy is uncommon in AFE
e) The majority of cases occur in the immediate post-partum period

Answer: c

Short Explanation
Young maternal age is relatively protective of AFE. There is no diagnostic test available at present, and diagnosis is made on clinical grounds. Coagulopathy is seen in the majority of patients with AFE. More than 70% of cases occur during labour.

Long Explanation
Amniotic fluid embolism (AFE) is a rare but potentially fatal syndrome that is unique to pregnancy. It is an obstetric emergency and most commonly presents in the intrapartum or immediate post-partum period. More than 70% of cases occur during labour. AFE classically presents as a sudden cardiovascular collapse associated with respiratory compromise and hypoxaemia, fetal distress and the development of a coagulopathy or disseminated intravascular coagulation (DIC). This is not always the presentation, and it is important to consider AFE as a diagnosis in any unwell obstetric patient.

Initially it was felt that AFE was due to mechanical obstruction of the maternal circulation by amniotic fluid. It has more recently been suggested that the clinical picture of AFE is due to an immune process whereby the fetal antigens in amniotic fluid initiate a cascade immune response similar to that seen in anaphylaxis.

There are no proven risk factors for AFE, but some associations include: maternal age >35 years; multiparity; placenta praevia and placental abruption; polyhydramnios; caesarean section or instrumental delivery; eclampsia; fetal distress and intrauterine fetal death; and induction or augmentation of labour.

As already mentioned, there are a number of different ways AFE can present, and symptoms in the obstetric patient may be preceded by fetal distress. Haemodynamic changes seen include left ventricular failure and pulmonary oedema. The amniotic fluid causes an increase in pulmonary vascular resistance and pulmonary vasospasm, which along with ventricular failure causes the hypoxaemia seen. Acute respiratory distress syndrome (ARDS) can occur as a result of the initial lung injury. The majority of patients with AFE develop some form of coagulopathy, because amniotic fluid contains procoagulant factors and hence activation of the coagulation cascade can be triggered.

The important points in the management of AFE are early recognition, resuscitation and delivery of the fetus. Haemodynamic stability should be maintained by using fluid filling and vasopressors. Treatment of the coagulopathy should include early involvement of a haematologist. The baby should be delivered early, within 5 minutes if the mother is undergoing CPR.

The morbidity and mortality associated with AFE is high, and the majority of patients who survive will require ICU care. There are no specific pharmacological or other therapies that prevent or treat AFE at present, and treatment on the ICU is generally targeted at organ support. A number of treatment options have been used, with varying success, including cardiopulmonary bypass and plasma exchange.

Dedhia JD, Mushambi MC. Amniotic fluid embolism. *Contin Educ Anaesth Crit Care Pain* 2007; **7**: 152–6. Available online at ceaccp.oxfordjournals.org/content/7/5/152 (accessed 30 June 2012).

MTF Question 39: Botulism

Regarding botulism, which of the following are true?

a) *Clostridium botulinum* is a Gram-negative anaerobic rod
b) Patients with botulism caused by wound infections should be treated with penicillin
c) Botulinum toxin blocks presynaptic release of acetylcholine
d) Patients present with flaccid paralysis and autonomic dysfunction
e) Botulinum antitoxin should be given to reverse the muscle weakness

Answer: b, c, d

Short Explanation

Clostridium botulinum is an anaerobic Gram-positive rod and is sensitive to penicillin. The toxin blocks presynaptic release of acetylcholine, causing paralysis. Antitoxin will limit the disease but not reverse paralysis.

Long Explanation

Clostridium botulinum (CB) is an anaerobic Gram-positive spore-forming rod. It grows in soil and dust and poorly preserved food. Under anaerobic conditions it produces the botulinum toxin that causes the clinical manifestations. The toxin is denatured by normal cooking (boiling) but the spores are more resistant, requiring pressure-cooking (e.g. 120 °C). The toxin can also be produced in infected wounds, which require debridement and penicillin to prevent further production. It is also associated with skin injections in drug abuse.

The toxin is a very potent inhibitor of presynaptic acetylcholine release, causing both autonomic and motor dysfunction. Typical presentation is with a descending flaccid paralysis, diplopia, bulbar symptoms, dry mouth and postural hypotension. Respiratory muscle weakness and bulbar dysfunction can lead to respiratory failure and death unless respiratory support is instituted.

The diagnosis can be confirmed by detecting either the organism (in faeces or vomitus) or the toxin (in faeces or serum). The toxin is tested for using an in-vivo assay (injection into rat peritoneum), which takes several days. Treatment is largely supportive, and a low threshold for admission to intensive care and intubation is needed. The antitoxin binds to circulating toxin and will limit the severity and progression of weakness but will have no effect on established weakness. Mortality is approximately 10%, but if patients survive they should return to normal muscle power – although this may take over a year to achieve.

Wenham T, Cohen A. Botulism. *Contin Educ Anaesth Crit Care Pain* 2008; **8**: 21–5. Available online at ceaccp.oxfordjournals.org/content/8/1/21 (accessed 30 June 2012).

MTF Question 40: Pharmacokinetic variation and trauma

Which of the following statements about the pharmacokinetics of drugs in patients following major trauma are correct?

a) Drugs administered via nasogastric tube have the same absorption kinetics as if they were taken orally
b) Hepatic enzyme activity is decreased following major trauma by the activity of pro- and anti-inflammatory cytokines
c) A patient anticoagulated with warfarin can expect to require a lower dose to maintain the same INR after major trauma
d) The volume of distribution of water-soluble drugs increases after major trauma
e) After head injury, brain levels of most drugs will increase

Answer: b, c, d, e

Short Explanation

Crushing or dissolving tablets for administration through a nasogastric tube alters the absorption kinetics. The stress response reduces serum albumin, increasing the free fraction of warfarin. Water retention is due to the release of antidiuretic hormone. Head injury damages the blood–brain barrier, allowing increased drug passage into the brain.

Long Explanation

Major trauma interferes with absorption, distribution, metabolism and elimination of drugs. The stress response increases cardiac output and redistributes fluid toward core organs, decreasing blood flow to the gut and skin and affecting absorption from these sites. Gut absorption is also affected by altered gastric and intestinal pH, because of gut ischaemia or antacid medications given to reduce the risk of gastric ulceration.

Crushing or dissolving oral tablets to make them fit down a nasogastric tube markedly alters the absorption kinetics of some drugs (e.g. phenytoin), increasing the rate of drug uptake with potentially toxic effects.

Pro- and anti-inflammatory cytokines downregulate hepatic production of albumin and other proteins and inhibit liver enzymes, including the cytochrome P450 system. Decreased plasma protein levels increase the free fraction of highly protein-bound drugs (e.g. warfarin), an effect that is magnified by acidosis (which alters the binding sites of albumin to reduce their drug affinity). Fluid and sodium are retained because of antidiuretic hormone and steroids, but fluid is lost into the interstitial space as the capillaries become leaky because of widespread inflammation. The overall effect is to increase the volume of distribution (V_D) for water-soluble drugs. Hepatic blood flow is impaired, as is renal blood flow, reducing drug clearance and first-pass effects for drugs with a high extraction ratio.

The use of extracorporeal circuits (e.g. for renal replacement therapy or extracorporeal membrane oxygenation) increases the V_D again, as well as complicating elimination. Some drug binds to the circuit, effectively removing it from the body, but haemofiltration/diafiltration has a variable effect on drug clearance. Some (usually smaller) drugs are cleared very efficiently and need to be given in higher doses to maintain an effective plasma concentration, while others are largely unaffected by renal replacement.

Renal function can also change rapidly, so frequent monitoring of drug levels needs to be maintained. The blood–brain barrier usually excludes all except highly lipid-soluble drugs from the brain, but its disruption by head injury or the use of hyper-osmolar agents (e.g. mannitol) in the treatment of raised intracranial pressure leads to higher than expected drug concentrations in the brain.

Peck T, Hill S, Williams M. *Pharmacology for Anaesthesia and Intensive Care*, 3rd edn. Cambridge: Cambridge University Press, 2008.
Smith T, Pinnock C, Lin T. *Fundamentals of Anaesthesia*, 3rd edn. Cambridge: Cambridge University Press, 2009.

MTF Question 41: Impact of occupational, environmental and socioeconomic factors on critical illness

Regarding the impact of occupational, environmental and socioeconomic factors on critical illness:

a) Alcohol-related deaths are more frequent in males than in females
b) Patients from lower socioeconomic backgrounds have a higher incidence of obstructive sleep apnoea than the general population
c) Low socioeconomic status is associated with worse long-term survival after critical illness, after adjusting for effects of age, severity of illness and comorbidities
d) Patients with a history of drug dependence are at increased risk of delirium in intensive care
e) Where patients with alcohol dependence require supplemental enteral nutrition, protein restriction is recommended to reduce the risk of hepatic encephalopathy

Answer: a, b, c, d

Short Explanation
Protein restriction used to be recommended in patients with alcohol dependence to reduce the risk of encephalopathy, but this practice has been abandoned as it was found to cause muscle wasting. Where encephalopathy is present, branched chain amino acid feeds may be preferred.

Long Explanation
Despite significant improvements in population health, the differences in health outcomes between patients of different socioeconomic status (health inequalities) have increased over time in many Western countries. Low socioeconomic status is associated with more comorbidities, higher acuity of critical illness, worse hospital outcomes and greater long-term mortality. The long-term mortality difference has been found to persist even after adjustment for acuity of critical illness and comorbidities.

Alcohol-related deaths are increasing in the UK, having doubled in the last 15 years. Alcohol-related deaths are more common in males, but are increasing in both sexes and across all age groups. The Alcohol Reduction Strategy for England estimates that up to 22 000 premature deaths per year are associated with alcohol misuse. Hospital admissions where alcohol-related disease was either the primary or secondary diagnosis are also increasing, with an estimated cost to the NHS of £1.7 billion per year.

Malnutrition is common in alcoholic patients and is associated with poor outcome. Nutrition should be commenced early, with enteral nutrition preferred over total parenteral nutrition (TPN). In the past, low-protein feeds have been recommended to reduce the risk of encephalopathy, but this is no longer the case, and routine enteral feeds can be used in most cases.

Department of Health. Alcohol statistics. Available online at www.dh.gov.uk/en/Publichealth/Alcoholmisuse (accessed 30 June 2012).

MTF Question 42: Lymphatic system

Regarding human lymphatics, which of the following statements are true?

a) The adult flow of lymph is 2–4 L/h
b) Collecting lymphatics have smooth muscle in their walls and have valves
c) Entrainment promotes lymph flow
d) Radical mastectomy and axillary node clearance results in upper-limb lymphoedema in 50% of patients
e) In a test tube, pure lymph will clot

Answer: b, c, e

Short Explanation

Lymph may be considered to be an ultrafiltrate of plasma – that which is not reabsorbed into the capillary. It contains coagulation factors and, in total, 7–9 g/dL of protein. Its flow rate is 2–4 L/day. Axillary lymph node clearance results in upper-limb oedema in 20% of patients.

Long Explanation

The flux of fluid across capillary endothelium is fairly well balanced (by Starling forces) such that net loss is of the order of 2–4 L per day into the interstitium. This excess passes into the lymphatics and is returned to the circulation by separate vessels. As the fluid arrives in the interstitium by virtue of an excess of pressure on one side of a semipermeable membrane, it can be regarded as an ultrafiltrate.

The fluid accumulates in initial lymphatics, which are devoid of smooth muscle and valves. Lymph flows through initial lymphatics under the influence of pulsatile muscles or arteries in the vicinity. Initial lymphatics coalesce into collecting lymphatics, which have valves and muscular walls that via peristaltic waves propel lymph towards rejoining the intravascular compartment at the subclavian veins (at the junctions with the internal jugular vein). The rapid flow of venous blood here produces an entrainment suction effect that further encourages lymph flow.

Just as an imbalance in Starling forces at the capillary may result in interstitial oedema, obstruction of lymph flow can result in a back-pressure sufficient to cause accumulation of lymph in the tissues – lymphoedema. Collecting lymphatics regularly traverse lymph nodes as they are also responsible for returning immune cells to the circulation. Lymphadenopathy (or surgical disruption of the lymphatics, as in radical mastectomy) can cause this obstruction and lead to lymphoedema. This occurs in the ipsilateral arm of 20% of patients who have had an axillary lymph node clearance.

Lymph does contain proteins (including coagulation factors) but in lower concentration than in plasma.

MTF Question 43: Treatment of migraine

Regarding drug prophylaxis in migraine, which of the following are considered first-line treatment?

a) Atenolol
b) Propanolol

c) Bisoprolol
d) Amitriptyline
e) Nortripyline

Answer: a, b, c, d, e

Short Explanation
The treatment of migraine is either by active or by preventive means. A combination of techniques can be implemented depending on attack frequency and severity. Second-line treatments include topiramate and sodium valproate. Gabapentin and methysergide are considered third line.

Long Explanation
Headache has been described as the most common medical complaint known to man. Primary headache accounts for more than 90% of headache complaints. This includes migraine, tension-type headache, cluster headache and the trigeminal autonomic cephalalgias, none of which is associated with demonstrable organic disease or structural neurological abnormality.

Migraine is characterised by various combinations of neurological, autonomic and gastrointestinal symptoms. It is divided into two types: migraine without aura (70%) and migraine with aura (30%). The International Classification of Headache Disorders (ICHD-II) has specific criteria for diagnosing migraine with or without aura.

Migraine with aura, previously termed classic migraine, has a reversible preceding aura comprising one or more of the following visual disturbances: homonymous hemianopsia, tunnel vision, scotoma, photopsia. Additionally, patients may experience photophobia, phonophobia, paraesthesia, hemiplegia, aphasia, nausea, vomiting, abdominal discomfort, diarrhoea. Migraine headache can be unilateral (60%) or bilateral (40%), located anywhere about the head or neck, and it may last for 4–72 hours. It has a throbbing, pulsating quality with moderate to severe intensity, and numerous accompanying features including nausea (90%), vomiting (33%), vertigo, fatigue, confusion, ataxia, drowsiness, photophobia, phonophobia and nasal congestion. Migraine is aggravated by postural change, activity and raised intracranial pressure. The recovery phase is one of irritability or malaise, although some feel refreshed or euphoric. Migraine attacks are triggered by stress, menses, pregnancy, dietary habit (e.g. red wine, cheese, chocolate and nuts), odours, light, and poor sleep.

Acute treatment: a stepped management has been recommended

* Step 1: Simple oral analgesic + antiemetic. Aspirin, ibuprofen, tolfenamic acid. Paracetamol alone is not efficacious. Prochlorperazine, domperidone or metoclopromide as indicated.
* Step 2: Rectal analgesic + antiemetic. Diclofenac suppository + rectal domperidone.
* Step 3: Specific anti-migraine drugs + antiemetic. Sumatriptan, zolmitriptan, rizatriptan, naratriptan. Ergotamine in cases of recurrent relapse.
* Step 4: Combination therapy of steps 1, 2, 3. Opioids provide small additional benefit.

Drug prophylaxis

* First line: atenolol, propanolol, bisoprolol, amitriptyline, nortriptyline
* Second line: topiramate, sodium valproate
* Third line: gabapentin, methysergide
* Other: pizotifen, clonidine, verapamil and fluoxetine have unproven efficacy

Non-drug interventions: exercise, physiotherapy, relaxation, stress reduction, biofeedback.

Farooq K, Williams P. Headache and chronic facial pain. *Contin Educ Anaesth Crit Care Pain* 2008; **8**: 138–42. Available online at ceaccp.oxfordjournals.org/content/8/4/138 (accessed 30 June 2012).

Olesen J, Steiner TJ. The international classification of headache disorders, 2nd edn (ICDH-II). *J Neurol Neurosurg Psychiatry* 2004; **75**: 808–11.

MTF Question 44: Ultrasound principles including Doppler

Which of the following are true in relation to the use of ultrasound in clinical practice?

a) Increased frequency of ultrasound during B-mode scanning results in higher-resolution scans
b) There is no risk of damage to red blood cells with Doppler ultrasound scanning
c) The use of Doppler in conjunction with standard ultrasound imaging reduces the risk of damage to tissues by cavitation
d) Increased frequency of ultrasound results in greater depth of tissue penetration
e) The heating effect of ultrasound fields is more marked in bone compared to soft tissues

Answer: a, e

Short Explanation

Small objects such as red blood cells can be agglomerated by the mechanical effects of Doppler ultrasound. Doppler ultrasound increases the risk of damage by cavitation. Increased frequency of ultrasound improves the resolution of images.

Long Explanation

Ultrasound has become a widely available modality of imaging in clinical medicine. Its applications also extend to treatment for various conditions. Ultrasound is a non-invasive, portable and low-risk modality of imaging.

There are factors that must be considered when using ultrasound, and some potential harmful effects. The frequency of ultrasound needs to be high enough to ensure that enough detail is seen in the image for the task in hand. Ultrasound with shorter wavelengths has higher frequencies, and this is also a factor. The depth of penetration is increased with lower-frequency ultrasound. A trade-off is necessary to achieve a detailed image at the correct depth.

The harmful effects of ultrasound include the heating effect, cavitation and mechanical effects. These effects are all more pronounced, and more likely to cause tissue damage, during continuous modes of ultrasound scanning. The use of Doppler increases the risk of harm again.

Smith T, Pinnock C, Lin T. *Fundamentals of Anaesthesia*, 3rd edn. Cambridge: Cambridge University Press, 2009; pp. 762–70.

MTF Question 45: Systemic inflammatory response syndrome

Which of the following are part of the definition of the systemic inflammatory response syndrome (SIRS)?

a) Heart rate > 100 beats/minute
b) Systolic blood pressure < 100 mmHg
c) Respiratory rate > 20 breaths/minute

d) Temperature $< 36\,^{\circ}\text{C}$
e) White blood cell count < 4000 cells/mm^3

Answer: c, d, e

Short Explanation
Systolic blood pressure is not part of the definition of SIRS. Heart rate is, but the criterion is a rate > 90 beats/minute.

Long Explanation
The systemic inflammatory response syndrome (SIRS) is the systemic response to a local inflammatory process, and it can therefore be triggered by a wide variety of pathological insults. The recognition of SIRS is important for identifying early critical illness and those who may require critical care. First described in 1992 at a joint meeting of the American College of Chest Physicians and the Society of Critical Care Medicine, this formal definition has been used in countless research publications and trials.

SIRS is defined by the presence of two or more of the following:

- temperature $> 38\,^{\circ}\text{C}$ or $< 36\,^{\circ}\text{C}$
- heart rate > 90 beats/minute
- respiratory rate > 20 breaths/minute or $PaCO_2 < 4.3$ kPa (or ventilator dependence)
- white blood cell count $> 12\,000$ cells/mm^3, < 4000 cells/mm^3, or $> 10\%$ band forms

Bersten AD, Soni N. Multiple organ dysfunction syndrome. In: *Oh's Intensive Care Manual*, 6th edn. Philadelphia, PA: Butterworth-Heinemann, 2009; pp. 123–9.

Bone RC, Balk RA, Cerra FB, *et al.* Definitions for sepsis and organ failure and guidelines for the use of innovative therapies in sepsis. The ACCP/SCCM Consensus Conference Committee. American College of Chest Physicians/Society of Critical Care Medicine. *Chest* 1992; **101**: 1644–55. Available online at chestjournal.chestpubs.org/content/101/6/1644.full.pdf (accessed 30 June 2012).

MTF Question 46: Sphincters

Regarding sphincters:

a) The lower oesophageal sphincter maintains a tonic constriction producing intraluminal pressure of 30 mmHg
b) Pre-capillary sphincters are located at the junction of arterioles and metarterioles
c) The pyloric sphincter poses little resistance to the passage of fluids
d) The sphincter of Oddi is located at the junction between the cystic duct and the duodenum
e) The internal bladder sphincter is innervated by the pudendal nerve

Answer: a, c

Short Explanation
Pre-capillary sphincters are located at the junction of metarterioles and capillaries. The sphincter of Oddi is found between the common bile duct and the duodenum. The internal bladder sphincter remains contracted under the influence of parasympathetic sacral nerves.

Long Explanation
Sphincters consist of annular arrangements of smooth muscle around a conduit. They limit the flow of fluid through them according to their tone, modifying the resistance posed. Some are in a state of tonic contraction; some contract when specifically stimulated.

The lower oesophageal sphincter is simply the terminal 5 cm of the oesophagus. It does not differ morphologically from the rest of the oesophagus but functionally it maintains a state of tonic contraction preventing reflux of gastric contents into the oesophagus, thereby protecting the oesophageal mucosa from the acid stomach contents. If incompetent, acid reflux not only risks metaplastic change of the mucosa but also increases the chance of regurgitation under anaesthesia.

Pre-capillary sphincters are located at the junction between metarterioles and capillaries and are under direct nervous control of the sympathetic nervous system. Alteration of tone here will regulate the resistance posed to blood flow through the particular vascular bed and will also influence the Starling forces across that capillary, changing the hydrostatic pressure and consequently affecting the flux of fluid across the endothelium.

The pyloric sphincter regulates the rate of passage of particulate stomach contents into the duodenum. Its tone is influenced by a number of paracrine hormones released by the duodenum in response to constituents of the chyme admitted. Furthermore, duodenal distension elicits enterogastric nervous reflexes that inhibit gastric emptying until the duodenum has emptied. The sphincter of Oddi is located at the junction between the common bile duct and the duodenum and it regulates the flow of bile into the duodenum. It probably gains more prominence than is warranted because of the fact that morphine can be shown to cause spasm of the sphincter. For this reason, it has been classically described that pethidine is a superior analgesic for pain of biliary origin. However, the clinical importance of the sphincter spasm caused by morphine is disputed and certainly not invariable. Also, pethidine is not without an unpleasant side-effect profile.

The internal bladder sphincter is in a state of tonic contraction under the influence of motor nerves of sacral parasympathetic origin, without voluntary control. This explains why patients do not become incontinent under anaesthesia. The external bladder sphincter is skeletal muscle under voluntary control via the pudendal nerves. The innervation of the genitourinary system is complex, with motor contributions from the parasympathetic, sympathetic and somatic nervous systems and sensory innervation from parasympathetic and sympathetic nerves. This is relevant when considering regional anaesthesia for urological surgery.

MTF Question 47: Antiemetics

In combined data from placebo versus drug trials, which of the following produced no significant risk reduction for postoperative nausea and/or vomiting (PONV)?

a) Magnesium
b) Glycopyrrolate
c) Metoclopramide
d) Ginger
e) Clonidine

Answer: c

Short Explanation
All the drugs stated were investigated in a 2006 Cochrane review. All were found to reduce the risk of PONV, but metoclopramide was the only one demonstrating statistical significance.

Long Explanation
In a Cochrane review of agents for PONV carried out in 2006 and looking at trials containing over 103 000 patients, of the drugs listed above, only metoclopramide demonstrated a significant effect.

Metoclopramide was included in 158 trials, and the risk of nausea or vomiting compared to placebo was 0.76, with 95% confidence intervals (CI) of 0.70–0.82.

Magnesium was in two trials with a risk of 0.79 (95% CI 0.36–1.72); glycopyrrolate in nine trials with a risk of 0.67 (95% CI 0.35–1.29); ginger in six trials with a risk of 0.79 (95% CI 0.55–1.14); clonidine in 30 trials with a risk of 0.73 (95% CI 0.52–1.02). All the $5HT_3$ antagonists were found to be effective, as were cyclizine, dexamethasone, dimenhyrdinate, droperidol, hyoscine, prochlorperazine and promethazine.

Carlisle JB, Stevenson CA. Drugs for preventing postoperative nausea and vomiting. *Cochrane Database Syst Rev* 2006; (**3**): CD004125. Available online at mrw.inter-science.wiley.com/cochrane/clsysrev/articles/CD004125/frame.html (accessed 30 June 2012).

MTF Question 48: Inflammation

Regarding inflammation:

a) Vasodilation is mediated by bradykinin
b) Increased vascular permeability inhibits the inflammatory response
c) Histamine increases vascular permeability
d) Chemotaxis is the process that limits the inflammatory response
e) Prostaglandin E_2 mediates vasodilation

Answer: a, c, e

Short Explanation

Vasodilation and increased vascular permeability enhance the inflammatory response. Chemotaxis is the chemical attraction of inflammatory cells to the site of infection/injury, and is part of the acute-phase response.

Long Explanation

Inflammation clinically manifests as rubor (erythema), tumor (swelling), calor (heat) and dolor (pain). Inflammatory responses occur at a local level and also at a systemic level. Local inflammatory changes occur at the site of infection/injury. These include vasodilation, increased vascular permeability, adhesion of molecules to vascular endothelium, chemotaxis, immobilisation of certain cells and activation of other cells.

Vasodilation is mediated by bradykinin and prostaglandin E_2. Increased vascular permeability is mediated by many factors including histamine, bradykinin, platelet activating factor and complement. This local vasodilation and increased vascular permeability allows other activated cells and mediators to reach the site of infection/injury and thus enhances the inflammatory response.

The inflammatory mediators interleukin-1, tumour necrosis factor, platelet activating factor and lipopolysaccharide are some of the mediators which promote the adhesion of leucocytes to vascular endothelium. This complicated process ultimately results in the capture of circulating leucocytes in the blood and strong adhesion to the endothelium. Leucocytes can then pass between endothelial junctions and into the tissues.

Chemotaxis is the chemical attraction of inflammatory cells to the site of infection/injury. Chemotactic mediators from the damaged site guide the leucocytes from the vascular endothelium toward the site of injury. The chemotactic mediators include various chemotactic factors, migration inhibition factor and interferon.

As described above, each process in the local inflammatory response has several mediators acting at each stage. There is a crossover in actions by these mediators, which is important for providing an efficient inflammatory response, as well as inflammatory responses at multiple sites or in multiple infections.

Reeves G, Todd I. *Lecture Notes on Immunology*, 3rd edn. Oxford: Blackwell, 1996; pp. 153–9.

MTF Question 49: Hereditary angio-oedema

Regarding hereditary angio-oedema:

a) It results from a disorder with complement
b) It has an autosomal dominant inheritance pattern
c) The majority of attacks occur spontaneously
d) Treatment options include administration of fresh frozen plasma
e) Upper airway obstruction is rarely a problem

Answer: a, d

Short Explanation

Hereditary angio-oedema results from congenital C1 esterase inhibitor deficiency. It has an autosomal recessive inheritance pattern. This condition is often triggered spontaneously but may follow trauma. Fresh frozen plasma contains C1 esterase inhibitor and may be included in treatment. Laryngeal oedema can cause upper airway obstruction, which can be fatal.

Long Explanation

Hereditary angio-oedema results from congenital C1 esterase inhibitor deficiency. It has an autosomal recessive inheritance pattern. The majority of patients with this condition are heterozygous for C1 esterase inhibitor deficiency, but inhibitor levels are usually well below 50% of normal. C1 esterase inhibitor usually inactivates various kinins, proteases and plasmins and kallikrein. Deficiency of C1 esterase inhibitor leads to activation of these components and also complement activation. This leads to inflammation and oedema of the face, mouth, larynx, skin and gastrointestinal tract, which can last for 2–3 days.

Hereditary angio-oedema usually presents by the age of 10 years. It may be triggered spontaneously (approximately two-thirds of cases) or may follow trauma (one-third of cases). Oedema of the gastrointestinal tract may present with severe abdominal pain. Laryngeal oedema may cause upper airway obstruction and can be fatal.

An acquired form of C1 esterase inhibitor deficiency does exist, occurring in association with lymphoproliferative disease.

Management of acute episodes of hereditary angio-oedema focuses first on the management of upper airway obstruction. Intravenous adrenaline, corticosteroids and antihistamines may be useful. Other treatments include inhibitors of fibrinolysis such as tranexamic acid and androgenic steroids such as danazol, which increase the synthesis of C1 esterase inhibitor. Treatment with danazol for 10 days preoperatively has been suggested as a way of boosting C1 esterase inhibitor levels. Synthetic purified C1 esterase inhibitor is available as an intravenous injection for the termination of acute episodes, but not for long-term use. Fresh frozen plasma contains C1 esterase inhibitor and may also be useful in treatment of acute episodes.

Reeves G, Todd I. *Lecture Notes on Immunology*, 3rd edn. Oxford: Blackwell, 1996; pp. 192–3.

Yentis S, Hirsch N, Smith G. *Anaesthesia and Intensive Care A-Z: an Encyclopaedia of Principles and Practice*, 3rd edn. Edinburgh: Butterworth-Heinemann, 2004; p. 246–7.

MTF Question 50: Asthma

A 48-year-old asthmatic patient a is reviewed in preoperative assessment clinic prior to admission for cholecystectomy in 4 weeks. He has spirometry showing FEV_1 1.2 L, FVC 2.5 L (predicted 2.6/3.2). He has had nightly symptoms for a week, but on clinical examination he is not distressed. His medication includes fluticasone 250 g bd and salmeterol 50 g bd. The likely management needed prior to surgery includes:

a) Admission for intravenous hydrocortisone
b) Addition of a leukotriene receptor antagonist to his medication
c) Specialist review
d) Commencement of antibiotics
e) Increase in his inhaled steroid medication

Answer: c, e

Short Explanation

Increasing inhaled steroids would be the first step for this patient, with a maximum dose of fluticasone of 2000 g/day. If this fails to control symptoms then one can consider the addition of another drug such as leukotriene receptor antagonists, slow-release theophylline or β_2-agonist tablets. If appropriate, oral steroids starting 1 week prior to surgery can be used to optimise respiratory function. Specialist advice will ensure patient optimisation for the operation. There is no infection, so antibiotics will not help.

Long Explanation

British Thoracic Society guidelines published in 2011 divided patients into low, intermediate and high probability of asthma depending on symptoms and spirometry. Clinical features that increase the probability of asthma are wheeze, shortness of breath, chest tightness, cough, symptoms worse at night or during exercise, worsened by non-steroidal anti-inflammatory drugs (NSAIDs). Other factors include atopic disorder, family history of asthma, unexplained low FEV_1 or PEF, or an unexplained peripheral blood eosinophilia.

Management of patients with asthma is based on a stepwise approach and escalating if there is no response. Initial treatment includes short-acting β_2-agonist inhaler as required, then low-dose steroid inhaler followed by long-acting β_2-agonists, high-dose inhaled steroids, addition of a fourth drug such as leukotriene receptor antagonists, slow-release theophylline or β_2-agonist tablets, and finally oral steroids and other treatments.

Acute asthma can be separated into mild, moderate, severe and life-threatening. This is determined by severity of symptoms and investigations. PEF > 50–75% signifies moderate exacerbation and 33–50% is severe. Life-threatening asthma is indicated by any one of the following: PEF < 35%, saturations < 92%, PaO_2 < 8 kPa, silent chest, cyanosis, poor respiratory effort, exhaustion, altered conscious level, arrhythmias. Intravenous steroids are indicated if oral or inhaled routes of administration are not possible due to the severity of the symptoms.

British Thoracic Society. *British Guideline on the Management of Asthma*, May 2008; revised May 2011. Available online at www.brit-thoracic.org.uk/guidelines/asthma-guidelines.aspx (accessed 30 June 2012).

National Institute for Health and Clinical Excellence (NICE). Inhaled corticosteroids for the treatment of chronic asthma in adults and in children aged 12 years and over, 2008. Available online at guidance.nice.org.uk/TA138 (accessed 30 June 2012).

MTF Question 51: Management of open fractures

Concerning open fractures:

a) Approximately 25% of tibial fractures are open fractures
b) Intravenous antibiotics should be commenced within 6 hours of the acute injury
c) All open fractures should be debrided within 6 hours of the injury
d) Up to 30% of patients with an open fracture will develop a significant infection following the injury
e) Definitive skeletal stabilisation of an open fracture should occur within 48 hours of the injury

Answer: a, d

Short Explanation
Intravenous antibiotics should be commenced within 3 hours of an open fracture injury. Current guidelines are that open fractures should be debrided within 24 hours; fractures with agricultural or marine contamination should be debrided within 6 hours. Ideally, skeletal stabilisation should be performed within 72 hours of the injury.

Long Explanation
Tibial fractures carry a high risk of being open (formerly known as compound) fractures, the incidence being in the region of 25%. All patients suffering an open fracture should be commenced on intravenous antibiotics within 3 hours of the injury; current guidelines advise co-amoxiclav, or clindamycin if the patient has penicillin allergy. Antibiotics should be given for 72 hours post injury, or up until definitive wound cover is achieved. Tetanus status in these patients should also be addressed.

Previous guidelines stated that all open fractures should undergo debridement within 6 hours of the injury, regardless of contamination; current guidelines advise debridement within 24 hours for 'clean' injuries, the emphasis being that surgery should be performed by a senior surgeon, on a dedicated trauma list, within normal working hours. If there is agricultural or marine contamination, patients should have debridement within 6 hours.

Injuries with concurrent vascular compromise should undergo surgery to ensure perfusion of the limb, with an absolute maximum delay of 6 hours of warm ischaemia. Adherence to best practice management guidelines can decrease the incidence of significant infection to 10%, but up to 30% of patients will develop an infection following an open fracture.

Patients who cannot undergo definitive skeletal stabilisation as a one-stage procedure should undergo debridement, with application of external fixation if necessary, and use of vacuum-assisted closure (VAC) therapy to keep the wound clean following debridement. Patients should have definitive skeletal stabilisation with wound cover, ideally within 72 hours of the injury. No patient should wait longer than 7 days for this definitive management, unless there are extenuating circumstances.

British Association of Plastic, Reconstructive and Aesthetic Surgeons (BAPRAS). New standards for the treatment of open fractures of the lower limb, 2009. Available online at www.bapras.org.uk/news.asp?id=357 (accessed 30 June 2012).

British Orthopaedic Association. *BOA Standards for Trauma (BOAST): BOAST 4: Management of Severe Open Lower Limb Fractures.* Available online at www.boa.ac.uk/en/publications/boast (accessed 30 June 2012).

MTF Question 52: Ischaemic heart disease and beta-blockers

The following are properties of bisoprolol in ischaemic heart disease:

a) Bisoprolol is a selective β_2-adrenoreceptor blocker

b) It reduces the activity of the heart muscle, reducing oxygen demand
c) It has a half-life of 12 hours and is therefore administered once daily
d) Bisoprolol has a higher cardioselectivity than atenolol
e) A dose of 20 mg should be started after a myocardial infarction as prophylaxis against recurrent infarction

Answer: b, c, d

Short Explanation
Bisoprolol is a selective β_1-adrenoreceptor blocker, inhibiting adrenergic stimulation of the heart. The 12-hour half-life makes a once-daily dose ideal. Bisoprolol is more cardioselective than atenolol. Bisoprolol is beneficial in prophylaxis against recurrent infarction, at a dose of 2.5–5 mg.

Long Explanation
Bisoprolol selectively and competitively blocks stimulation of β_1-adrenoreceptors (β_1-adrenergic receptors) by adrenaline and noradrenaline, reducing myocardial contractility, heart rate and cardiac oxygen demand. This reduces the rate of myocardial infarction.

Bisoprolol has a half-life of 10–12 hours, is metabolised by the liver, and is renally eliminated. These factors make once-daily administration appropriate. Bisoprolol is more highly selective for β_1-receptors than atenolol, metoprolol and betaxolol.

Addition of a β-blocker post-infarction can reduce 3-year mortality by up to 20% and reduce re-infarction rates by up to 25%. The optimum dose to improve cardiac oxygenation is 2.5–5 mg. Increasing the dose above 5 mg has minimal improvement in beneficial effects and the side-effect profile increases significantly.

All patients with evidence of cardiac failure (New York Heart Association class I, II, III, IV) should be taking a cardioselective β-blocker such as bisoprolol, unless contra-indicated. These β-blockers have a beneficial effect on morbidity and mortality.

Coats AJ. CAPRICORN: a story of alpha collection and beta-blockers in left ventricular dysfunction post-MI. *Int J Cardiol* 2001; **78**: 109–13.
Leopold G. Balanced pharmacokinetics and metabolism of bisoprolol. *J Cardiovasc Pharmacol* 1986; **8** (Suppl 11): S16–20.

MTF Question 53: ALS algorithms

The following drugs and doses are correctly stated parts of the algorithm for the routine ALS management of cardiac arrest:

a) Adrenaline, 1 mg
b) Atropine, 3 mg
c) Sodium bicarbonate, 50 mmol
d) Amiodarone, 300 mg
e) Magnesium, 2 g

Answer: a, d

Short Explanation
All the doses stated are correct. Atropine, sodium bicarbonate and magnesium may have a role in the management of cardiac arrests, but are not included for routine use in the ALS algorithm.

Long Explanation

Drug treatment in cardiac arrest is controversial, as there is very little evidence for any of the treatments recommended.

Regarding adrenaline, there are some animal data and some evidence for improved short-term survival in humans with its use, so it has been retained in the algorithm. In the presence of shockable rhythm, 1 mg is recommended after the third shock, then every alternate shock. In non-shockable rhythm, 1 mg of adrenaline should be given as soon as intravenous access is achieved, then every 3–5 minutes after that.

The balance of evidence is in favour of the use of antiarrhythmic agents in shock-refractory VF/VT. Amiodarone is recommended on the basis of expert consensus, and 300 mg should be administered after the third shock. A further 150 mg may be given in the event of recurrent or refractory VF/VT. If amiodarone is not available, lidocaine 1 mg/kg is a reasonable alternative (lidocaine should not be administered if amiodarone has been given).

Atropine used to be recommended in the management of asystole or slow pulseless electrical activity (PEA) arrest. However, there is a complete absence of evidence to support its use in either in- or out-of-hospital cardiac arrest, so its routine use is no longer recommended. However, if there is a specific indication, it may still be considered. Some have suggested that as it is a relatively safe drug it should be used 'just in case', but its use increases the chance of drug error (additional drug being administered in an emergency), makes prognostication more unreliable after return of spontaneous circulation (ROSC) due to pupillary dilation, and may cause undesirable tachycardia after ROSC.

Cardiac arrest is a profoundly acid-generating condition, rapidly causing profound acidaemia. This has in the past been treated with sodium bicarbonate. However, sodium bicarbonate can cause intracellular acidosis, has a negatively inotropic effect, causes an osmotic load to the compromised brain, and causes left shift of the oxygen dissociation curve. Its routine use is therefore not recommended, although it may be considered in certain situations such as arrest due to hyperkalaemia or tricyclic anti-depressant overdose.

Magnesium is only recommended in the treatment of refractory VT/VF associated with possible hypomagnesaemia, torsade-de-pointes VT and digoxin toxicity.

Resuscitation Council UK. Adult advanced life support. Resuscitation Guidelines 2010. Available online at www.resus.org.uk/pages/guide.htm (accessed 30 June 2012).

MTF Question 54: Sepsis management

A previously well 48-year-old female is admitted to the emergency department with acute onset of productive cough, fever to 39.8 °C, heart rate of 130 bpm (sinus tachycardia) and a blood pressure of 75/40 mmHg. Chest x-ray shows opacification of the right lung field with air-bronchogram. Which of the following statements about her initial management are correct?

a) Antibiotic administration should be delayed until after a sample of cerebrospinal fluid has been obtained for microscopy and culture
b) Antibiotic administration should be delayed until after blood samples have been collected for culture
c) Antibiotic administration should be delayed until after laboratory evidence of leucocytosis is available to confirm presence of infection
d) Fluid resuscitation should be delayed until central venous pressure monitoring is in situ in order to assess the haemodynamic response to fluid boluses
e) Noradrenaline is an appropriate initial vasopressor if the haemodynamic parameters fail to respond to fluid boluses

Answer: b, e

Short Explanation

The scenario suggests severe sepsis secondary to pneumonia. Intravenous antibiotics should be administered as soon as possible. Appropriate cultures should be obtained before starting antibiotics, provided this does not significantly delay antimicrobial therapy, as might occur with a lumbar puncture. Fluid resuscitation should begin immediately in patients with hypotension.

Long Explanation

The Surviving Sepsis Campaign is an international collaboration aimed at improving the diagnosis, survival and management of patients with sepsis. Severe sepsis is defined as sepsis-induced tissue hypoperfusion or organ dysfunction. Guidelines include recommendations for initial resuscitation, diagnosis, antibiotic therapy, fluids, vasopressors, glucose control, steroids and ventilation.

Intravenous antibiotics should be administered as soon as possible, and always within the first hour of recognising severe sepsis. Cultures should be obtained before starting antibiotics provided this does not cause significant delay. Appropriate cultures would include two or more blood cultures, and cultures from other sites where clinically indicated. Lumbar puncture would not be clinically indicated in this case, and may significantly delay antibiotic administration.

Fluid resuscitation with colloid or crystalloid should be started immediately in patients with hypotension or raised serum lactate levels. Invasive monitoring should be inserted as soon as practical, but should not delay resuscitation. Vasopressors are indicated where fluid boluses cause a rise in central venous pressure without concomitant improvement in heart rate or blood pressure. If vasopressors are required, noradrenaline or dopamine are the initial vasopressors of choice.

Adrenaline or vasopressin may be indicated where the blood pressure is poorly responsive to noradrenaline or dopamine.

Surviving Sepsis Campaign Guidelines. Available online at www.survivingsepsis. org/Guidelines (accessed 30 June 2012).

MTF Question 55: Amiodarone

The following are recognised adverse effects of treatment with amiodarone:

a) Steatohepatitis
b) Perception of everything tasting bitter
c) Yellowing of axillary skin
d) Epiphora
e) Peripheral myopathy

Answer: a, b, e

Short Explanation

Skin discolouration is usually blue or green and involves parts of the body regularly exposed to the sun such as the hands or feet. Amiodarone produces dry eyes rather than epiphora (watery eyes).

Long Explanation

Questions about the adverse effects of amiodarone are as frequent as the adverse effects of amiodarone! Examiners will want you to be able to reel off corneal microdeposits, thyroid disease and lung fibrosis, but with amiodarone it doesn't just end there.

Cumulative doses of amiodarone may harm the liver; the usual effect is to produce steatohepatitis (fatty liver). The perception of everything tasting bitter is commonly seen, as is skin discolouration. The discolouration is usually blue or green and involves parts of the body more regularly exposed to the sun such as the hands or feet. Epiphora, the production of excess tears or watery eyes, is the opposite of what generally occurs with amiodarone. Patients often complain of dry eyes. Peripheral myopathy and neuropathy may occur. This is usually reversible if treatment is discontinued. Other side effects include nausea, vomiting, bradycardia, tremor and sleep disturbances.

Bennett PN, Brown MJ. *Clinical Pharmacology*, 10th edn. Edinburgh: Churchill Livingstone Elsevier, 2008; pp. 454, 585.
British National Formulary. Available online at www.bnf.org (accessed 30 June 2012).

MTF Question 56: Thalassaemia

Regarding the thalassaemias:

a) Red blood cell destruction occurs intravascularly
b) A complete absence of β-globin (β°/β°) is associated with intrauterine death (Bart's hydrops)
c) The same patient can have both α- and β-thalassaemia
d) Inadequate transfusion is known to result in frontal bossing
e) Splenomegaly is common in β-thalassaemia minor

Answer: c, d

Short Explanation
Unmatched globin chains precipitate, resulting in red blood cell membrane damage. Red blood cell destruction is therefore in the marrow. Complete absence of α-globin results in Bart's hydrops. Splenomegaly is rare in β-thalassaemia minor.

Long Explanation
The thalassaemias are genetic diseases resulting in the under- or non-production of one globin chain of haemoglobin. These unmatched globin chains precipitate, causing red cell membrane damage and subsequent haemolysis in the bone marrow. They are commonly seen in families from the Mediterranean to the Far East. Thalassaemia may be α or β depending on the genetic defect, and thalassaemia may coexist with sickle cell anaemia or with another thalassaemia, resulting in a more severe clinical picture than either alone.

Patients with thalassaemia may be heterozygous or homozygous. For α-thalassaemia the homozygous state is called Bart's hydrops and is incompatible with life. Heterozygous α-thalassaemia patients have only a mild anaemia. β-Thalassaemia minor (heterozygous) also presents with a mild anaemia and is usually clinically insignificant. β-Thalassaemia major (homozygous) presents with moderate to severe anaemia depending on the genetic defect and the resulting levels of β-globin chains.

Patients are often transfusion-dependent, and normal development correlates with this – frontal bossing and other skeletal abnormalities occur with bone marrow hyperplasia from undertransfusion. Long-term transfusion requires treatment with iron chelators to avoid endocrine, liver and cardiac failure from iron overload. Splenectomy should be considered in patients with hypersplenism.

Wilson M, Forsyth P, Whiteside J. Haemoglobinopathy and sickle cell disease. *Contin Educ Anaesth Crit Care Pain* 2010; **10**: 24–8. Available online at ceaccp.oxfordjournals.org/content/10/1/24 (accessed 30 June 2012).

MTF Question 57: Patient-controlled analgesia

Concerning patient-controlled analgesia (PCA):

a) Adding ketamine into a morphine PCA improves postoperative analgesia
b) Giving low-dose ketamine IV perioperatively will improve analgesia when PCA is used postoperatively
c) The main proven advantage of PCA is improved patient satisfaction
d) PCA decreases the total morphine dose the patient requires perioperatively when compared with conventional analgesia
e) PCA produces a clinically small but statistically significant improvement in perioperative analgesia compared with conventional analgesia

Answer: b, c, e

Short Explanation

PCA is associated with improved patient satisfaction, but its other clinical benefits (including improved analgesia) are modest. It is not associated with increased risk of adverse events or outcomes compared with conventional analgesia. Ketamine is used perioperatively in conjunction with PCA, but there is no benefit in adding it into the PCA morphine. There is conflicting evidence on the impact of PCA on opioid consumption.

Long Explanation

Perioperative low-dose ketamine in the range 0.15–1.0 mg/kg intravenously, used in conjunction with patient-controlled analgesia (PCA) morphine, is opioid-sparing and reduces the incidence of nausea and vomiting. There is level 1 evidence to support this statement, as described in a Cochrane review on ketamine. However, adding ketamine into the PCA morphine neither spares opioid nor improves analgesia, nor improves nausea and vomiting.

The number needed to treat (NNT) to gain one more patient satisfied with his/her analgesia is between 1.9 and 8. Improvement in analgesia with PCA is clinically small but statistically significant. It has been hypothesised that the conventional administration of analgesia is unlikely to be as efficient in the real world as it is in research trials, possibly leading to an understatement of the analgesic benefit of PCA.

Evidence regarding PCA opioid consumption is contradictory. Unchanged, increased and decreased consumption have been reported when PCA is compared with conventional treatment.

See Macintyre *et al.* (reference below) for a comprehensive review of current evidence in acute pain.

Bell RF, Dahl JB, Moore RA, Kalso E. Perioperative ketamine for acute postoperative pain. *Cochrane Database Syst Rev* 2006; (1): CD004603. Available online at onlinelibrary.wiley.com/doi/10.1002/14651858.CD004603.pub2/abstract (accessed 30 June 2012).

Macintyre PE, Schug SA, Scott DA, Visser EJ, Walker SM. *Acute Pain Management: Scientific Evidence*, 3rd edn, Melbourne: Australian and New Zealand College of Anaesthetists and Faculty of Pain Medicine, 2010. Available online at www.anzca.edu.au/resources/college-publications/Acute%20Pain%20Management/books-and-publications/acutepain.pdf (accessed 30 June 2012).

Bandolier reviews on PCA available online at www.medicine.ox.ac.uk/bandolier/booth/painpag/Acutrev/Other/AP050.html and www.medicine.ox.ac.uk/bandolier/booth/painpag/Acutrev/Other/PCAup.html (accessed 30 June 2012).

MTF Question 58: Rocuronium

It is true to say of rocuronium that:

a) It is less potent than vecuronium
b) It is 10% protein-bound
c) The dose for modified rapid sequence induction is 0.5 mg/kg
d) Its effects can be reversed by administration of γ-cyclodextrin
e) It can be administered via the intramuscular route

Answer: a, d, e

Short Explanation
Rocuronium is 30% protein-bound. The dose for modified rapid sequence induction is 0.9–1.2 mg/kg. A dose of 0.5 mg/kg is not sufficient for the speed of onset required for rapid sequence induction.

Long Explanation
Rocuronium is an aminosteroid neuromuscular blocking drug. It is used for elective intubations (dose 0.6 mg/kg) in addition to more recently being used in modified rapid sequence inductions. It has an intermediate duration of action of around 20–35 minutes. It is structurally different from vecuronium at only four positions but is less potent. This reduced potency means that it has a rapid onset of action. This is because a less potent drug requires administration of a higher dose, resulting in an increased number of molecules present at the neuromuscular junction. When the large doses required for rapid sequence induction are administered its duration of action is prolonged. For this reason neuromuscular blockade monitoring must be used before waking the patient.

Rocuronium can be administered intramuscularly, but the duration of action is very long in this situation. Up to 50% of the drug is excreted in the bile. It has a small antivagal effect which can be useful in procedures which cause vagal stimulation.

The recent emergence of sugammadex, a γ-cyclodextrin, has encouraged its use in rapid sequence induction. This molecule effectively reverses the effects of rocuronium by encapsulating the rocuronium molecules. This means that molecules of rocuronium at the neuromuscular junction diffuse away and its effect there is reduced. The dose of sugammadex required to reverse rocuronium within 3 minutes when it has been administered for a rapid sequence induction is 16 mg/kg. A 5 mL vial of sugammadex contains 500 mg. This could potentially be used in the 'can't intubate can't ventilate' scenario.

Gordon M. Medical pharmacology. Chapter 20: neuromuscular blocking drugs. Available online at www.cybermedicine2000.com/pharmacology2000/Central/NMJ/NMJobj1.htm#Nondepolarizing Blockers (accessed 30 June 2012).
Peck T, Hill S, Williams M. *Pharmacology for Anaesthesia and Intensive Care*, 3rd edn. Cambridge: Cambridge University Press, 2008; p. 196.

MTF Question 59: Endotracheal drugs

During an adult cardiac arrest, which of the following drugs are recommended as being suitable to be administered down an endotracheal tube?

a) Amiodarone
b) Vasopressin
c) Calcium gluconate
d) Adrenaline
e) Sodium bicarbonate

Answer: all false

Short Explanation
In the 2010 Resuscitation Guidelines the tracheal administration of drugs was abandoned in favour of interosseous as a second tactic if intravenous access cannot be secured.

Long Explanation
The 2010 guidelines for adult advanced life support clearly state that tracheal administration of drugs in resuscitation is no longer recommended. The ease of gaining intraosseous access and the complications of giving tracheal drugs, which include unpredictable response and impairment of gas exchange, have led to this technique now being abandoned.

Prior to these latest recommendations, adrenaline was administered down a tracheal tube in adults at a dose of 3 mg diluted in a volume of 10 mL. Other drugs that previously had been administered and were thought to be effective via the endotracheal route included atropine, lidocaine, naloxone and vasopressin. Calcium gluconate, sodium bicarbonate and amiodarone were never recommended via the endotracheal route. Amiodarone would be a local irritant to the lung.

Resuscitation Council UK. Resuscitation Guidelines 2010. Available online at www.resus.org.uk/pages/guide.htm (accessed 30 June 2012).

MTF Question 60: Aortic aneurysm
Regarding aortic aneurysms:

a) Patients with an abdominal aortic aneurysm with a diameter > 55 mm should be offered surgical repair
b) In patients fit for either EVAR (endovascular aneurysm repair) or open aneurysm repair, EVAR has lower 30-day postoperative mortality than open repair
c) In patients unfit for open repair, EVAR demonstrates a lower long-term mortality than non-operative measures
d) The majority of abdominal aortic aneurysms are suprarenal
e) During dissection of an abdominal aneurysm, blood dissects between the tunica media and tunica adventitia

Answer: a, b

Short Explanation
The majority of abdominal aortic aneurysms (AAA) are infrarenal. Patients with aneurysms > 55 mm in diameter are offered repair. EVAR is beneficial for patients who are fit for either repair in terms of 30-day postoperative mortality, but long-term mortality is not decreased by EVAR in patients who are not fit for open surgery. During dissection, blood tracks between the tunica intima and tunica media.

Long Explanation
Screening for abdominal aortic aneurysms (AAA) is being rolled out across the NHS in the UK, with ultrasounds being offered to men in their 65th year. Patients found to have an aneurysm greater than 55 mm in diameter are offered surgery, because of the increased risk of rupture at this size.

The majority of aneurysms are infrarenal, in that they arise below the level of the renal arteries at L1. Suprarenal aneurysms are technically more difficult in terms of operative management because of the involvement of the renal vasculature.

The randomised controlled trial EVAR 1 compared EVAR with open repair, and demonstrated 30-day postoperative mortality to be 1.7% in the EVAR group, compared with 4.7% in the open repair group. The EVAR 2 trial studied patients who were unfit for open repair, and compared EVAR with non-operative management and found no benefit of EVAR, stating that conservative measures were of highest importance in this patient population.

Aneurysms may be complicated by rupture, infection, thrombosis, emboli or dissection. When dissection occurs, a tear in the tunica intima allows blood to flow between the tunica intima and tunica media (innermost and middle layers, respectively). The tunica adventitia is the outermost layer.

EVAR trial participants. Endovascular aneurysm repair and outcome in patients unfit for open repair of abdominal aortic aneurysm (EVAR Trial 2): randomised controlled trial. *Lancet* 2005; **365**: 2187–92.

Greenhalgh RM, Brown LC, Kwong GP, *et al.* Comparison of endovascular aneurysm repair with open repair in patients with abdominal aortic aneurysms (EVAR Trial 1) 30 day operative mortality results: a randomised controlled trial. *Lancet* 2004; **364**: 843–8.

SBA Question 61: Pacemakers

A patient is fitted with a VVI pacemaker. Which one of the following is INCORRECT regarding the functions of this pacemaker?

a) An intrinsic rhythm of a P wave transmitted to the ventricles will result in inhibition of pacing output
b) An ectopic of ventricular origin will result in inhibition of pacing output
c) A supraventricular tachycardia (SVT) transmitted to the ventricles will result in inhibition of pacing output
d) Polyfocal ectopics as a result of a wire introduced during insertion of a central venous catheter result in activation of pacing output
e) Administration of glycopyrronium bromide is more likely to increase than decrease the rate of pacing output

Answer: e

Short Explanation

VVI pacemakers are inhibited by intrinsic ventricular activity. Polyfocal ectopics caused by wire insertion may result in significant compensatory pauses, thus resulting in activation of pacing (if only temporarily). Glycopyrronium will increase sinoatrial node activity, thus increasing intrinsic heart rate, and this will decrease rather than increase the rate of pacing output.

Long Explanation

The classification of pacemakers is essential knowledge for the FRCA. The table below details the five-letter abbreviation (sometimes, as here, abbreviated to the first three letters):

Code	Indication	Function
AAI	Sinus node disease Normal A-V conduction	Demand atrial pacing
VVI	Bradycardia without need for preserved A-V conduction (e.g. AF)	Demand ventricular pacing
DDD	Bradycardia Impaired A-V conduction	Maintains A-V concordance
DDDR	Bradycardia Impaired A-V conduction	Maintains A-V concordance Exercise response

(Table reproduced from Mackay J, Arrowsmith JE. *Core Topics in Cardiac Anaesthesia*. Cambridge University Press, 2004)

A VVI pacemaker therefore paces the ventricle, senses the ventricle, and its activity is inhibited by the presence of intrinsic activity. In a patient in sinus rhythm with normal atrioventricular (AV) conduction, therefore, pacemaker activity will be inhibited (although if the intrinsic rate is lower than the set rate of the pacemaker there will still be some pacing activity). This equally applies to a supraventricular tachycardia (SVT) with normal AV conduction. A premature ventricular complex ('ectopic') will be sensed in the same way as the transmitted atrial impulses are – as ventricular activity – and the result will again be inhibition.

A Seldinger wire inserted too far during central venous catheterisation may elicit ectopic electrical activity from either the atrium or the ventricle. Initiation of a premature ventricular complex may result in a fully compensatory pause which exceeds the duration of the normal interval between QRS complexes. So, while the ectopic itself will inhibit pacemaker activity, its presence may result in a subsequent activation of pacemaker function secondary to a prolonged delay afterwards. The chances of this occurring are potentially increased by the presence of multiple ectopics.

Glycopyrronium bromide is an anticholinergic, and in the presence of normal AV conduction this will result in an increase in heart rate. In the absence of normal AV conduction, there may be little change in the heart rate, but regardless there will be either a decrease or little change in pacemaker activity.

Allen M. Pacemakers and implantable cardioverter defibrillators. *Anaesthesia* 2006; **61**: 883–90.

Mackay J, Arrowsmith JE. *Core Topics in Cardiac Anaesthesia*. Cambridge: Cambridge University Press, 2004.

SBA Question 62: The choking child

After a long day, you quickly stop in the hospital shop to grab a snack for the drive home. Whilst waiting to pay, your attention is drawn to a frantic woman calling for help for her choking child. She is kneeling over a 3-year-old girl who is conscious and appears to be coughing, but no noise is made. Which of the following is the single most appropriate immediate action?

a) Deliver five back blows
b) Continue to encourage coughing
c) Call for help and deliver up to five abdominal thrusts
d) Perform a finger sweep to dislodge the object
e) Place the child in the recovery position

Answer: a

Short Explanation

This is a case of choking in a child with an ineffective cough. As the child is conscious, the most appropriate immediate action is to deliver up to five back blows. If this fails, up to five abdominal thrusts should be performed. Encouraging the child to cough is appropriate if the child is coughing effectively.

Long Explanation

When you are presented with the scenario of a choking child, the first step is to assess the severity by determining if an effective cough is present or absent. Signs of an effective cough include crying or verbal response to questions, loud cough, able to take a breath before coughing and fully responsive. In this setting, the child should be encouraged to continue coughing, as 'a spontaneous cough is likely to be more effective and safer than any manoeuvre a rescuer might perform.'

Signs of an ineffective cough include inability to vocalise, quiet/silent cough, inability to breathe, cyanosis or decreasing level of consciousness. In this setting, the child will become asphyxiated rapidly, so help should be sent for immediately. If the child is conscious, up to five back blows should be delivered, checking to see if each blow has relieved the obstruction. If this fails and the child is still conscious, give up to five chest thrusts for an infant or abdominal thrusts for a child. If this still fails and the victim remains conscious, alternate five back blows with five chest/abdominal thrusts.

If the victim becomes unconscious, the airway should be opened. Look for an obvious object and, if one is visible, remove it with a single finger sweep. Do not attempt blind or repeated finger sweeps, as this may further impact the object. Proceed as per the Resuscitation Council's paediatric basic life support algorithm.

Resuscitation Council UK. Paediatric basic life support. Resuscitation Guidelines 2010. Available online at www.resus.org.uk/pages/guide.htm (accessed 30 June 2012).

SBA Question 63: POSSUM risk scoring

Regarding POSSUM risk scoring, which of the following is the LEAST correct?

a) POSSUM provides an estimation of both morbidity and mortality, to guide appropriateness of surgery
b) The POSSUM equation was modified to the P-POSSUM equation, as the former was deemed to over-predict death in low-risk patients
c) The P-POSSUM risk scoring includes 12 preoperative physiological parameters
d) Peritoneal contamination is an operative parameter included in the P-POSSUM risk estimation
e) The white blood cell count is a physiological parameter included in the P-POSSUM risk estimation

Answer: a

Short Explanation
The P-POSSUM version of the POSSUM (Physiological and Operative Severity Score for the enUmeration of Mortality and Morbidity) risk scoring system requires 12 physiological and 6 operative parameters to estimate surgical morbidity and mortality. It was developed as a tool for surgical audit, not to determine the appropriateness of surgery. In fact, as operative parameters are not known until surgery is complete, it should not be used alone to guide the appropriateness of surgery.

Long Explanation
POSSUM is the most internationally validated individual risk scoring system, and it has been applied to a number of surgical specialties including orthopaedics, vascular, head and neck and gastrointestinal/colorectal surgeries. It was originally developed to facilitate surgical audit and the comparison of outcome measures, as the calculation is adjusted in respect to the patient's preoperative physiological condition. There are a number of different POSSUM scores, including CR-POSSUM for colorectal patients, P-POSSUM for general surgical patients, O-POSSUM for oesophagogastric surgery and vascular-POSSUM for vascular surgery patients. The calculation of P-POSSUM uses 12 physiological and 6 operative parameters to provide an estimation of both morbidity and mortality.

Physiological parameters	Operative parameters
Age	Operative magnitude (minor, moderate, major, complex)
Cardiac signs or symptoms	Number of operations within 30 days
Respiratory signs or symptoms	Operative blood loss per operation
	Peritoneal contamination
Systolic BP	Malignancy status
Heart rate	Timing of operation (elective, urgent, emergency)
Glasgow Coma Scale	
Urea	
Sodium	
Potassium	
Haemoglobin	
White blood cell count	
ECG (AF or other abnormality)	

A disadvantage of the POSSUM risk scoring system is that the calculation includes operative variables. These parameters will not be known until after the surgery is complete. This presents some obvious difficulties if POSSUM is to be used for estimating preoperative risk and the appropriateness of surgery.

The original POSSUM calculation was criticised as overestimating the risk of mortality in low-risk groups. Therefore, the equation was modified to the Portsmouth predictor equation for mortality (P-POSSUM), which utilises an alternative statistical approach.

Subsequent studies have shown P-POSSUM to both over- and under-predict mortality in different setting. P-POSSUM does not have a morbidity calculator, so the POSSUM morbidity equation is still used. There have also been reports of overprediction of mortality in different surgical specialties. This has led to the development of specific risk scoring tools such as V-POSSUM for elective vascular surgery and CR-POSSUM in colorectal surgery.

Barnett S, Moonesinghe S. Clnical risk scores to guide perioperative management. *Postgrad Med J* 2011; **87**: 535–41. Available online at pmj.bmj.com/content/87/1030/535 (accessed 30 June 2012).

Smith J, Tekkis P. Risk prediction in surgery. 2011. Available online at www.riskprediction.org.uk (accessed 30 June 2012).

SBA Question 64: Prolonged neuromuscular blockade

Having performed a rapid sequence induction using 5 mg/kg thiopental and 1 mg/kg suxamethonium for an appendectomy, you attach a nerve stimulator to monitor degree of neuromuscular blockade. After 20 minutes there are no twitches seen in response to a supramaximal stimulus. Which of the following statements would NOT explain the observed phenomenon?

a) The patient is mildly hypermagnesaemic (plasma magnesium 2.8 mmol/L)
b) The patient is 30 weeks pregnant
c) The patient has chronic hepatic failure
d) The patient is taking regular cyclophosphamide
e) The patient is clinically malnourished

Answer: a

Short Explanation

Hepatic failure, pregnancy and malnutrition cause acquired deficiency of normal plasma cholinesterase, while cyclophosphamide can inhibit cholinesterase, and all of them may potentially prolong the action of suxamethonium.

Long Explanation

This question is simply testing your knowledge of factors that can cause prolonged paralysis following the administration of suxamethonium.

Hypermagnesaemia may cause potentiation of non-depolarising neuromuscular blockade, but not of suxamethonium. Hypermagnesaemia may cause flaccidity in its own right, but the plasma level given here is only mild and is the least likely reason in this scenario for the paralysis.

There are a number of conditions that can cause acquired deficiency of normal cholinesterase, leading to reduced hydrolysis of suxamethonium and hence prolonged paralysis following its use. These include hepatic failure, hypoproteinaemia, pregnancy, malnutrition, burns, or following plasmapheresis. Some drugs (e.g. cyclophosphamide, echothiophate) can cause prolonged paralysis via inhibition of cholinesterase.

Butyrylcholinesterase (pseudocholinesterase, plasma cholinesterase) is a glycoprotein enzyme produced by the liver, circulating in the plasma. Butyrylcholinesterase deficiency results in delayed metabolism of only a few compounds of clinical significance, including suxamethonium, mivacurium, procaine and cocaine.

In individuals with normal plasma levels of normally functioning butyrylcholinesterase enzyme, hydrolysis and inactivation of approximately 90–95% of an intravenous dose of suxamethonium occurs before it reaches the neuromuscular junction. The remaining 5–10% of the suxamethonium dose acts as an acetylcholine receptor agonist at the neuromuscular junction, causing prolonged depolarisation of the postsynaptic junction of the motor end-plate. This depolarisation initially triggers fasciculation of skeletal muscle. As a result of prolonged depolarisation, endogenous acetylcholine released from the presynaptic membrane of the motor neurone does not produce any additional change in membrane potential after binding to its receptor on the myocyte. Flaccid paralysis of skeletal muscles develops within 1 minute.

In normal subjects, skeletal muscle function returns to normal approximately 5 minutes after a single bolus injection of suxamethonium as it passively diffuses away from the neuromuscular junction. Butyrylcholinesterase deficiency can result in higher levels of intact suxamethonium molecules reaching receptors in the neuromuscular junction, causing the duration of paralytic effect to continue for as long as 8 hours.

Alexander DR. Pseudocholinesterase deficiency clinical presentation. *Medscape Reference*. Available online at emedicine.medscape.com/article/247019-clinical (accessed 30 June 2012).

Yentis S, Hirsch N, Smith G. *Anaesthesia and Intensive Care A–Z: an Encyclopaedia of Principles and Practice*, 4th edn. Edinburgh: Butterworth-Heinemann, 2009.

SBA Question 65: Gate control theory of pain

Which ONE of the following treatment modalities is best explained by the gate control theory of pain?

a) Capsaicin cream
b) Lidocaine patches
c) Transcutaneous electrical nerve stimulation

d) Guanethidine block

e) Gabapentin

Answer: c

Short Explanation

Capsaicin cream causes depletion of substance P. Lidocaine is a sodium channel blocker. Guanethidine blocks the re-uptake of noradrenaline and depletes stores in the postganglionic nerve terminals. Gabapentin is an anticonvulsant.

Long Explanation

The mode of action of transcutaneous electrical nerve stimulation (TENS) is complex, but it is based on the gate control theory. Electrical stimulation excites A afferent nerve fibres connected to tactile receptors. A fibres enter the spinal cord and ascend in the dorsal columns, but also give collaterals in the spinal cord which synapse with short interneurones ending near C fibre terminals. These interneurones release γ-aminobutyric acid (GABA) which causes presynaptic blockade of the C afferents, preventing them from exciting the substantia gelatinosa cells and hence closing the gate to nociceptive input.

Capsaicin is an alkaloid derived from chillies. It first entered European knowledge after Columbus's second voyage to the New World in 1494. There is evidence that capsaicin can deplete substance P in local nerve sensory terminals. Substance P is thought to be associated with initiation and transmission of painful stimuli, as well as with a number of diseases including arthritis, psoriasis and inflammatory bowel disease.

Lidocaine patches are used to relieve the pain of post-herpetic neuralgia (the burning, stabbing pains, or aches that may last for months or years after a shingles infection). Lidocaine is an amide local anaesthetic that acts as a sodium channel blocker. It was first synthesised under the name Xylocaine by Swedish chemist Nils Löfgren in 1943.

Guanethidine is an antihypertensive agent that acts by selectively inhibiting transmission in postganglionic adrenergic nerves. It is believed to act mainly by preventing the release of noradrenaline at nerve endings and causing depletion of noradrenaline in peripheral sympathetic nerve terminals.

Gabapentin was originally developed for the treatment of epilepsy, and currently is also used to relieve neuropathic pain.

Lynch L, Simpson K. Transcutaneous electrical nerve stimulation and acute pain. *Br J Anaesth CEPD Rev* 2002; **2**: 49–52. Available online at ceaccp.oxfordjournals.org/content/2/2/49 (accessed 30 June 2012).

SBA Question 66: Anaesthesia for carcinoid syndrome

A 74-year-old man is admitted to hospital with abdominal pain and distension. He gives a 3-month history of weight loss and diarrhoea. His past medical history is unremarkable except for recently diagnosed asthma. A CT scan shows an obstructive lesion at the rectosigmoid junction, with a single hepatic metastasis. He undergoes a Hartmann's procedure. During manipulation of the tumour he becomes slightly hypotensive and tachycardic, and develops marked facial erythema and a significant wheeze. Which one of the following is the best treatment in this situation?

a) Intravenous (IV) hydrocortisone and nebulised salbutamol

b) IV fluids and IV chlorpheniramine

c) IV fluids, IV magnesium sulphate, IV hydrocortisone

d) IV fluids and IV octreotide

e) IV adrenaline infusion

Answer: d

Short Explanation

The history is consistent with carcinoid syndrome, and the mainstay of the management of a carcinoid crisis is the use of octreotide, a somatostatin analogue, which reduces tumour secretion. Salbutamol, magnesium sulphate and hydrocortisone help to treat bronchoconstriction due to asthma, but do not help the underlying cause in this situation. Peripheral adrenaline would be useful if anaphylaxis were suspected, but catecholamines can aggravate carcinoid syndrome. Chlorpheniramine is not used intravenously.

Long Explanation

Carcinoid tumours are rare, affecting up to 4.5 per 100 000 in some populations, although this incidence may be increasing. They are derived from enterochromaffin cells, and are found in the distribution of the embryological fore- (including the lungs), mid- and hindgut. As neuroendocrine cells they release a wide range of hormones and biogenic amines, including serotonin, corticotrophin, histamine, dopamine, prostaglandins and kallikrein, among others.

Carcinoid tumours are often found coincidentally, during surgery for other conditions. They may cause vague or few symptoms, but may conversely present with obstructive features (gastrointestinal or pulmonary). Carcinoid syndrome may also be a feature of the tumours – but is only present in about 10% of cases. In gastrointestinal tumours, the vasoactive hormones released travel in the portal venous system and are metabolised by the liver, and therefore do not result in systemic effects. These systemic effects only occur for tumours that arise in the lungs or liver, or those that metastasise to or beyond the liver. Systemic features include flushing, diarrhoea, lacrimation and rhinorrhoea, and right heart valvular fibrosis can result over time. More severe features, including bronchospasm, tachycardia, wide blood pressure variations (hypo- or hypertension), termed carcinoid crises, can be provoked by anaesthetic, radiological and surgical procedures, as in the case presented here.

Anaesthetic management of a patient with carcinoid syndrome is based around avoiding precipitants of tumour secretion. Interestingly these precipitants include some of the very features of tumour secretion – drugs causing histamine release (e.g. morphine, atracurium), hypo- and hypertension, stimulation of the autonomic nervous system. Handling of the tumour intraoperatively can also elicit hormone release. Noradrenaline use in the context of a carcinoid crisis may paradoxically cause increasing vasodilation by eliciting tumour release of bradykinin. The mainstay of the management of a carcinoid crisis is the use of octreotide, a somatostatin analogue, which reduces tumour secretion. Some have also advocated ondansetron for its antiserotonergic effects. Management of intraoperative blood pressure includes the use of short-acting intravenous agents such as remifentanil, labetalol and esmolol, and phenylephrine.

Farling PA, Durairaju AK. Remifentanil and anaesthesia for carcinoid syndrome. *Br J Anaesth* 2004; **92**: 893–5.

Powell B, Al Mukhtar A, Mills GH. Carcinoid: the disease and its implications for anesthesia. *Contin Educ Anaesth Crit Care Pain* 2011; **11**: 9–13.

SBA Question 67: Mechanisms of pain

Which of these is the current International Association for the Study of Pain (IASP) definition of 'neuropathic pain'?

a) Pain caused by a lesion or disease of the somatosensory nervous system
b) Pain initiated or caused by a primary lesion or dysfunction in the nervous system
c) Pain caused by a lesion or disease of the central somatosensory nervous system
d) Pain caused by a lesion or disease of the peripheral somatosensory nervous system
e) Pain defined by a specific series of clinical parameters in the presence or absence of demonstrable damage to nerve tissue

Answer: a

Short Explanation
The other four definitions are: (b) neuropathic pain (1994 version); (c) central neuropathic pain; (d) peripheral neuropathic pain; (e) neuropathic pain (prior to 1994).

Long Explanation
The International Association for the Study of Pain (IASP) is an international organisation of professionals involved in research, diagnosis or treatment of pain. Its mission is 'to bring together scientists, clinicians, health care providers, and policy makers to stimulate and support the study of pain and to translate that knowledge into improved pain relief worldwide'. It was formed in 1973 and is responsible for the international definition of pain: 'an unpleasant sensory or emotional experience associated with actual or potential tissue damage and expressed in terms of such damage'. It publishes the monthly journal *Pain*.

The current (2008) definition of neuropathic pain is 'pain caused by a lesion or disease of the somatosensory nervous system'. The 1994 definition was 'Pain initiated or caused by a primary lesion or dysfunction in the nervous system'. Until 1994 the definition was 'pain defined by a specific series of clinical parameters in the presence or absence of demonstrable damage to nerve tissue'.

The 1994 definition of neuropathic pain was revised because it was regarded as too broad. The term *nervous system* does not illustrate that neuropathic pain requires some interaction with the *somatic* nervous system. The term *somatosensory* refers to received information about the body, including visceral organs, not merely information about the outside world. The term *lesion* means an abnormality demonstrated by diagnostic investigations (imaging, biopsy, laboratory tests). The term *disease* is used when the cause of the lesion is known.

Central neuropathic pain is defined as 'pain caused by a lesion or disease of the central somatosensory nervous system'. Peripheral neuropathic pain is 'pain caused by a lesion or disease of the peripheral somatosensory nervous system'.

IASP Taxonomy available online at www.iasp-pain.org/Content/NavigationMenu/GeneralResourcelinks/PainDefinitions (accessed 30 June 2012).
IASP Clinical Updates available online at www.iasp-pain.org/AM/Template.cfm?Section=Clinical_Updates (accessed 30 June 2012).

SBA Question 68: Patient positioning

You are called to see a postoperative patient in the recovery room, whom you find has developed a corneal abrasion. The most likely position the patient was in during the procedure is:

a) Lateral
b) Lithotomy with reverse Trendelenburg
c) Prone knees/chest

d) Prone jack-knife
e) Supine

Answer: a

Short Explanation

The lateral position is associated with the greatest number of ocular complications. These are primarily corneal abrasions, but they occur with equal frequency in both the dependent and non-dependent eyes.

Long Explanation

The frequency of eye injury during anaesthesia and surgery is very low (< 0.1% of anaesthetics), but the spectrum of injury ranges from mild discomfort to permanent loss of vision. Corneal abrasions are reported most commonly. They are caused by direct trauma to the cornea by foreign objects (facemasks, surgical drapes, etc.) combined with decreased basal tear production secondary to general anaesthesia.

These injuries are largely preventable by application of eye tape but are not influenced by the use of eye ointment. The lateral position is associated with the greatest number of ocular complications. These are primarily corneal abrasions, and they occur with equal frequency in both the dependent and non-dependent eyes.

Special consideration should also be given to the prone position, where a head ring or horseshoe headrest is often utilised. In this position, the head may move significantly during a surgical procedure, resulting in direct pressure on the eye. If this pressure exceeds arterial pressure then arterial inflow may be reduced dramatically, resulting in potentially devastating retinal ischaemia.

Knight DJW, Mahajan RP. Patient positioning in anaesthesia. *Contin Educ Anaesth Crit Care Pain* 2004; **4**: 160–3. Available online at ceaccp.oxfordjournals.org/content/4/5/160 (accessed 30 June 2012).

SBA Question 69: Pyloric stenosis

A 4-week-old boy presents with projectile vomiting and weight loss. He is clinically dehydrated and a diagnosis of pyloric stenosis is confirmed by ultrasound scan. Blood chemistry taken at the time of presentation is likely to show:

a) Na^+ 129 mmol/L, K^+ 2.9 mmol/L, Cl^- 110 mmol/L, HCO_3^- 24 mmol/L, pH 7.38
b) Na^+ 145 mmol/L, K^+ 3.0 mmol/L, Cl^- 111 mmol/L, HCO_3^- 34 mmol/L, pH 7.32
c) Na^+ 140 mmol/L, K^+ 4.4 mmol/L, Cl^- 84 mmol/L, HCO_3^- 31 mmol/L, pH 7.49
d) Na^+ 127 mmol/L, K^+ 2.8 mmol/L, Cl^- 85 mmol/L, HCO_3^- 33 mmol/L, pH 7.54
e) Na^+ 128 mmol/L, K^+ 2.9 mmol/L, Cl^- 88 mmol/L, HCO_3^- 21 mmol/L, pH 7.52

Answer: d

Short Explanation

Hypochloraemic alkalosis with low potassium is typical of pyloric stenosis. Sodium levels can be variable. This is a metabolic rather than a respiratory alkalosis so the bicarbonate will be normal or high.

Long Explanation

Pyloric stenosis is a functional stomach outlet obstruction caused by hypertrophy of the muscles of the pyloric sphincter. It is more common in first-born, Caucasian males and has a hereditary element. It presents with vomiting after feeds, weight loss and dehydration. The vomiting is non-bilious and may be projectile. The child is usually ravenous and will eagerly feed. Keen surgical registrars will tell you they can feel an olive-shaped mass in the right upper quadrant and see visible peristalsis when the child feeds.

The biochemical abnormalities are a result of the persistent emesis causing loss of hydrochloric acid and fluid. Hydrochloric acid is produced by the parietal cells of the stomach. To produce this acid, bicarbonate is transported out of the cell in exchange for chloride ions. This causes an alkalosis. In response to the dehydration the kidney tries to retain sodium. However, chloride in the filtrate is low, limiting sodium reabsorption in the proximal convoluted tubule. In the distal convoluted tubule this higher concentration of sodium is reabsorbed in exchange for potassium and hydrogen ions, leading to hypokalaemia and worsening alkalosis and causing paradoxical acidic urine. Loss of acid from the urine and vomitus will produce the characteristic metabolic acid which from the Siggaard-Andersen nomogram we know will be associated with a normal or raised plasma bicarbonate level.

The patient should be given intravenous maintenance fluid and have all nasogastric or vomiting losses replaced with intravenous 0.9% saline with potassium. Although managing this hungry child can be distressing for the parents, the biochemistry should be corrected by the fluid regime before surgery.

Association of Paediatric Anaesthetists of Great Britain and Ireland. *APA Consensus Guideline on Perioperative Fluid Management in Children*, v 1.1, September 2007. Available online at www.apagbi.org.uk/sites/default/files/ Perioperative_Fiuid_Management_2007.pdf (accessed 30 June 2012).

Pyloric stenosis. PubMed Health. Available online at www.ncbi.nlm.nih.gov/pub-medhealth/PMH0001965 (accessed 30 June 2012).

SBA Question 70: Neurosurgical techniques in pain management

A 79-year-old woman with a metastatic pelvic tumour complains of pain on her left hip and leg secondary to a pathological fracture. It is intense on movement but can be absent at rest. The prognosis is poor, and survival at 1 year is minimal. Because of other comorbidities it is not amenable to surgery. Which ONE intervention is most likely to produce long-lasting pain relief with minimal side effects?

a) Femoral nerve block
b) Sciatic nerve block
c) Guanithidine block
d) Percutaneous cordotomy
e) Systemic opioids

Answer: d

Short Explanation
Regional techniques are unlikely to have a long-lasting effect and may not cover hip pain. Guanithidine block is generally used in complex regional pain syndrome. The amount of opioid needed to treat incident pain will often over-sedate the patient when at rest.

Long Explanation
Percutaneous cordotomy is a technique primarily useful for cancer pain management. It interrupts transmission through the spinothalamic tract by creating a radiofrequency lesion in the anterolateral quadrant of the spinal cord. The best indication is unilateral cancer pain below the shoulder, especially neuropathic or incident pain. Patients with brachial plexopathy from Pancoast tumour or sacral plexopathy from pelvic malignant disease are excellent candidates. It is generally performed at C1–C2. At this level, the

spinothalamic tract is in the anterolateral quadrant of the cord. Pain fibres enter the cord through the dorsal horn and then may ascend several levels before crossing over and taking their final position in the spinothalamic tract. A lesion at C1–C2 will produce analgesia bellow C4 or C5 on the contralateral side.

Neuropathic pain responds poorly to medical therapy. Brachial and sacral plexopathy can be particularly challenging. Better responses can be obtained with intrathecal opioid techniques, especially when local anaesthetics are added. Even then, pain relief may be unsatisfactory.

Incident pain occurs when the patient is comfortable at rest but develops severe pain on movement. Examples are pelvic, femur, humerus or vertebral body fractures that may not be amenable to surgical stabilisation.

Neuropathic pain must be differentiated from deafferentation pain (post-herpetic pain, thalamic pain, spinal cord lesions), which would not be relieved by cordotomy. Deafferentation pain is related to the loss of afferent sensory input and accounts for the relatively poor results in non-cancer patients.

The benefits of cordotomy tend to decrease with time. Although nerve regeneration has not been demonstrated, pain recurrence can appear years later. By the end of 1 year, almost 40% of patients no longer have absolute pain relief and around 15% will develop post-cordotomy dysaesthesia. Good to excellent results should be achieved in 90% of patients, with minimal morbidity.

Waldman S. *Interventional Pain Management*. Philadelphia, PA: Saunders, 1996; pp. 527–40.

SBA Question 71: One-lung ventilation

When considering your choice of anaesthetic for thoracic surgery, which ONE of the following operations is an absolute indication for using a double-lumen endotrachael tube?

a) Oesophagectomy
b) Right upper lobectomy
c) Open surgery on the left main bronchus
d) Left total pneumonectomy
e) Open thoracic aortic aneurysm repair

Answer: c

Short Explanation

The relative indications for use of a double-lumen tube (DLT) are generally to improve surgical access, which is true for all of the above apart from open surgery on the left main bronchus. In this case single lung isolation is necessary to assist with control of ventilation.

Long Explanation

This subject is a favourite of the examiners and can be asked at any stage during the final FRCA examination. It is a good idea to have seen a double-lumen tube (DLT) used, or at least to have handled one and to understand how they work. It is also useful to have an understanding of how they are sized. There are a number of subjects that can be discussed when talking about DLTs and one-lung ventilation, so it is worth having a good general overview of these topics.

The indications for being able to provide one-lung anaesthesia (and the commonest technique used in this country is by means of a DLT) can be split into absolute and relative. The absolute indications are generally to facilitate the isolation of one lung from another to assist with ventilation (such as in a bronchopleural fistula or surgical repair of a main bronchus) or to avoid contamination (from haemorrhage or infection). Another absolute indication is unilateral bronchopulmonary lavage.

The relative indications are generally related to improving surgical access in thoracic surgery (such as oesophagectomy, lobectomy, mediastinal surgery or pneumonectomy) or non-thoracic surgery (such as spinal surgery). Another relative indication is in a patient with severe hypoxaemia due to unilateral lung disease.

As well as the indications for one-lung anaesthesia, you may be asked about the physiology of one-lung anaesthesia, the complications (especially hypoxaemia) and the preoperative assessment of the thoracic surgical patient.

Eastwood J, Mahajan R. One-lung anaesthesia. *Br J Anaesth CEPD Rev* 2002; **2**: 83–7. Available online at ceaccp.oxfordjournals.org/content/2/3/83 (accessed 30 June 2012).

SBA Question 72: Myofascial/musculoskeletal pain syndromes

A patient presents to the pain clinic complaining of pain in the right suprascapular area. On examination a palpable taut band within the skeletal muscle is found. It has a hypersensitive spot that is able to reproduce referred pain when stimulated. Which of the following interventions is MOST likely to produce immediate pain relief?

a) Systemic opioids
b) Anticonvulsants
c) Antidepressants
d) TENS
e) Psychotherapy

Answer: d

Short Explanation

Transcutaneous electrical nerve stimulation (TENS) has shown moderate evidence for immediate effects over myofascial trigger points. Myofascial pain tends to be opioid-resistant. The onset of anticonvulsants and antidepressants is slow, and they may not work for this condition. Psychotherapy does not produce immediate pain relief.

Long Explanation

Myofascial pain syndrome (MPS) is a musculoskeletal pain condition characterised by local and referred pain perceived as deep and aching, and by the presence of myofascial trigger points in any part of the body. It is a common condition that may account for 30% of patients complaining of pain in primary care.

The pathophysiology of myofascial trigger points is incompletely understood, and a number of morphological changes, neurotransmitters, neurosensory features, electrophysiological features and motor impairments have been implicated in their pathogenesis.

Clinical features include: trigger points characteristically elicit referred pain when stimulated; the duration of the referred pain is variable (seconds, hours, days); the referred pain is perceived as a deep, aching, and burning pain, although sometimes it may be perceived as superficial pain; the referred pain may spread caudally or cranially and the intensity and expanded area of referred pain are positively correlated with the degree of trigger point activity (irritability).

Management of myofascial trigger points is multimodal. The most commonly used interventions are:

- Massage, ischemic compression, pressure release, and other soft tissue interventions (such as muscle energy) have shown moderately strong evidence for immediate pain relief.
- Dry needling of trigger points has shown clinical benefits, but more studies are needed. Laser therapy shows strong evidence of effectiveness for pain relief.
- Transcutaneous electrical nerve stimulation (TENS) and magnet therapy have shown moderate evidence for immediate effects over myofascial trigger points.
- Exercise has shown moderate benefit; this can include stretching and range of motion, strengthening, endurance, or coordination exercises.
- Ultrasound therapy has weak evidence for effectiveness in management of trigger points.

International Association for the Study of Pain (IASP). *Myofascial Pain.* Available online at www.iasp-pain.org/AM/AMTemplate.cfm?Section=Home&TEMPLATE=/CM/ContentDisplay.cfm&CONTENTID=9288 (accessed 30 June 2012).

SBA Question 73: Use of mechanical assist devices

Which of the following is the most appropriate indication for use of intra-aortic balloon pump (IABP) therapy in critical care?

a) A confused 76-year-old gentleman, 2 days post admission following an acute myocardial infarction who has developed cardiogenic shock and is oliguric
b) A 56-year-old lady who has developed hypotension and chest pain, 2 days after admission for a fractured humerus following a road traffic accident
c) A 66-year-old gentleman who had an acute myocardial infarction and developed cardiogenic shock 2 days post femoral–popliteal bypass for severe peripheral vascular disease
d) A 54-year-old hypotensive gentleman with a history of ischaemic heart disease, admitted under the surgeons with a suspected leaking abdominal aortic aneurysm, whom they want to stabilise preoperatively
e) A 23-year-old intravenous drug user in septic shock who has developed worsening shortness of breath and hypotension despite 2 weeks of intravenous antibiotics

Answer: a

Short Explanation

IABP therapy is considered a class I indication for managing cardiogenic shock not rapidly reversed by pharmacological therapy. Absolute contraindications to IABP therapy include aortic dissection, which is a possibility in the case of the 56-year-old. Relative contraindications include severe peripheral vascular disease (the 66-year-old), abdominal aortic aneurysm (the 54-year-old), and uncontrolled sepsis (the 23-year-old).

Long Explanation

The intra-aortic balloon pump (IABP) is the most widely used circulatory assist device in critically ill patients with cardiac disease. The aim of IABP treatment is to improve ventricular performance of the failing heart by increasing myocardial oxygen supply and decreasing myocardial oxygen demand. The haemodynamic effects are to reduce systolic pressure, increase diastolic pressure, reduce afterload and preload, increase cardiac output and improve coronary blood flow.

Indications for the use of IABP therapy include acute myocardial infarction, cardiogenic shock, acute mitral regurgitation (MR) and ventricular septal defect (VSD), refractory unstable angina, refractory left ventricular failure, refractory ventricular arrhythmias, cardiomyopathies, catheterisation and angioplasty, infants and children with complex cardiac anomalies, cardiac surgery, weaning from cardiopulmonary bypass and sepsis. The aim of IABP is to achieve haemodynamic stability until a definitive course of treatment or recovery occurs.

Absolute contraindications to IABP therapy are aortic regurgitation, aortic dissection, end-stage heart failure with no anticipation of recovery, and aortic stents. Relative contraindications are uncontrolled sepsis, abdominal aortic aneurysm, tachyarrhythmias, severe peripheral vascular disease, and major arterial reconstructive surgery.

Complications associated with the use of IABPs arise from problems with insertion (vascular injury, limb ischaemia, aortic dissection, cardiac tamponade, malposition causing cerebral or renal compromise), problems associated with use (balloon rupture, gas embolus, haemolysis) and problems associated with anticoagulation and infection. Suboptimal timing of inflation and deflation of the balloon can also worsen haemodynamic instability.

Krishna M, Zacharowski K. Principles of intra-aortic balloon counterpulsation. *Contin Educ Anaesth Crit Care Pain* 2009; **9**: 24–8. Available online at ceaccp.oxfordjournals.org/content/9/1/24 (accessed 30 June 2012).

SBA Question 74: Failed intubation

An 80 kg 64-year-old man is scheduled for an elective laparoscopic right hemicolectomy to remove an adenocarcinoma. Following induction of anaesthesia, and neuromuscular blockade using 40 mg atracurium, you are unable to visualise the vocal cords via direct laryngoscopy, after four attempts using a variety of laryngoscope blades. You are also unable to pass a bougie but can still ventilate easily. Assistance is on the way but will take some time to arrive. Select the most suitable course of action from the following:

a) Continue oxygenation via facemask and inform the surgeon of the problem. Wake the patient up once four twitches are visible on train of four and plan an elective awake fibreoptic intubation
b) Insert a standard LMA and, if oxygenation is adequate, proceed with the case and ask the surgeon to limit the pressure of gas used for laparoscopy to 10 mmHg
c) Give a further 10 mg of atracurium, continue bag-mask oxygenation, ask the anaesthetic assistant to fetch the intubating bronchoscope and perform an asleep fibreoptic intubation
d) Insert a standard LMA and, if oxygenation is adequate, attempt to perform a fibreoptic intubation, proceeding with surgery if successful
e) Perform an emergency cricothyroidotomy using either an open or Seldinger technique and proceed with surgery

Answer: d

Short Explanation
As you can oxygenate the patient easily then the last option is incorrect, as it runs the risk of worsening what is, at present, a safe situation. The first option is not incorrect, but it is not as suitable as other options. Insertion of a laryngeal mask airway (LMA) is a safe 'next step', as it allows you to continue to ventilate the patient, attach to monitoring to display end-tidal volatile, O_2, CO_2 etc., and importantly provides a route for intubation. An LMA, in general, makes fibreoptic intubation easier, so the third option is incorrect. The patient in this situation needs intubating – which allows elimination of the second option and leaves you with the fourth as the most suitable course of action.

Long Explanation

The priority in this situation is ensuring the patient remains oxygenated and stable. It would not be 'wrong' to continue to ventilate the patient via a bag and mask, wait for the muscle relaxant to wear off and wake the patient up, but this would not be the most pragmatic of options. At this stage the Difficult Airway Society (DAS) sensibly advocates insertion of a laryngeal mask airway (LMA).

The importance of the laryngeal mask in this situation is that it will generally allow:

- good ventilation
- attachment to the breathing system
- attachment of monitoring to display end-tidal volatile agent, O_2 and CO_2 levels
- a route for intubation

Both the classic (LMA) and intubating (iLMA) laryngeal masks are suitable, although initially the classic will be available in all places and will be most familiar.

At this point in time it is important to check the following:

- check that the patient is oxygenated
- check that the patient is anaesthetised
- check that the patient is properly paralysed
- check that the cardiovascular system is stable
- check that the CO_2 is at a reasonable level

Once these checks have been made, the secondary intubation can be attempted. This is intubation through the LMA. DAS recognises that blind intubation through the iLMA has a high success rate, but promotes a visual fibreoptic technique through the iLMA or classic LMA according to the anaesthetist's preference.

If intubation is successful, the position of the tube in the trachea is confirmed by capnography. If intubation by this technique fails, or if ventilation by the LMA is not possible, then at this point it is appropriate to either remove the LMA and ventilate using a bag and mask or ventilate through the LMA and allow the patient to wake up when muscle relaxation can be antagonised. The procedure is a laparoscopic one, and likely to take a reasonable amount of time, so managing the patient on an LMA throughout rather than using it solely as an aid to entotracheal intubation would be inappropriate.

Difficult Airway Society guidelines are available online at www.das.uk.com/guide lines/ddl.html (accessed 30 June 2012).

SBA Question 75: Methaemoglobinaemia

A 28-year-old male is brought into the emergency department (ED) unconscious. His partner tells you that as well as consuming alcohol and cocaine, he saw him drink from a bottle of amyl nitrate, having mistaken it for a 'shot'. He is deeply cyanosed and tachypnoeic. The pulse oximeter shows a haemoglobin saturation of 52%. An arterial blood sample is chocolate-brown in colour. His arterial blood gas analysis is as follows: pH 7.46; PaO_2 18 kPa; $PaCO_2$ 2.3 kPa; HCO_3 16.4 mmol/L; base excess −8 mmol/L; oxygen saturation 96%. What is the most appropriate treatment?

a) Preoxygenate the patient, intubate and transfer to ICU for ventilation and haemofiltration
b) Give high-flow oxygen and telephone the nearest centre providing hyperbaric oxygen therapy
c) Intubate the patient and give 10 mL of 1% methylene blue solution
d) Intubate the patient and contact the nearest centre with the facility for ECMO (extracorporal membrane oxygenation).
e) Intubate the patient in the ED, send a toxicology screen and give N-acetyl cysteine

Answer: c

Short Explanation

The history and findings are consistent with a diagnosis of methaemoglobnaemia. Most arterial blood gas analysers calculate the oxygen saturation based on the PaO_2 and hence give 'false high' values in such cases. The treatment requires supportive care while reducing the oxidised haemoglobin from its ferric state back to the ferrous state with methylene blue.

Long Explanation

Methaemoglobinaemia is rare but its clinical presentation is classic and early recognition can speed up treatment and avoid unnecessary investigations and invasive treatment, reducing morbidity and mortality.

Methaemoglobinaemia occurs when the ferrous haem moiety of haemoglobin is oxidised to the ferric state. It can occur due to either a genetic defect in red cell metabolism or haemoglobin structure, or ingestion of a variety of drugs and toxins. Substances causing acquired methaemoglobinaemia include nitrates, prilocaine, dapsone, antimalarials, sulphonamides and dyes.

The condition may cause diagnostic confusion because of low oxygen saturation on the pulse oximeter in the presence of a normal saturation on the blood gas. Standard pulse oximeters give spuriously low readings in the presence of excess methaemoglobin (MetHb), whereas most arterial blood gas analysers calculate the oxygen saturation based on the PaO_2 and hence give falsely high readings in a case of methaemoglobinaemia. Co-oximetry is required to give an accurate measure of the percentage of MetHb present.

Clinical features depend on the MetHb levels in blood. The clinical picture of cyanosis and classical chocolate colour of the blood first appear when the MetHb levels reach 15–20%. Levels between 20–45% are associated with dyspnoea, lethargy, dizziness and headaches. When MetHb levels rise above 45% an impaired conscious level is seen, and levels above 55% can cause seizures, cardiac arrhythmias and complete loss of consciousness.

Treatment is supportive in the first instance. Methylene blue in a dose of 1–2 mg/kg causes reduction of the oxydised haem to its reduced ferrous state, allowing normal oxygen carriage and reversing the anaemic hypoxia seen.

Falkenhahn M, Kannan S, O'Kane M. Unexplained acute severe methaemoglobinaemia in a young adult. *Br J Anaesth* 2010; **86**: 278–80.

SBA Question 76: Pathophysiology, diagnosis and management of pneumothorax

A previously fit 43-year-old is brought into the emergency department following a fall from a height of 15 metres. He was unconscious at scene with obvious facial injuries and bruising over his left flank and pelvis and an open fracture of his left femur. The paramedics inserted a laryngeal mask airway (LMA) at the scene and are ventilating him with increasing difficulty. He has an 18 gauge cannula in situ and has received 500 mL of crystalloid en route. He was initially cardiovascularly stable but the crew report that he has been getting progressively more hypotensive with a BP on arrival of 73/46 mmHg, although his pulse rate has dropped from 110 to 65 bpm and he is centrally cyanosed. On examination he has poor air entry, much worse on the left. Which of the following is the most urgent initial management strategy?

a) Obtain urgent chest, abdominal and pelvic x-rays in the emergency department
b) Remove the LMA, preoxygenate, then proceed to urgent rapid sequence intubation and ventilation
c) Arrange an urgent trauma series CT scan (head, CTL spine, chest, abdomen and pelvis)

d) Insert an intercostal drain

e) Insert two large-bore intravenous access, arrange urgent cross-match and commence cautious fluid resuscitation titrated against a palpable radial pulse and apply a pelvic binder

Answer: d

Short Explanation

All of these interventions are required, and in a well-functioning trauma resuscitation most of them would be expected to happen simultaneously. But urgent decompression of a potential tension pneumothorax has the highest priority, as it is quickly diagnosed and treated with a thoracostomy, which is life-saving when performed quickly.

Long Explanation

There are several potential differential diagnoses as to the cause of this patient's deterioration. He has obvious external head, abdominal, pelvic and long bone fractures on one side. As these injuries are apparently so severe the likelihood of a significant chest injury is high, even if there is no external evidence.

The order of management of this patient should follow a CABC route (catastrophic bleeding, airway, breathing, circulation). There is no obvious catastrophic bleeding, although it is possible from abdominal, pelvic or long bone injury. A pneumothorax is caused by the passage of air from the respiratory tract into the pleural space from which it cannot escape, causing collapse of the lung as the intrathoracic pressure increases. This effect is potentiated by positive-pressure ventilation. Progression of the pneumothorax can lead to obstruction of venous return, with a fall in cardiac output and subsequent cardiac arrest.

The worsening compliance to hand ventilation, hypotension, hypoxia and brady-cardia, along with poor left-sided air entry, are highly suggestive of a tension pneumo-thorax. Hyper-resonance and tracheal deviation are unreliable clinical signs, and their absence should not deter the clinician from decompressing the chest. The rate of his clinical deterioration makes waiting for radiological confirmation unwise. The relative bradycardia can sometimes be seen paradoxically in hypovolaemic shock, and it may be a response to hypoxia or a sign of raised intracranial pressure.

The traditional way of excluding a tension pneumothorax is a needle decompres-sion (usually with a large-bore venous cannula) in the second intercostal space, mid-clavicular line. This can be performed if there is no other equipment available in the emergency situation, but the insertion of a formal intercostal drain is then required regardless of the result – because if there was previously no pneumothorax, one may now have been created. In a trauma scenario it should be a very rapid procedure to perform finger thoracostomy (classically fifth intercostal space, mid-axillary line) and insertion of a drain, which should then be connected to an underwater seal.

Chest trauma: tension pneumothorax. Available online at www.trauma.org/archive/thoracic/CHESTtension.html (accessed 30 June 2012).

MacDuff A, Arnold A, Harvey J; BTS Pleural Disease Guideline Group. Management of spontaneous pneumothorax: British Thoracic Society Pleural Disease Guideline 2010. *Thorax* 2010; **65** (Suppl 2): ii18–31.

SBA Question 77: Fluids administered in theatre

A 45-year-old insulin-dependent diabetic presents first on your list for an inguinal hernia repair. He tells you his glucose levels are well controlled with twice-daily injections of Novomix30 and that, as advised by the pre-assessment nurse, he has halved his morning dose. His HbA1c is 7.8% and capillary blood glucose this morning is 8.9 mmol/L. Which one of the following is the most suitable intraoperative fluid regimen for this person?

a) 0.45% sodium chloride with 5% glucose and 0.15% potassium chloride
b) 0.45% sodium chloride with 5% glucose and 0.3% potassium chloride
c) 0.9% sodium chloride with 5% glucose and 0.15% potassium chloride
d) 0.9% sodium chloride
e) Hartmann's solution

Answer: e

Short Explanation
This is a well-controlled diabetic patient (HbA1c < 8.5%) presenting for a short operation. Current guidelines recommend that in such patients who are on twice-daily Novomix30 (or similar), their morning dose should be halved and provided that their blood glucose level can be maintained in the range 6–10 mmol/L, no variable-rate intravenous insulin infusion (VRIII) regimen is needed and Hartmann's solution is the intraoperative fluid of choice.

Long Explanation
In April 2011, a guideline endorsed by many organisations including the Royal College of Anaesthetists was published to highlight the management of adults with diabetes undergoing surgery and elective procedures. In particular, the guideline provides recommendations on which patients require a variable-rate intravenous insulin infusion (VRIII), previously known as a sliding scale, as well as which fluids are best used in the intraoperative period. The document also provides recommendations regarding which long-term treatment regimens (insulin and non-insulin diabetic medications) need altering during the perioperative period (see reference for more details).

With regard to the VRIII, it is recommended that this is avoided if the starvation period for the operation is short (only one missed meal) and the patient has good glycaemic control (HbA1c <8.5% and a capillary blood glucose between 6 and 10 mmol/L), as was the case in this question. It is recommended that in these cases, VRIII should only be commenced if it is proving difficult to maintain the blood glucose levels in the range 4–12 mmol/L.

Which fluids to use in the intraoperative period depends on whether a VRIII is needed. In those who do not require a VRIII, Hartmann's solution is now the fluid of choice. Previously, 0.9% sodium chloride was the fluid of choice in type 2 diabetic patients for fear that Hartmann's solution might lead to hyperglycaemia due to the lactate contained within the solution being converted to glucose by the liver. However, it has been shown that 1 litre of Hartmann's solution would yield a maximum of 14.5 mmol of glucose, and even if 1 litre was rapidly infused it would only raise the blood glucose by 1 mmol/L. Also, the recent GIFTASUP consensus paper has advocated that Hartmann's should replace 0.9% sodium chloride solutions to reduce the risk of inducing hyperchloraemic acidosis.

For patients requiring a VRIII, the guidelines advocate the use of 0.45% sodium chloride with 5% glucose and 0.15% potassium chloride as first-choice solution.

Joint British Diabetes Societies Inpatient Care Group. *Management of Adults With Diabetes Undergoing Surgery and Elective Procedures: Improving Standards*. April 2011. Available online at www.diabetes.org.uk/Documents/Professionals/ Reports and statistics/Management of adults with diabetes undergoing surgery and elective procedures – improving standards.pdf (accessed 30 June 2012).

British consensus guidelines on intravenous fluid therapy for adult surgical patients (GIFTASUP). Available online at www.bapen.org.uk/pdfs/bapen_ pubs/giftasup.pdf (accessed 30 June 2012).

SBA Question 78: Obesity and anaesthesia

Regarding the use of intravenous anaesthetic agents in obese patients, all of the following statements are correct, EXCEPT which one?

a) Induction dose of propofol should be calculated using ideal body weight
b) Initial dose of midazolam should be calculated using total body weight
c) Remifentanil dose should be calculated using ideal body weight
d) Suxamethonium dose should be calculated using ideal body weight
e) Morphine dose should be calculated using ideal body weight

Answer: d

Short Explanation

Suxamethonium should be dosed to total body weight (TBW) up to 140 kg. Propofol should be dosed according to ideal body weight (IBW) for induction bolus, but TBW or corrected weight for maintenance. Morphine and remifentanil should both be dosed by IBW, whereas a bolus of midazolam should be calculated according to TBW.

Long Explanation

Obesity provides the anaesthetist with a pharmacokinetic challenge. Data on drug doses are often drawn from studies on individuals with normal body mass index. However, differences in pharmacokinetic values such as volume of distribution (V_D), protein binding and clearance (Cl) can be significant in the morbidly obese. Lipophilic drugs tend to show a significant increase in V_D, whereas hydrophilic drugs may show little or no change. Remifentanil is an exception – despite its being highly lipophilic there is little change in the V_D in obesity.

Unfortunately the clinical reality is rarely as simple as this, and other factors dictate the extent and duration of drug action – including organ dysfunction related to obesity.

In clinical practice, what this usually means is a decrease in the dose given. In terms of specifics, this can be guided by the following calculated weight adjustments:

- total body weight in kg (TBW) = the actual weight/mass of the patient
- ideal body weight in kg (IBW) = height (cm) – 100 (105 for women)
- lean body mass in kg (LBM) = 1.1(weight) – 128 (weight/height)^2 (substitute 1.07 and 148 respectively for female calculations)

It is important to note that these calculations are not infallible. In particular, a graph showing the change in LBM with weight for a person of any given height is an n-shaped curve that tends to increase up to a point, and then actually decreases above a certain weight. (Note that the Schnider model for propofol target-controlled infusions uses LBM in calculations – if the calculated LBM is on the decreasing aspect of the curve it defaults to the maximum value – the apex of the curve.)

In terms of specific drugs, the halogenated volatile agents show no significant changes in dose requirements, but may undergo increased metabolism. This may result in increased inorganic fluoride concentrations – the clinical relevance of which is unclear. Thiopental as a bolus has an increased V_D, but the increased cardiac output associated with obesity means potentially lower peak plasma concentrations. An increased dosage (e.g. 7.5 mg/kg) using the IBW is therefore recommended. Propofol can be bolused using IBW, but for maintenance infusions, given that there is no significant increase in accumulation in obesity, an adjustment increase of 40% of the excess weight (that above IBW) is recommended. Midazolam, which is again highly lipophilic, when given as a bolus should be given in terms of TBW, but because of accumulation should be adjusted to IBW for infusion. Muscle relaxants are a hydrophilic group, generally associated with a small V_D. However, in spite of this, data from studies concerning clinical effect show variation in recommendations, with the aminosteroids tending to favour the use of IBW, and the benzylisoquinoline agents the use of TBW.

The Society of Bariatric Anaesthetists has produced an excellent factsheet that describes the modifications needed for drug dosing in the obese.

Anaesthesia for the obese patient. Available online at www.sobauk.com/index. php?option=com_phocadownload&view=file&id=3:single-sheet-guidelines&Itemid=61 (accessed 30 June 2012)

De Baerdemaeker LEC, Mortier EP, Struys MMRF. Pharmacokinetics in obese patients. *Contin Educ Anaesth Crit Care Pain* (2004) **4**: 152–5. Available online at ceaccp. oxfordjournals.org/content/4/5/152 (accessed 6 January 2012).

SBA Question 79: Principles of physiotherapy in the critically ill

A 72-year-old male with a history of chronic obstructive pulmonary disease (COPD) is 7 days post emergency laparotomy. He remains intubated and ventilated on pressure-controlled ventilation with an inspired pressure of 26 cm/H_2O, a PEEP of 8 cm/H_2O and an FiO_2 of 0.5. He has recently developed a secondary ventilator-associated pneumonia and has been restarted on antibiotics and noradrenaline infusion (0.1 g/kg/h) to maintain his mean arterial pressure (MAP). He is currently stable, lightly sedated but cooperative. A tracheostomy is planned after the weekend in view of his likely protracted clinical course. The physiotherapist comes to you, as the registrar on the unit, for advice about her management of this patient. Which ONE of the following describes the best approach to this patient's physiotherapy?

a) All physiotherapy should be delayed until after the tracheostomy
b) His vasopressors should be weaned off before any aggressive physiotherapy is undertaken
c) Chest physiotherapy alone should be undertaken regularly to improve secretion clearance and oxygenation
d) Passive mobilisation and positioning are more important than chest physiotherapy
e) A combination of regular chest physiotherapy and early passive and then active mobilisation (as tolerated) should be undertaken

Answer: e

Short Explanation
Physiotherapy input in the critically ill patient is an integral part of multidisciplinary management. A combination of chest and musculoskeletal physiotherapy can and should be delivered throughout the course of a patient's stay in a critical care unit, with neither one being more important/useful than the other. Vasopressor use does not preclude the delivery of physiotherapy.

Long Explanation
A combination of chest physiotherapy, positioning, early passive and then active mobilisation, aiming to optimise cardiopulmonary and functional status, has been shown to improve outcomes in the critically ill, and these interventions are particularly important in longer-term patients. Although caution should be exercised in unstable patients, treatment can usually be tailored on an individual risk–benefit assessment.

The physiotherapist has an important role as part of the multidisciplinary team in the ICU setting. Critically ill patients commonly have respiratory dysfunction and can have prolonged periods of immobility with associated deconditioning, muscle weakness, dyspnoea, depression/anxiety and reduced health-related quality of life. Appropriate physiotherapy can improve patient outcomes and reduce the risks associated with intensive care by optimising cardiopulmonary function and functional abilities. There is an increasing appreciation of the need for rehabilitation from the early stages of critical illness, throughout its course and as a continuum thereafter.

Chest physiotherapy aids secretion clearance, and improves V/Q matching, lung compliance and work of breathing. It can also help prevent pulmonary complications. A combination of recruitment manoeuvres, manual techniques, suctioning, positioning and mechanical adjuncts are commonly used on an individualised basis.

Early physical activity has been shown to improve outcomes in critical illness. Combinations of positioning, passive stretching and range-of-motion exercise, resistive muscle training and active mobilisation are effective at various stages of critical illness.

The physiotherapist should be responsible for individual assessments and implementation of cardiopulmonary and mobilisation plans, ensuring that treatments are effective, safe and continually re-evaluated. There is an associated contribution to the patient's overall well-being by providing emotional support and enhancing communication.

Bersten AD, Soni N. *Oh's Intensive Care Manual*, 6th edn. Philadelphia, PA: Butterworth-Heinemann, 2009; pp. 43–51.

Gosselink R, Bott J, Johnson M, *et al.* Physiotherapy for adult patients with critical illness: recommendations of the European Respiratory Society and European Society of Intensive Care Medicine Force on Physiotherapy for Critically Ill Patients. *Intensive Care Med* 2008; **34**: 1188–99.

SBA Question 80: Acute kidney injury

A 68-year-old man with a past medical history of hypertension (treated with atenolol 50 mg daily and ramipril 10 mg daily) underwent an elective right hemicolectomy for colonic adenocarcinoma 5 days ago. He has suffered significant pain (treated with paracetemol, diclofenac and a morphine PCA), and has an ongoing ileus with abdominal distension. Over the last 24 hours, his creatinine has doubled from his baseline of 130 mmol/L to 270 mmol/L, accompanied by a reduced urine output. As the ICU registrar, you have been asked to see him regarding his acute kidney injury (AKI). Which of the following statements is LEAST correct?

a) Hypovolaemia is likely to be contributing significantly to his AKI
b) His past medical history is likely to be relevant
c) Medication administered for his pain is likely to have contributed to his AKI
d) He is likely to have raised intra-abdominal pressure contributing to his AKI
e) The single dose of gentamicin he received as routine prophylaxis interoperatively is likely to be contributing to his AKI

Answer: e

Short Explanation
A single dose of gentamicin given perioperatively in a well-hydrated elective patient is unlikely to cause acute kidney injury 5 days later.

Long Explanation
Postoperative renal failure is commonly multi-factorial. This patient's past medical history may well be relevant – he had preoperative renal dysfunction, and hypertension is associated with renal artery atheroma and stenosis, as well as direct damage. The diclofenac he received for pain management may also have contributed to his acute kidney injury (AKI).

Hypovolaemia is common after major laparotomies. With his ongoing ileus, his bowel may have become oedematous, resulting in further volume loss. This bowel oedema may result in a rise in intra-abdominal pressure, which can further contribute to his renal failure.

Aminoglycosides do cause AKI, but most commonly in hypovolaemic patients, or where high doses are used over prolonged periods, where sustained high serum levels are seen. AKI would be unlikely 5 days after administration of a normal prophylactic dose of gentamicin in a patient who at the time should have been relatively euvolaemic.

Bersten AD, Soni N. Acute renal failure. In: *Oh's Intensive Care Manual*, 6th edn. Philadelphia, PA: Butterworth-Heinemann, 2009; pp. 509–14.

Renal Association. Acute kidney injury guidelines. Available online at www.renal.org/clinical/GuidelinesSection/AcuteKidneyInjury.aspx (accessed 30 June 2012).

SBA Question 81: Laryngospasm

You have just extubated a 5-year-old girl following tonsillectomy. She has coughed once but you now cannot ventilate her. You think she is in complete laryngospasm. Which of the following best describes the afferent (sensory) and efferent (motor) pathways involved in this reflex arc?

a) Afferent: external branch of superior laryngeal nerve. Efferent: recurrent laryngeal nerve.

b) Afferent: recurrent laryngeal nerve. Efferent: internal branch of superior laryngeal nerve.

c) Afferent: internal branch of superior laryngeal nerve and recurrent laryngeal nerve. Efferent: external branch of superior laryngeal nerve and recurrent laryngeal nerve.

d) Afferent: internal branch of superior laryngeal nerve. Efferent: pharyngeal branches of vagus.

e) Afferent: external branch of superior laryngeal nerve. Efferent: pharyngeal branches of vagus.

Answer: c

Short Explanation
Sensory innervation of the larynx above the vocal cords is via the internal branch of the superior laryngeal nerve. Below the cords it is via the recurrent laryngeal nerve. Motor supply is via the recurrent laryngeal nerve to all intrinsic muscles except cricothyroid muscle, which is supplied by the external branch of the superior laryngeal nerve.

Long Explanation
Laryngospasm typically involves three structures: the aryepiglottic folds, the false vocal cords and the true vocal cords. Laryngeal cartilages are manipulated by the intrinsic muscles of the larynx, particularly the lateral cricoarytenoid (cord adduction), thyroarytenoid (cord adduction) and cricothyroid (cord tensioning) muscles. A multitude of mechanoreceptors, chemoreceptors and thermoreceptors are located throughout the larynx, being most abundant around the laryngeal inlet. The posterior aspect of the true vocal cords has a greater density of receptors than the anterior aspect.

Stimulation of these receptors results in afferent signalling via the superior laryngeal nerve when structures above the true vocal cords are involved. Sensory innervation below the level of the true vocal cords is provided by the recurrent laryngeal nerve, which serves as the afferent pathway in this instance. Efferent pathways are provided by the external branch of the superior laryngeal nerve, which supplies the cricothyroid muscle, and the recurrent laryngeal nerve, which supplies the rest of the intrinsic muscles.

The pharyngeal branch of the vagus nerve is the principal motor nerve of the pharynx, innervating all muscles of the pharynx (except stylopharyngeus) and the soft palate. It also provides sensation. Pharyngeal constriction may contribute to glottic closure. Stimulation of nasal mucosa, soft palate and pharynx in animals has demonstrated that major afferent pathways lie within the pharyngeal branch of the vagus. It is not, however, the major efferent pathway in laryngospasm.

Hampson-Evans D, Morgan P, Farrar M. Pediatric laryngospasm. *Paediatr Anaesth* 2008; **18**: 303–7. Available online at www.cairnsanaes.org/downloads-2/files/Hampson-Evans.pdf (accessed 30 June 2012).

Head & neck anatomy. *Anaesthesia* UK 2007. Available online at www.frca.co.uk/article.aspx?articleid=100712 (accessed 30 June 2012).

SBA Question 82: Anaesthesia in the elderly

Spinal anaesthesia is administered to a 52 kg 89-year-old undergoing hip hemiarthroplasty. Her only medical condition is well-controlled hypertension, for which she takes atenolol and ramipril. Following the block her blood pressure drops from 130/70 mmHg to 65/40 while her heart rate remains stable at 80 bpm. She has received 500 mL crystalloid in the past 30 minutes. What is the most appropriate action?

a) Position the patient slightly head down, raising her legs and give the remaining 500 mL of crystalloid, rechecking the blood pressure every 1–2 minutes
b) Give 3 mg incremental boluses of ephedrine
c) Give the remaining 500 mL of crystalloid and recheck the blood pressure every 1–2 minutes
d) Give 0.5 mg incremental boluses of metaraminol and recheck the blood pressure every 1–2 minutes
e) Give 250 mL colloid and 3 mg incremental boluses of ephedrine, rechecking the blood pressure

Answer: d

Short Explanation
Hypotension occurs commonly following both regional and general anaesthesia in the elderly. It should be treated by cautious use of fluids and early use of a vasopressor. Ephedrine may be ineffective in the elderly; α-agonists such as metaraminol or phenylephrine could be used in preference.

Long Explanation
Spinal anaesthesia causes a reduction in blood pressure due to loss of sympathetic tone and therefore a reduction in systemic vascular resistance. The required compensatory increase in heart rate and stroke volume are less effective in the elderly, who may be on β-blockers and whose ventricles are stiffer and less compliant. The concomitant use of an ACE inhibitor in this patient further compounds the problem, and there is much debate as to whether these drugs should be withheld before surgery.

Attempts to maintain preload by administering fluids should be limited to 8 mL/kg, given while the block is evolving. Fluid overload is a real risk in this population. The choice of vasopressor is again open to debate. β-Receptor sensitivity is reduced in the elderly, limiting the use of β-agonists such as the mixed α- and β-agonist ephedrine. Pure α-agonists such as metaraminol and phenylephrine, however, produce a response comparable with that seen in the younger adult population.

Murray D, Dodds C. Perioperative care of the elderly. *Contin Educ Anaesth Crit Care Pain* 2004; 4: 193–6. Available online at ceaccp.oxfordjournals.org/content/4/6/193 (accessed 30 June 2012).

SBA Question 83: *Clostridium difficile*-associated diarrhoea

Five patients in different wards within your hospital have developed watery diarrhoea. Stool samples are sent for detection of *Clostridium difficile* toxin. In which patient's sample is the toxin most likely to be present?

a) The 52-year old male with chronic renal failure, otherwise fit, who attends the hospital three times weekly for intermittent haemodialysis; on day 3 of a short course of trimethoprim for a urinary tract infection
b) The 82-year-old female, day 1 post primary total hip replacement, who has a penicillin allergy and was given 24 hours of perioperative clindamycin as prophylaxis against operative site infection
c) The 68-year-old male, on a general surgical ward, day 11 after anterior resection for colonic carcinoma, on day 5 of intravenous vancomycin for a methicillin-resistant *Staphylococcus aureus* (MRSA) wound infection
d) The 5-year-old male, admitted to a general paediatric ward 7 days previously with lobar pneumonia, on day 7 of co-amoxiclav
e) The 68-year-old male, day 8 in intensive care after sustaining thoracic injuries in a road traffic collision, intubated and ventilated; has received 6 days' ciprofloxacin therapy for a urinary tract infection; also receiving proton-pump inhibitor therapy

Answer: e

Short Explanation

Strongly associated risk factors for development of *Clostridium difficile*-associated diarrhoea include use of broad-spectrum antibiotics (particularly fluoroquinolones, cephalosporins and clindamycin, with longer treatment periods conferring greater risk), gastric acid suppression (e.g. using proton-pump inhibitors), and age over 65 years. The combination of risk factors puts the 68-year-old at greatest risk.

Long Explanation

Many studies have identified risk factors for development of *Clostridium difficile*-associated diarrhoea (CDAD). However, strain variability, heterogeneity between patient populations and other confounding factors have made it difficult to reproduce the findings of any one study.

Antibiotic administration is the most significant and frequently reported predisposing factor in development of CDAD. Disruption of normal endogenous bowel flora allows *C. difficile* to proliferate. While most antibiotics have been associated with the disease at some point, fluoroquinolones, cephalosporins (especially third-generation), clindamycin and aminopenicillins have been implicated most commonly. A large retrospective study identified a strong association with the use of cephalosporins and fluoroquinolones for > 7 days, with odds ratios ranging from 2.5 (fluoroquinolones) to 9.2 (third-generation cephalosporin). One study examining the use of carbapenems for prophylaxis against surgical site wound infection in elective colorectal surgery found a significant increase in CDAD rates. Concurrent use of multiple antimicrobials is thought to increase risk further.

Antibiotics observed to be less commonly implicated are gentamicin, antipseudomonal penicillins and vancomycin. The UK Health Protection Agency (HPA) highlights that clindamycin is no longer the most frequently implicated antibiotic, possibly because of a decline in its usage following the notoriety it has received in the aetiology of CDAD. Routes of administration which spare the endogenous gut flora may minimise risk; however, cases have been reported that implicate topical antimicrobials!

The same retrospective study referred to above found that both H_2-receptor blockers and proton-pump inhibitors were independent risk factors for the disease. However, other studies have failed to demonstrate such a relationship, and the issue remains contentious.

Age is an important factor in the development of CDAD. The HPA reported a total of 10 846 cases from a 3-month period in 2008, of which 8663 were observed in patients over 65 years.

Underlying disease conditions probably play a role. For example, oncology patients have a higher risk of developing CDAD, possibly due to the use of chemotherapy, numerous courses of antibiotics in both disease prophylaxis and treatment, and frequent hospital attendance. Outbreaks have been seen in hospital renal units, where patients may be at increased risk due to comorbidity and impaired immunity.

Dubberke ER, Reske KA, Yan Y, *et al. Clostridium difficile*-associated disease in a setting of endemicity: identification of novel risk factors. *Clin Infect Dis* 2007; **45**: 1543–9. Available online at cid.oxfordjournals.org/content/45/12/1543 (accessed 30 June 2012).

Health Protection Agency. Clostridium difficile *Infection: How to Deal with the Problem*. London: Department of Health, 2009. Available online at www.hpa.org.uk/webc/HPAwebFile/HPAweb_C/1232006607827 (accessed 30 June 2012).

SBA Question 84: Symptom control in terminal illness

Which one of the following is LEAST appropriate in the management of pancreatic pain?

a) Eating low-fat meals
b) Radiofrequency ablation of the coeliac plexus
c) Opioids
d) Pancreatic enzyme supplementation
e) Splanchnic nerve block

Answer: b

Short Explanation
Radiofrequency ablation of the coeliac plexus is not possible, as the plexus surrounds the aorta and cannot therefore be reached with radiofrequency. Coeliac plexus block, however, may play an important role in the management of pancreatic pain.

Long Explanation
Pain due to pancreatitis or pancreatic carcinoma is often a visceral pain which is mediated via the coeliac plexus. This is an autonomic plexus sitting posterior to the aorta at the level of the L1 vertebra. The plexus is formed from the splanchnic nerves, which can be targeted further up, anterolateral to the T11 vertebra, with the same analgesic effect. The coeliac plexus is a fairly diffuse collection of nerves and can be blocked by diffusion of a bilateral injection of a 10 mL volume of solution placed anterolaterally to the L1 vertebra. The splanchnic nerves are discrete and can be targeted by radiofrequency ablation at the T11 level with good effect. For this reason, a splanchnic nerve block may be effective where a coeliac plexus block has failed to relieve pain.

Coeliac plexus blocks are performed using local anaesthetic alone for non-malignant disease, or alcohol for longer-lasting effect in malignant disease. The coeliac plexus provides the autonomic supply to the upper abdominal organs from stomach down to transverse colon. The descending colon and rectum are supplied by the inferior mesenteric plexus; the other pelvic organs are supplied by the inferior and superior hypogastric plexuses.

The procedure for coeliac plexus block involves fluoroscopic guidance. With the patient prone and sedated, a long (spinal) needle is introduced 7 cm lateral to the spinous process of the L1 vertebra, until the needle tip is anterolateral to the L1 vertebral body. Radio-opaque dye confirms that there is no intravascular spread and the solution is injected. The procedure is repeated on the other side.

The procedure can also be performed using endoscopic ultrasound to guide the needle through the gut wall.

Contraindications to coeliac plexus block include abdominal aortic aneurysm. Side effects include those of sympathetic blockade, e.g. hypotension and diarrhoea, as well as damage to intra-abdominal viscera, sexual dysfunction and irritation of lumbar nerve roots. Intravascular injection of phenol into the spinal arteries can cause paraplegia.

Pancreatic enzyme supplementation in pancreatic cancer treatment is a controversial area with a number of contradictory trial results, with some suggesting benefit and others suggesting no alteration in survival. There is further work being done in this area, investigating both pancreatic enzyme supplementation in isolation and as a part of a wide range of complementary therapies. A low-fat diet may reduce pain severity, and opioids have an important role in pain relief in pancreatic cancer as in many other types of cancer pain.

Coeliac plexus block. *Anaesthesia UK* 2009. Available online at www.frca.co.uk/article. aspx?articleid=100539 (accessed 30 June 2012).

Wong GY, Schroeder DR, Carns PE, *et al.* Effect of neurolytic celiac plexus block on pain relief, quality of life, and survival in patients with unresectable pancreatic cancer: a randomized controlled trial. *JAMA* 2004; **291**: 1092–9. Available online at jama. ama-assn.org/content/291/9/1092 (accessed 30 June 2012).

SBA Question 85: Antenatal assessment of the pregnant woman

You are asked to see a woman who is 34/40 weeks gestation in the antenatal clinic. She is a primigravida who is morbidly obese with a body mass index (BMI) of 52 (weight 126 kg, height 1.55 m). What would be the best piece of advice that you could give her in order to prepare for labour?

a) Advise her to avoid gaining weight in the last 4–6 weeks of pregnancy
b) Advise her that it may not be possible to deliver her baby safely within 30 minutes should a category 1 caesarean section be needed
c) Advise her to request an epidural early in labour so that operative procedures can be more easily dealt with under epidural top-up
d) Advise her that the incidence of failed or difficult intubation rises from 1 in 280 to approximately 1 in 3 in the obese obstetric population
e) Advise her to avoid an epidural if possible as she would have a four times greater risk of suffering a severe headache afterwards

Answer: c

Short Explanation
There would be little point advising the obese parturient about weight management at this late stage. The obstetricians should ideally initiate discussion about adverse obstetric and neonatal outcomes. Whilst it is necessary to discuss difficulties associated

with obesity, the take-home message should not be statistics on headaches and failed intubation.

Long Explanation

In an ideal world all obese women who were thinking about conceiving would receive weight management counselling. The main emphasis of management for obese parturients is to advise them at the initial 8–10 week booking appointment to avoid weight gain or lose a few kilos under guidance from midwives and dieticians.

Obese pregnant women present both physiological and practical challenges. The role of the anaesthetist in the antenatal clinic is to make the parturient aware of the anaesthetic risks associated with obesity (difficult epidural, intravenous cannulation, general anaesthesia), but at 34 weeks gestation it is important not to lose the confidence and trust of the woman by alienating her even more because of her weight.

In view of the well-established fact that the incidence of both emergency caesarean section and assisted delivery rates increases with obesity, women are generally advised to have an epidural early on in labour. The early epidural is easier to insert, and it then allows time for failed insertions and requesting assistance if difficult. Ultrasound assessment may facilitate insertion by identifying the vertebral spaces. There is a higher rate of epidural re-insertion amongst obese women, and this increases in a linear fashion with BMI. Due to the technical challenge of epidural insertion in obese parturients, the chance of dural tap increases from about 0.5–1% in normal-weight women to about 4%.

The prevalence of obesity amongst the obstetric population in 2007 was estimated to be approximately 24%, an increase from 16% in 1993. The 2006–08 Confidential Enquiry into Maternal Deaths showed that obesity was a common feature among the women who died. Of those women who died from direct causes 47% were overweight or obese, as were 50% among those who died from indirect causes.

A 1-year national cohort study undertaken by the UK Obstetric Surveillance System (UKOSS) in 2007–08 showed that the prevalence of extreme morbid obesity (BMI > 50) was 87 per 100 000 maternities. Compared with the rest of the obstetric population, these women had a risk of pre-eclampsia that was 4 times greater, and the risks were 3.8 times greater for intensive care admissions, 3.5 times greater for caesarean section, and 6 times greater for requiring general anaesthesia.

Centre for Maternal and Child Enquiries (CMACE). Saving Mothers' Lives: reviewing maternal deaths to make motherhood safer: 2006–08. The Eighth Report on Confidential Enquiries into Maternal Deaths in the United Kingdom. *BJOG* 2011; **118** (Suppl. 1): 1–203. Available online at onlinelibrary.wiley.com/doi/10.1111/j.1471–0528.2010.02847.x/pdf (accessed 30 June 2012).

Gupta A, Faber P. Obesity in pregnancy. *Contin Educ Anaesth Crit Care Pain* 2011; **11**: 143–6. Available online at ceaccp.oxfordjournals.org/content/11/4/143 (accessed 30 June 2012).

SBA Question 86: Tachycardia

You are called to review your patient in the recovery room who has developed a tachycardia with a regular rate of 145 beats per minute. Blood pressure is recorded as 75/40 mmHg. An ECG shows a QRS of duration 0.14 s. Preoperatively, you noted a left bundle branch block. Which is the single most appropriate immediate action?

a) Give amiodarone 300 mg intravenously followed by a 900 mg infusion
b) As known bundle branch block, give adenosine 6 mg as a rapid intravenous bolus
c) Control rate with β-blocker
d) DC cardioversion with 150 J biphasic shock
e) Synchronised DC cardioversion with 100 J monophasic shock

Answer: d

Short Explanation

This patient has a tachycardia with adverse features. Therefore, the most appropriate action is synchronised DC cardioversion. As this is a broad-complex rhythm, a higher energy is required. The Resuscitation Council (UK) recommends starting with 120–150 J biphasic shock (200 J monophasic) and incrementally increasing if this fails.

Long Explanation

In this scenario, the first step is to assess the patient using the ABC approach. Consider the potential cause for the tachycardia and treat as appropriate. In addition, look for signs of the following adverse features: shock (including hypotension – systolic blood pressure < 90 mmHg, pallor, sweating, confusion or impaired consciousness), syncope, myocardial ischaemia or heart failure. These adverse features have been modified from the 2005 Resuscitation Council (UK) guidelines for peri-arrest arrhythmias and represent a single set of features common to both brady- and tachyarrhythmias.

If adverse features are present, as seen with this patient, synchronised DC cardioversion is indicated. If the rhythm is broad-complex, the Resuscitation Council (UK) recommends starting with 120–150 J biphasic shock (200 J monophasic) and incrementally increasing if this fails. Regular narrow-complex tachycardia will often terminate with lower energies (begin with 70–120 J biphasic, 100 J monophasic). If DC cardioversion fails after three attempts, give amiodarone 300 mg intravenously and repeat shock. Follow this with a 900 mg amiodarone infusion.

If no adverse features are present, the next step is to determine if the rhythm is broad- or narrow-complex and regular or irregular. It is worthwhile to review the Resuscitation Council (UK) tachycardia algorithm. With reference to the options above:

- Amiodarone 300 mg IV followed by a 900 mg infusion is the treatment for a regular broad-complex tachycardia without adverse features.
- Adenosine 6 mg as a rapid intravenous bolus is the treatment for a previously confirmed supraventricular tachycardia with bundle branch block without adverse features. You treat this scenario as for a regular narrow-complex tachycardia. This would have been an appropriate treatment for this patient if he was normotensive.
- Rate control with a β-blocker is the treatment for an irregular narrow-complex tachycardia without adverse features. The most probable arrhythmia of this kind is atrial fibrillation. In this setting, the duration of arrhythmia must be considered to determine if rate control versus chemical cardioversion is the most appropriate option.

Resuscitation Council UK. Peri-arrest arrhythmias. Resuscitation Guidelines 2010. Available at www.resus.org.uk/pages/guide.htm (accessed 30 June 2012).

SBA Question 87: Day-case anaesthesia

A 60-year-old man presents for hernia repair on your day-case general surgical list. He has a history of type 2 diabetes, asthma and hypertension. As you make your preoperative assessment you note that he is overweight with a potentially difficult airway. He volunteers that he has not taken his morning medication in order to be nil by mouth for the procedure. In which ONE of the following circumstances would this patient be unsuitable for discharge on the day of the procedure?

a) He has a history of obstructive sleep apnoea with nasal CPAP at home
b) Following the procedure he suffers postoperative nausea that is resistant to antiemetics
c) His preoperative blood pressure is 157/93 mmHg

d) He has a body mass index of $42 \, kg/m^2$

e) He experiences an episode of laryngospasm in the recovery room

Answer: b

Short Explanation

Obstructive sleep apnoea and morbid obesity are only relative contraindications to day-case surgery. The borderline hypertension is probably explained by omission of antihypertensives and preoperative anxiety. Provided the patient recovers well following the laryngospasm, discharge the same day is reasonable. Nausea interferes with the resumption of normal diet and should be controlled prior to discharge, especially in a diabetic.

Long Explanation

Advances in surgical and anaesthetic technique have led to an increase in the variety of procedures considered suitable for day-case surgery, but overall rates of day-case surgery remain variable across the UK. The NHS plan published in 2000 identified a target of 75% of elective surgery to be performed as day case. Effective preoperative assessment and preparation with protocol-driven nurse-led discharge are fundamental to safe and effective day and short-stay surgery. It is now accepted that the majority of patients are suitable for day-case procedures unless there is a valid reason why an overnight stay would be to their benefit.

Patient assessment for day surgery falls into three categories: social factors, medical factors and surgical factors.

The patient must understand the planned procedure and postoperative care, and must consent to day-case surgery. Following procedures under general anaesthetic a responsible adult must escort the patient home and provide support for the first 24 hours. The patient's domestic circumstances must be appropriate for postoperative care.

Fitness for procedure relates to the patient's health as determined at preoperative assessment, and is not limited by arbitrary criteria such as ASA status, age or body mass index (BMI). Patients with stable chronic disease are often managed better as day cases because of minimal disruption to their daily routine. Obesity per se is not a contraindication, and even morbidly obese patients can be safely managed in expert hands, with appropriate resources. The incidence of complications during the operation or early recovery phase increases with increasing BMI. However, these complications would still occur with inpatient care and have usually resolved or been successfully treated by the time a day-case patient is discharged. In addition, obese patients benefit from the short-duration anaesthetic techniques and early mobilisation associated with day surgery.

The procedure should not carry significant risk of serious complications requiring immediate medical attention such as haemorrhage or cardiovascular instability. Postoperative symptoms should be controllable by a combination of oral medications and local anaesthetic techniques. The procedure should not prevent the patient from resuming oral intake within a few hours. Patients should usually be able to mobilise before discharge, although full mobilisation is not always essential.

Verma R, Alladi R, Jackson I, *et al.* Day case and short stay surgery: 2. *Anaesthesia* 2011; **66**: 417–34.

SBA Question 88: TENS

Regarding transcutaneous electrical nerve stimulation (TENS), which type of nerve fibres are said to be stimulated?

a) Aα
b) Aβ
c) Aδ
d) B
e) C

Answer: b

Short Explanation
Electrical stimulation excites Aβ afferent nerve fibres connected to tactile receptors. Aα are motor fibres and primary receptors to muscle spindle. Aδ are free nerve endings to touch and temperature. B are preganglionic autonomic fibres. C are unmyelinated nociceptor fibres and postganglionic autonomic fibers.

Long Explanation
Transcutaneous electrical nerve stimulation (TENS) is a well-established technique in the pain management armamentarium. The equipment consists of a battery-operated stimulator with connecting leads and skin electrodes. The mode of action is complex but it is based on the gate control theory. Electrical stimulation excites Aβ afferent nerve fibres connected to tactile receptors. Aβ fibres enter the spinal cord and ascend in the dorsal columns but also give collaterals in the spinal cord which synapse with short interneurones ending near C-fibre terminals. These interneurones release γ-aminobutyric acid (GABA) which causes presynaptic blockade of the C afferents, preventing them from exciting the substantia gelatinosa cells and hence closing the gate to nociceptive input.

The physiological effect depends on the type of stimulation applied. Low-frequency TENS (2 Hz) may be mediated via pro-enkephalin-derived peptides acting on μ receptors. High-frequency stimulation (100 Hz) may release dynorphin-like substances with analgesic effects via κ receptors.

TENS can be delivered in different modes (continuous, pulsed and acupuncture-like) by altering the frequency and intensity of the electrical current. Continuous TENS causes a non-painful paraesthesia in the stimulated area. Pulsed TENS produces non-painful paraesthesia felt as bursts. Acupuncture-like TENS is similar to pulsed TENS but is associated with non-painful muscle twitch. Duration and timing of TENS stimulation is another variable to consider. Intermittent stimulation for short intervals may be more effective than prolonged or continuous stimulation.

Lynch L, Simpson KH. Transcutaneous electrical nerve stimulation and acute pain. *Br J Anaesth CEPD Rev* 2002; **2**: 49–52. Available online at ceaccp.oxfordjournals.org/content/2/2/49 (accessed 30 June 2012).

SBA Question 89: Arterial tourniquets

A 32-year-old man is undergoing open reduction and internal fixation of a distal forearm fracture. An arterial tourniquet is inflated at the mid-humeral level. The surgeons do not want to deflate the tourniquet. Which of the following provides the best reason for allowing the tourniquet to stay inflated?

a) The patient received ketamine preoperatively to reduce the hypertension caused by tourniquet use
b) Every 30 minutes of tourniquet inflation only increases the risk of nerve damage by 50%
c) The patient is at a lower risk of neurological injury as he is relatively young
d) The tourniquet will help to reduce anaesthetic requirements by reducing physiological sensory nerve conduction from the surgical site

e) The tourniquet had only been inflated for 2 hours

Answer: a

Short Explanation
Ketamine has been shown to reduce 'tourniquet hypertension'. The risk of nerve damage is increased threefold every 30 minutes, and younger age predicts nerve damage following prolonged usage. Pain transmission from distal to the tourniquet will be absent after 1 hour but pain from the tourniquet site itself will take over.

Long Explanation
Tourniquet use is widespread, and largely occurs without complication. However, the consequences of tourniquet-related complications can be severe. Most literature recommends a maximum inflation time of 1.5–2 hours, after which time a break of 10–15 minutes should be used to allow regeneration of muscle ATP.

After between 15 and 45 minutes a physiological conduction block affecting both motor and sensory nerve fibres prevents nerve transmission to and from distal to the tourniquet site. However, pain from the tourniquet site itself may be the cause of the 'tourniquet hypertension' seen with increasing duration of tourniquet inflation. This may be attenuated with ketamine (low dose), clonidine, and even topical local anaesthetic cream.

Each 30 minutes a tourniquet is inflated there is a threefold increase in the incidence of neurological damage. Somewhat surprisingly, younger age is an independent predictor of neurological damage following prolonged tourniquet times, potentially because of the lower normal systolic pressures (and a standardised 'one pressure suits all' approach to tourniquet inflation). Following deflation of the tourniquet, there is an elevation of arterial CO_2 tensions, which has been shown to increase middle cerebral blood flow velocity of up to 50%.

Deloughry JL, Griffiths, R. Arterial tourniquets. *Contin Educ Anaesth Crit Care Pain* 2009; **9**: 56–60. Available online at ceaccp.oxfordjournals.org/content/9/2/56 (accessed 30 June 2012).

SBA Question 90: Preoxygenation

You are anaesthetising an obese 45-year-old man for an emergency laparotomy to investigate a suspected bleeding duodenal ulcer. He has a BMI of 40 and Hb of 9.5 g/dL. With regard to oxygenation in this patient, which one of the following statements is true?

a) Impending hypoxaemia will be detected by monitoring his arterial oxygen saturations
b) He will desaturate at the same rate as a patient matched for age and size who is not critically ill
c) Because he is anaemic, there will be a reduction in the time to critical hypoxia despite adequate preoxygenation
d) Preoxygenating obese patients in a head-up position reduces the time to critical hypoxaemia
e) As an adult, he will remain oxygenated longer during apnoea than an equivalently unwell 5-year-old child, principally due to his relatively larger functional residual capacity

Answer: c

Short Explanation

Oximetry can detect a decrease in sats before any clinical signs are present, but it is a poor tool for *predicting* hypoxaemia. Critically ill patients desaturate more rapidly. Preoxygenating obese patients head-up will increase the time to critical hypoxaemia. Children have a greater VO_2 than adults, and this is the main reason why children develop critical hypoxia more quickly.

Long Explanation

Preoxygenation is a simple procedure, and it can have a significant influence on time to desaturation. The aim of preoxygenation is to replace nitrogen in the functional residual capacity (FRC) with oxygen.

During apnoea the arterial partial pressure of oxygen (PaO_2) decreases in direct relation to the alveolar partial pressure of oxygen (PaO_2), and the arterial haemoglobin oxygen saturation (SaO_2) remains 90% as long as the haemoglobin can be reoxygenated in the lungs. The SaO_2 only starts to decrease when the store of oxygen in the lungs is depleted and the PaO_2 is around 6–7 kPa. Its subsequent decline is rapid (about 30% every minute). At the start of this rapid decline, the SaO_2 is still 90–95%. This point can be defined as 'critical hypoxia'. It is for this reason that oximetry is not a good tool for predicting impending hypoxaemia.

The importance of haemoglobin is not in the storage of oxygen but in its effective transport from the lungs to the tissues. Anaemia will cause a small reduction in the time to critical hypoxia, although this effect will be more noticeable in patients who also have a reduced FRC.

Critically ill patients suffer arterial desaturation more rapidly than healthy patients because of one or several of the following: cardiopulmonary pathology, anaemia, low cardiac output, hypermetabolic states, ventilation/perfusion imbalances, pain, airway obstruction, and depressed respiratory effort.

Various factors significantly influence the time period from the onset of apnoea to critical hypoxia. The FRC is the most important store of oxygen, and the greater the FRC the longer the time before critical hypoxia develops. Patients with a reduced FRC include the obese, the pregnant and those with lung disease.

The supine positioning of obese patients further reduces the FRC. For severely obese patients, preoxygenation in the 25° head-up position achieves oxygen tensions 20% higher than when preoxygenation is applied in the supine position.

Children have smaller FRC and greater VO_2 per unit weight than healthy adults. Critical hypoxia develops more quickly after the onset of apnoea, and this is more pronounced in younger children. The biggest component of this is the relatively greater VO_2.

Sirian R, Wills J. Physiology of apnoea and the benefits of preoxygenation. *Contin Educ Anaesth Crit Care Pain* 2009; **9**: 105–8. Available online at ceaccp.oxfordjournals. org/content/9/4/105 (accessed 30 June 2012).

Paper 2

MTF Question 1: Advance decisions and living wills

Regarding advance decisions made by competent patients, which of the following are true?

a) They may be ignored by a healthcare worker as they are not legally binding in the UK
b) They can authorise doctors to carry out a specific form of treatment
c) They should only be applied to a specific set of circumstances and pathologies
d) They should be disregarded in patients with dementia
e) They allow patients to refuse any type of treatment

Answer: c, e

Short Explanation

Advance Decisions (advance directives, living wills) allow patients to refuse any treatments but they cannot authorise doctors to carry out a specific form of treatment. They apply to certain very defined circumstances. Competent patients who anticipate future incompetence (e.g. dementia) may indicate their preferences for future treatment by completing an Advance Decision.

Long Explanation

Competent patients who anticipate future incompetence through illness may indicate their preferences for future treatment by completing an Advance Decision. For example, patients may indicate that they do not wish to undergo life-saving surgery if they suffer from dementia when they are older. Many Jehovah's Witnesses carry with them an Advance Decision forbidding the administration of blood or blood components. Advance Decisions are legally binding on healthcare workers if they are made voluntarily by a competent, adequately informed patient who expresses an explicit refusal of treatment under certain defined circumstances.

When a situation falls fully within the terms of the Advance Decision, clinicians should respect the terms unless there is evidence that the patient may have changed his or her mind since signing it.

Advance Decisions cannot authorise doctors to do anything outside the law, or compel them to carry out a specific form of treatment.

The Mental Capacity Act 2005 has entered the statute books for England and Wales. It formalises the role of the 'Advance Decision', which would become legally binding if the patient has lost capacity and the situation which he/she has anticipated then develops. In the case of predictable incapacity, where their competence is likely to be lost through future illness (Alzheimer's disease, Huntington's dementia), patients may choose to prepare an Advance Decision stating which treatments they would accept and refuse, if needed.

AAGBI. *Consent for Anaesthesia*. AAGBI Guidelines. London: Association of Anaesthetists of Great Britain and Ireland, 2006. Available online at www.aagbi. org/sites/default/files/consent06.pdf (accessed 30 June 2012).

MTF Question 2: Cystic fibrosis

A 25-year-old woman is admitted to hospital with recurrent chest infections. She is also known to have cystic fibrosis (CF). Which of the following statements are true?

a) The most likely organism causing the chest infection is *Pseudomonas aeruginosa*
b) Nebulised antibiotics are used in chronic infections
c) Physiotherapy is contraindicated in this patient, as it can increase the risk of pneumothorax
d) Restricted dietary intake is important in this case, to reduce bronchial secretions
e) The patient is likely to have had functionally abnormal lungs since birth

Answer: a, b

Short Explanation
The initial infecting organisms for CF patients are *Staphylococcus aureus* and *Haemophilus influenzae*. Eventually infection with *Pseudomonas aeruginosa* supervenes. Physiotherapy is an essential part of this patient's treatment, as thick secretions trap bacteria within the small airways of the lungs. *P. aeruginosa* infection can sometimes be eradicated by the early use of nebulised antibiotics. Any septic patient requires good nutrition to optimise immune function. Newborn babies with CF have normal lungs.

Long Explanation
Cystic fibrosis (CF) is an autosomal recessive disorder characterised by abnormal transport of chloride and sodium across epithelium. This leads to thick, viscous secretions in the lungs, liver, intestine, pancreas and reproductive tract. Symptoms often present within the first year. Diagnosis is by sweat test, genetic testing and neonatal screening. Further tests are used to determine pancreatic insufficiency.

A neonate with CF has normal lungs, but repeated chest infections lead to bronchiectasis as well as pulmonary hypertension and respiratory failure. The initial infecting organisms for CF patients are *Staphylococcus aureus* and *Haemophilus influenzae*. Eventually infection (and colonisation) with *Pseudomonas aeruginosa* supervenes.

The main stems of treatment involve a multidisciplinary team approach. This can be further divided into systems. Most of the morbidity and more than 90% of the mortality of CF is related to chronic pulmonary sepsis and its complications. Treatment includes physiotherapy to clear secretions, aerosols and nebulisers, antibiotics (sometimes for life), mucus thinners, anti-inflammatories, bronchodilators, nutritional support, exercise and monitoring for complications. As respiratory function worsens, bilevel positive airway pressure (BiPAP) ventilators can improve oxygenation and when combined with physiotherapy can help sputum clearance. Chronic *Pseudomonas aeruginosa* lung infections can be treated with inhaled antibiotics. Allergic bronchopulmonary aspergillosis needs to be considered, especially when there is a lack of response to standard antibiotics.

Diabetes mellitus is the most common non-pulmonary complication, giving mixed features of type 1 and type 2. CF patients often develop nasal polyps, severely limiting airflow and reducing the sense of smell. Infertility in males is due to the absence of the vas deferens, although the sperm themselves function normally. Median predicted age of survival for CF is in the mid-30s. This chronic illness can be very difficult to manage, requiring time-consuming daily treatment routines.

Cystic Fibrosis Trust. *Consensus Documentation: Standards for the Clinical Care of Children and Adults with Cystic Fibrosis in the UK*. 2nd edn, December 2011. Available online at www.cftrust.org.uk/aboutcf/publications/consensusdoc (accessed 30 June 2012).

Flume PA, O'Sullivan BP, Robinson KA, *et al*. Cystic fibrosis pulmonary guidelines: chronic medications for maintenance of lung health. *Am J Respir Crit Care Med* 2007; **176**: 957–69. Available online at ajrccm.atsjournals.org/content/176/10/957 accessed 30 June 2012).

MTF Question 3: Electrocution

Regarding electrical hazards, which of the following are true?

a) A current of 5 mA will cause ventricular fibrillation if applied directly to the myocardium
b) Direct current is less likely to cause ventricular fibrillation than alternating current
c) The muscles present the highest impedance to current flow when current is applied to the patient
d) As current frequency increases above 50 Hz the risk of ventricular fibrillation increases linearly
e) Microshock can occur when external ECG leads are applied to the chest

Answer: a, b

Short Explanation
The skin presents the highest impedance to current flow when current is applied to a patient. Current frequency of 50 Hz is the most lethal current frequency. Microshock occurs when internal equipment comes into direct contact with the heart.

Long Explanation
The risk of electrocution is potentially high during the intraoperative period in view of the amount of electrical equipment used in close proximity to the patient. There are stringent safety requirements designed to reduce this risk and so there is a low reported incidence of patient harm from electrocution.

Current applied to the patient will flow through the patient if he or she is earthed. Different sizes of externally applied current will have different effects on the patient. 1 mA will cause tingling, 5 mA will cause pain, 15 mA will cause tonic muscle contraction and pain, 50 mA will cause tonic contraction of respiratory muscles and respiratory arrest, and 75–100 mA will cause ventricular fibrillation. The damage caused is also proportional to the duration of current application, the current pathway and the type of current.

The direct current required to cause ventricular fibrillation is much higher than the alternating current. Mains-current frequency (50 Hz) is the most lethal, and current frequencies much higher than this cause heating only.

The skin presents the highest impedance to flow. This impedance can be lowered if the skin is wet with sweat or inflamed.

Microshock occurs when intracardiac equipment such as central lines comes into direct contact with the heart. In this situation, current of only 150 μA will trigger ventricular fibrillation. This equipment must have almost undetectable current leakage to prevent harm to the patient.

Al-Shaikh B. *Essentials of Anaesthetic Equipment*, 3rd edn. Edinburgh: Churchill Livingstone, 2007; pp. 216–17.

Davis PD, Kenny GNC. *Basic Physics and Measurement in Anaesthesia*, 5th edn. Oxford: Butterworth-Heinemann, 2003; p. 183.

MTF Question 4: Back pain: steroid injections

Regarding epidural steroid injections for low back pain of > 6 months' duration, which of the following statements are true?

a) In 2009 NICE recommended the use of epidural steroids in the treatment of nerve root pain
b) Fluoroscopy is mandatory in all epidural steroid injections for low back pain
c) Caudal injection of epidural steroids in adults has an increased risk of accidental dural puncture
d) Congestive cardiac failure is a relative contraindication to epidural steroid injection
e) Particulate steroid preparations risk anterior spinal artery syndrome

Answer: d, e

Short Explanation

The National Institute for Health and Clinical Excellence (NICE) has not issued guidance about the management of patients with nerve root pain, only non-specific low back pain. The Royal College of Anaesthetists recommends, not mandates, the use of fluoroscopy for epidural injection for spinal pain. Caudal epidural injection, via the sacral hiatus at S5, reduces the risk of inadvertent dural puncture; the dural sac ends at S2 in adults.

Long Explanation

Low back pain and radicular pain (nerve root compression pain) is primarily due to inflammatory mediators irritating and sensitising free nerve endings supplying the annulus fibrosus (outer layer) of intervertebral discs, and spinal nerve roots. Phospholipase A_2 (PLA_2) releases arachidonic acid from phospholipid cell membranes, which increases the production of cyclooxygenase and lipoxygenase. This subsequently increases levels of prostaglandin, thromboxanes and leukotrienes, which are associated with inflammation, ischaemia and pain. Corticosteroids inhibit the action of PLA_2; other actions include carbohydrate, fat and protein metabolism (glucocorticoids) and regulation of electrolytes and water (mineralocorticoids). Possible fluid retention after steroid therapy gives rise to the relative contraindication of epidural injections in patients with congestive cardiac failure.

In the chronic pain setting, there are several methods used to deliver steroid directly to the source of the pathology and therefore reduce local inflammation. In low back pain, the most common procedures are caudal epidural injections, interlaminar and transforaminal approaches. The caudal approach via the sacral hiatus (if present), the developmental absence of the S5 lamina and spinous process, reduces the incidence of dural puncture; the dural sac ends at S2 in adults. The caudal approach is useful for lower lumbar nerves, the cauda equina, and can be imaged under fluoroscopy (and ultrasound).

There is ongoing debate with regard to the use of particulate (triamcinolone) and non-particulate steroid preparations (dexamethasone and methylprednisolone). Some evidence suggests that particulate suspensions result in greater improvement in pain scores after treatment, but there is the issue of the potential risks of using them. With particle sizes being greater than red blood cells (7.5–7.8 μm), inadvertent injection into a small artery may lead to the development of anterior spinal artery syndrome, the most devastating consequence of this being complete motor loss below the level of the lesion.

The Royal College of Anaesthetists issued its recommendations for good practice in the use of epidural injections for back pain in April 2011. It recognised that it is accepted practice to perform epidural injections without fluoroscopy for perioperative and obstetric analgesia, as the end point of effectiveness is clinically apparent. However, in the pain setting, the effectiveness of epidural injection of steroid is not immediately obvious, and the use of fluoroscopy is therefore recommended, although not mandatory, to confirm accurate needle placement and spread of injectate, using appropriate non-ionic water-soluble contrast medium.

The evidence for epidural steroids is very much a source of contention amongst pain specialists. The National Institute for Health and Clinical Excellence (NICE) does not recommend any epidural steroid injections for the treatment of non-specific low back pain of between 6 weeks' and 12 months' duration, but the guidance does not apply to patients suffering disabling symptoms for more than 12 months, or to those with nerve root pain.

Collighan N, Gupta S. Epidural steroids. *Contin Educ Anaesth Crit Care Pain* 2010; 10: 1–5. Available online at ceaccp.oxfordjournals.org/content/10/1/1 (accessed 30 June 2012).

National Collaborating Centre for Primary Care. *Low Back Pain: Early Management of Persistent Non-Specific Low Back Pain*. NICE Clinical Guideline 88. London: RCGP, 2009. Available online at www.nice.org.uk/nicemedia/live/11887/44334/44334. pdf (accessed 30 June 2012).

Royal College of Anaesthetists Faculty of Pain Medicine. *Recommendations for Good Practice in the Use of Epidural Injection for the Management of Pain of Spinal Origin in Adults*. London: Royal College of Anaesthetists, 2011. Available online at www. rcoa.ac.uk/docs/EpiduralInjections.pdf (accessed 30 June 2012).

MTF Question 5: Urinary electrolytes

Regarding urinary electrolytes:

a) Electrolytes usually found in urine include sodium, glucose and potassium
b) Urinary sodium levels can indicate volume status
c) Urinary sodium levels increase in syndrome of inappropriate antidiuretic hormone secretion (SIADH)
d) Urinary potassium levels increase with increased aldosterone levels
e) Values vary according to diet

Answer: b, c, d, e

Short Explanation

Glucose is not usually found in urine. Sodium is responsible for the distribution of total body water. When sodium is reabsorbed, water follows. Low urinary sodium levels may indicate hypovolaemia. In SIADH, urinary sodium is high and plasma sodium is low.

Long Explanation

Urinary electrolytes usually consist of sodium, potassium, calcium and chloride. Glucose is freely filtered at the glomerulus but then completely reabsorbed in the proximal tubule and hence is not usually found in the urine. Glucose may appear in the urine in diabetes mellitus, pregnancy, urinary tract infections and sepsis.

The amount of electrolytes excreted by the kidney is largely dependent on the daily intake, and so urinary electrolyte values do vary according to diet. This can make the interpretation of electrolyte values difficult. Analysis of urinary electrolytes should always be taken in the clinical context.

Sodium is the main extracellular cation and is responsible for the movement and distribution of total body water. When sodium is reabsorbed water follows, and therefore low urinary sodium levels may indicate that sodium is being reabsorbed to allow the reabsorption of water. This may indicate hypovolaemia. As mentioned above, analysis of these values should always be taken in the clinical context because there are many other reasons why urinary sodium may be low.

In the syndrome of inappropriate antidiuretic hormone secretion (SIADH), urinary sodium levels are high and plasma sodium levels or plasma osmolality is low, in the absence of hypovolaemia, oedema or diuretics. In other words, the secretion of anti-diuretic hormone is inappropriately high for the osmotic status of the patient.

Aldosterone, secreted from the adrenal cortex, acts to increase potassium secretion in the distal tubules. This results in potassium loss in the urine. Aldosterone has the opposite effect on sodium, acting to increase sodium reabsorption, hence reducing urinary sodium concentration.

Brandis K. *The Physiology Viva: Questions and Answers*, revised edn. [Australia], 2002; p. 159.

Sherwood L. *Human Physiology: From Cells To Systems*, 3rd edn. Belmont, CA: Wadsworth, 1997; pp. 488–93

MTF Question 6: Paget's disease of bone

Regarding Paget's disease of bone:

a) Serum alkaline phosphatase levels are raised in 85% of patients with untreated Paget's disease
b) The disease presents with increased serum calcium and phosphate
c) The risk of sarcoma is around 1%
d) Pain is worse in the morning but improves during the day
e) Bisphosphonates are first-line treatment

Answer: a, d, e

Short Explanation
There is an increase in serum alkaline phosphatase, but serum calcium and phosphate levels remain normal. The risk of malignant change is around 1%, but the risk of sarcoma is 1 in 1000.

Long Explanation
Paget's disease is a remodelling disorder of bone. It is an age-related condition affecting 1–2% of adults aged over 55 years, increasing to around 7% over the age of 80 years. It is thought to be caused by a combination of genetic and environmental factors. Bone pain is the most common symptom, most commonly affecting the pelvis or spine, and it is usually worse when lying down. The pain is caused by the high turnover of bone and by nerve compression. Other symptoms often include arthralgia, neural deafness, increased bone density, cardiac failure and pathological fractures. Diagnosis is made from the characteristic appearance on x-ray and/or elevated level of serum alkaline phosphatase with normal calcium and phosphate levels.

Treatment is aimed at relieving bone pain and preventing progression of the disease. First-line treatment consists of bisphosphonates, which slow the remodelling of the bone. Bisphosphonates work by attaching to hydroxyapatite binding sites on bony surfaces, especially surfaces undergoing resorption. When osteoclasts begin to reabsorb bone that is impregnated with bisphosphonate, the bisphosphonate released during resorption impairs the ability of the osteoclasts to form the ruffled border (a specialised cell membrane), to adhere to the surface of the bone and to produce the proteins necessary for continued bone resorption. Bisphosphonates also reduce osteo-clast activity by decreasing osteoclast progenitor development and recruitment and by promoting osteoclast apoptosis. Simple analgesia can improve bone pain, with some patients benefitting from low-dose tricyclic antidepressants. Medical treatment can be used prior to orthopaedic surgery to reduce bleeding.

Complications are uncommon but can potentially be fatal. These include fractured bones, deformed bone, sarcoma, hypercalcaemia, kidney stones, heart failure, deaf-ness. In those patients who develop malignant change 50% are osteosarcomas, 25% fibrosarcomas and 25% giant-cell tumours. The median survival following malignant change is less than 1 year.

Selby P, Davie M, Ralston S, Stone M. Guidelines on the management of Paget's disease of bone. *Bone* 2002; **31**: 366–73.

MTF Question 7: Management of tachyarrhythmias

Regarding the management of tachyarrhythmias:

a) It is generally easy to distinguish between supraventricular tachycardia (SVT) and ventricular tachycardia (VT) on the 12-lead ECG
b) Atrial fibrillation (AF) will normally cardiovert in response to an adequate dose of adenosine
c) New AF in critically ill patients is generally related to an underlying structural cardiac abnormality
d) Digoxin therapy is contraindicated in the treatment of AF in the presence of Wolff–Parkinson–White (WPW) syndrome
e) In the presence of an arterial blood pressure of 86/43 mmHg, VT should normally be treated with amiodarone in the first instance

Answer: a, d

Short Explanation

AF will not generally cardiovert with adenosine, but the ventricular rate may slow, allowing easier analysis of the rhythm strip. AF is not normally associated with under-lying cardiac disease when it occurs in critical illness. VT in the presence of hypotension should normally be treated with DC cardioversion first.

Long Explanation

Tachyarrhythmias can be divided into those originating within the ventricle (VT), and those from above the ventricle, in the bundle of His, AV node or atria (SVT). Common SVTs include atrial fibrillation (AF), atrial flutter, and nodal re-entry arrhythmias. Chronic AF is often associated with structural cardiac abnormalities, such as those induced by ischaemic heart disease or respiratory disease. In critical illness, the AF is often triggered by a combination of electrolyte abnormalities, circulating cytokines and raised catecholamine levels rather than structural heart disease. It is therefore harder to sustain sinus rhythm after cardioversion of critical-illness AF.

In general, SVT can be distinguished from VT on the ECG by examining the QRS complexes. SVT will have narrow QRS complexes, compared to the broad complexes of VT. This can be confused by the presence of an underlying bundle block, as this will cause SVT to have widened QRS complexes. In general, any tachyarrhythmia with broad complexes should be treated as VT unless a supraventricular origin is clear.

In SVT, adenosine can be used. This markedly increases the refractory period of the AV node, effectively terminating re-entry tachyarrhythmias. It will not, however, be successful in cardioverting AF or atrial flutter, although it may reduce the ventricular rate sufficiently for diagnosis to be made. Digoxin also slows AV nodal transmission, slowing the ventricular rate in AF. In Wolff–Parkinson–White (WPW) syndrome, slowing AV node transmission will cause preferential transmission through the aberrant pathway, contraindicating both digoxin and adenosine.

In general, all tachyarrhythmias causing significant haemodynamic compromise, such as hypotension or pulmonary oedema, should be treated by DC cardioversion. In the absence of compromise, pharmacological therapy can be attempted. Depending on the rhythm, the focus of treatment can be either reduction of the ventricular rate or cardioversion. Antiarrhythmic drugs effective in these situations include amiodarone, magnesium, β-blockers, calcium channel blockers and digoxin for rate control. Additionally, once structural cardiac disease has been excluded, other options for rhythm control include flecainide and sotalol.

Bersten AD, Soni N. Management of cardiac arrhythmias. In: *Oh's Intensive Care Manual*, 6th edn. Philadelphia, PA: Butterworth-Heinemann, 2009; pp. 204–16.

MTF Question 8: Measurement of pH

Regarding the measurement of pH with the pH electrode, which of the following are true?

a) The active (measuring) electrode is silver/silver chloride
b) Calibration is not necessary
c) The potential difference created is in the order of 60 mV per unit of pH
d) The system must be maintained at 37 °C
e) A linear relationship exists between the potential difference and the pH

Answer: a, c, d, e

Short Explanation
The active electrode is silver/silver chloride, surrounded by pH-sensitive glass. The system must be calibrated by two buffer solutions before use and maintained at 37 °C. A linear relationship exists between the potential difference and pH. For every unit of pH, the potential output is 60 mV.

Long Explanation
The pH electrode consists of a measuring electrode and a reference electrode. The measuring (active) electrode is a silver/silver chloride electrode inside a pH-sensitive glass bulb. The glass bulb contains a buffer, which keeps the pH inside the glass bulb constant. This ensures that the pH difference across the pH-sensitive glass is due to the pH of the sample.

The reference electrode is also silver/silver chloride, in contact with the blood sample via a saturated potassium chloride solution. This solution is in contact with the blood sample via a membrane, which protects the electrode from contamination. Any damage to the membrane or build-up of protein deposits can result in an inaccurate result. The reference electrode is in contact with the blood via the potassium chloride solution and the measuring electrode is in contact with the buffer within the pH-sensitive glass. This completes an electric circuit. A potential difference is produced between the two electrodes, which is proportional to the hydrogen ion concentration of the blood sample. For each unit of pH, there is an electrical output of approximately 60 mV.

The electrode system must be calibrated with two buffer solutions prior to use, and the system must be maintained at 37 °C for accurate results.

Al-Shaikh B, Stacey S. *Essentials of Anaesthetic Equipment*, 2nd edn. London: Churchill Livingstone, 2002; pp. 165–7.

Davies PD, Kenny GNC. *Basic Physics and Measurement in Anaesthesia*, 5th edn. Oxford: Butterworth-Heinemann, 2003; pp. 211–13.

MTF Question 9: Hepatitis C

Regarding hepatitis C:

a) It is a DNA virus
b) Early infection is often asymptomatic
c) Approximately 85% of patients develop cirrhosis by 20 years
d) On blood testing, the AST : ALT ratio is > 1 : 1 in the absence of cirrhosis
e) Interferon-α if given in acute infection can decrease progression to chronicity

Answer: b, e

Short Explanation
Hepatitis C is an RNA flavivirus. Approximately 85% of patients develop chronicity, and around 25% develop cirrhosis within 20 years. The AST : ALT ratio is < 1 : 1 until cirrhosis develops.

Long Explanation
Hepatitis C is an enveloped, single-stranded RNA virus in the family Flaviviridae. It is present worldwide, and most common in Africa and southern Europe. It is transmitted by sexual contact and blood, including intravenous drug use and tattoos.

In the first 12 weeks or so of infection most people are asymptomatic. Those that do show symptoms mostly show vague flu-like symptoms including jaundice (~20%), abdominal pain, urticaria and malaise. Around 85% develop chronic infection, around 25% develop cirrhosis within 20 years, and some will develop hepatocellular carcinoma. Diagnostic investigations include examining the aspartate aminotransferase to alanine aminotransferase (AST : ALT) ratio, which is < 1 : 1 in early infection, and the detection of anti-HCV antibodies. Antibodies may take up to 6 weeks to show after acute disease, and a negative reading early on therefore does not necessarily exclude infection. Patients with antibodies should undergo testing for Hepatitis C RNA present in serum. If Hepatitis C PCR testing is positive then liver biopsy should be carried out to assess the level of hepatocellular damage – to detect any level of cirrhosis and fibrosis.

Combination therapy with ribavirin and interferon-α should be given for between 6 and 12 months. These inhibit viral replication. The aim here is to reduce amino-transferase levels and eradicate viral RNA from serum. Treatment success depends a lot on viral load. Prognosis will be poor in patients with high alcohol consumption, and therefore it is important to discourage this.

Ballinger A, Patchett S. *Pocket Essentials of Clinical Medicine*, 4th edn. Edinburgh: Saunders, 2007; pp. 133–45.

Ryan KJ, Ray CG. *Sherris Medical Microbiology*, 4th edn. New York, NY: McGraw Hill, 2004; pp. 551–2.

MTF Question 10: Pre-hospital intubation

When considering intubation in the pre-hospital environment, which of the following statements are true?

a) All practitioners in the pre-hospital environment should be capable of tracheal intubation
b) Securing the airway should be the priority in the critically injured pre-hospital patient

c) Appropriately trained paramedics are permitted to use drugs to facilitate tracheal intubation and maintenance of anaesthesia
d) Standards governing a pre-hospital intubation are the same as those governing an in-hospital intubation
e) When outdoors, pre-hospital tracheal intubation is likely to be easier on a sunny day than at night

Answer: d

Short Explanation
Scene safety is the first priority in the pre-hospital environment. It is not necessary to intubate the trachea to provide an adequate airway. Only doctors are permitted to give anaesthetic agents or muscle relaxants. Pre-hospital intubation is held to exactly the same standards as hospital. Intubation is more difficult in bright sunlight. In pre-hospital care the management of life-threatening haemorrhage may take priority over securing the airway.

Long Explanation
The first consideration in pre-hospital care is scene safety, after which patients may be triaged and treated. The standard practice for checking vital signs, ABC (airway, breathing, circulation), has been updated (particularly in military circles) to CABC, with the first C standing for catastrophic haemorrhage.

The focus of airway care of the critically ill patient should always be to ensure an adequate airway and oxygenation, regardless of location or practitioner. Many pre-hospital practitioners have not been trained in laryngoscopy or do not have the opportunity to maintain the skill. Alternative techniques such as simple airway manoeuvres, airway adjuncts, laryngeal mask airways (LMAs) or bag-valve-mask (BVM) ventilation are all appropriate, depending on the situation.

Paramedics are very limited in their prescribing capability according to Joint Royal Colleges Ambulance Liaison Committee (JRCALC) guidelines and are not permitted to use anaesthetic agents or muscle relaxants to intubate or to maintain anaesthesia post intubation. Patients who have been administered drugs that are outside the prescribing capabilities of other practitioners should not be left by the doctor until there are other appropriately qualified personnel available.

Pre-hospital anaesthesia and intubation is held to exactly the same standards as that required for an emergency induction of anaesthesia in hospital. These include a trained intubator and assistant, equipment and monitoring.

Bright sunlight will cause the intubator's pupils to constrict and make it difficult to visualise structures in the relative dark of the patient's mouth. When intubating in daylight, it is advisable to create some form of shade by asking assistants to hold a sheet over yourself and the patient.

AAGBI Safety Guideline. *Pre-hospital Anaesthesia*. London: AAGBI, 2009. Available online at www.aagbi.org/publications/guidelines/docs/prehospital_glossy09.pdf (accessed 30 June 2012).

Joint Royal Colleges Ambulance Liaison Committee. JRCALC Guidelines. Available online at jrcalc.org.uk/guidelines.html (accessed 30 June 2012).

MTF Question 11: Transfer of the critically ill patient

With regard to the transfer of the critically ill patient, which of the following are correct?

a) The use of dedicated transfer teams improves the outcome of critically ill patients between hospitals

b) Routine transfers for capacity reasons alone are acceptable

c) The minimum personnel for the transfer team includes at least one attendant whose sole responsibility is care of the patient

d) The decision to transfer must be made by both the referring and the receiving consultant

e) Fixed-wing aircraft should be considered for transfer distances greater than 240 km (150 miles)

Answer: a, d, e

Short Explanation

Transfers for capacity reasons should only be considered as a last resort. Patients should be accompanied by two appropriately trained attendants. The decision to transfer must be made by the consultant responsible for intensive care, in conjunction with consultant colleagues from relevant specialties in both the referring and receiving hospitals.

Long Explanation

Studies have shown that the use of dedicated transport teams improves the outcome of critically ill patients transferred between hospitals. One study showed a reduction in physiological derangement and 12-hour mortality when it compared specialist retrieval teams with standard ambulance transport with a doctor from the referring hospital (7.7% vs. 3%).

The Department of Health has published guidelines on admission and discharge from intensive care. Hospitals should have contingency measures to ensure that transfers for capacity reasons alone are as a last resort. Any decision made should include full discussion with the patient (if able) and relatives. If the receiving hospital is outside the hospital's designated transfer group (a hospital network based on geographical location) it should be classified as an adverse event.

Two attendants should accompany the critically ill patient. One should be a medical practitioner with appropriate training in intensive care, anaesthesia or other acute medical specialty. They should also have had appropriate training in retrieval medicine. The other should ideally be a nurse with intensive care experience. Both should be familiar with intensive care procedures and transport equipment.

The referring intensive care consultant must make the decision to transfer. However, this should be done in consultation with the receiving consultant and consultant colleagues of relevant specialties. The decision is based on the benefits of transferring the patient, such as interventions available at the receiving hospital, weighed against the risks of transfer, such as the deleterious effects of movement (e.g. acceleration and deceleration forces).

Air transport should be considered for longer journeys, with fixed-wing aircraft being an option for distances over 240 km (150 miles). The benefits of flying (reduced journey time) must be considered against the potential difficulties, including need for inter-vehicle transfers and confined operating space.

Association of Anaesthetists of Great Britain and Ireland. *Recommendations for the Safe Transfer of Patients with Brain Injury.* London: AAGBI, 2006. Available online at www.aagbi.org/sites/default/files/braininjury.pdf (accessed 30 June 2012).

Department of Health. *Comprehensive Critical Care: a Review of Adult Critical Care Services.* London: Department of Health, 2000. Available online at www.dh.gov.uk/en/Publicationsandstatistics/Publications/PublicationsPolicyAndGuidance/DH_40065 85 (accessed 30 June 2012).

Intensive Care Society. *Guidelines for the Transport of the Critically Ill Adult*. London: ICS, 2002. Available online at www.ics.ac.uk/intensive_care_professional/stand-ards_and_guidelines/transport_of_the_critically_ill_ 2002 (accessed 30 June 2012).

MTF Question 12: Cytomegalovirus

An HIV-positive patient presents with sore throat, malaise with bloody diarrhoea, blurring of vision and pain around the eye. Fundoscopy shows a 'pizza pie' appearance and a presumptive diagnosis of cytomegalovirus (CMV) is made. Which of the following are true?

a) Were this the diagnosis, large intracytoplasmic/intracellular inclusions – 'owl's eye bodies' – would be expected on tissue biopsy examination
b) CMV is mostly asymptomatic in newborns if transmitted in utero, with few complications later
c) The preferred treatment for CMV is intravenous fluconazole
d) Pneumonitis is more common than retinitis in HIV patients with CMV
e) CMV can lead to acute viral hepatitis

Answer: a, e

Short Explanation
CMV is one of the TORCH infections that can be passed on in utero, can lead to severe congenital abnormalities and can be fatal. Treatment is with ganciclovir. Fluconazole is an antifungal agent. Retinitis is more common than pneumonitis in HIV patients with CMV.

Long Explanation
Cytomegalovirus (CMV) is an opportunistic virus common amongst HIV-positive and other immunocompromised patients (e.g. post-transplant). Specific IgM antibodies indicate acute disease, although these are unreliable in HIV. It is associated with a variety of complications including oesophagitis, colitis, cholecystitis and hepatitis as well as interstitial pneumonitis (which occurs much more in post-transplants than in HIV patients).

Around 65% of immunocompromised patients are infected with CMV. Most show no symptoms, with a small number having a glandular fever-type syndrome before latency develops. In post-transplant recipients, fever is more common than pneumonitis, with hepatitis and retinitis being less so. In HIV/AIDS patients retinitis is most common. 'Owl's eye bodies', seen as large intracytoplasmic/intracellular inclusions, are characteristic of CMV and are found on microscopic study of tissue biopsy.

CMV-negative irradiated blood will obviously be needed when transfusing all imunocompromised patients. In CMV retinitis exudates and haemorrhages follow the retinal vasculature, giving a 'pizza pie' or 'cottage cheese and ketchup' appearance on fundoscopy.

Treatment of CMV is with ganciclovir via central venous line, or with the prodrug valganciclovir or foscarnet. For post-transplant prophylaxis, ganciclovir 0.25 mg/kg/24 h via intravenous infusion for the first 2 weeks postoperatively can be used in patients who were seropositive preoperatively, and valaciclovir 2 g 6-hourly orally for ~90 days in the preoperatively seronegative patients.

Congenital CMV is one of the TORCH infections – toxoplasmosis, rubella, CMV and herpes simplex – that can lead to congenital defects in the newborn. For example jaundice, hepatosplenomegaly and a purpuric rash similar to the 'blueberry muffin' appearance of congenital rubella syndrome. Long-term defects include microcephaly, cerebral palsy, epilepsy, visual impairment and deafness. The virus can be detected in urine, saliva or blood within the first week. There is no specific treatment.

Ballinger A, Patchett S. *Pocket Essentials of Clinical Medicine*, 4th edn. Edinburgh: Saunders, 2007; pp. 53–4.
Offermanns S, Rosenthal W. *Encyclopedia of Molecular Pharmacology*, 2nd edn. Berlin: Springer, 2008; pp. 437–8.

MTF Question 13: Bicarbonate

Regarding bicarbonate:

a) It is the principal buffer in erythrocytes
b) It is the principal buffer in plasma
c) Of the bicarbonate filtered at the glomerulus, 95% is reabsorbed in the proximal convoluted tubule
d) Its concentration in cerebrospinal fluid is the same as that in plasma
e) It is the moiety responsible for the titratable acidity of urine

Answer: b, d

Short Explanation

Haemoglobin is the principal buffer in erythrocytes. Over 4 mol of bicarbonate is filtered by the kidneys every day, 85% of which is reabsorbed in the proximal convoluted tubule. Titratable acidity, where protons may be 'locked' in the tubular fluid and bicarbonate reabsorbed, is due to moieties such as phosphates, ammonium and sulphates.

Long Explanation

A buffer system is a combination of a weak acid and its conjugate base that will resist changes in pH despite the addition of an acid or alkali. This is achieved by the equilibrium that exists between the weak acid and base being displaced to favour the acid or the base, to compensate for the opposite moiety that has been added to the system. Carbonic acid (formed by the combination of carbon dioxide and water) with bicarbonate, its conjugate base, makes up an important physiological buffer. When considering the buffering capacity of whole blood, 56% is achieved by erythrocytes (35% haemoglobin, 18% bicarbonate, 3% phosphates) and 44% by plasma (35% bicarbonate, 7% plasma proteins, 2% phosphates). The concentration of bicarbonate in plasma is approximately 24 mmol/L, and as the glomerular filtration rate is 180 L/day it can be seen that 4320 mmol of bicarbonate (24 × 180) is filtered by the kidneys every day. 85% is reabsorbed in the proximal convoluted tubule, 10% in the thick ascending loop of Henle and 5% in the distal tubule and collecting ducts. The process by which bicarbonate is reabsorbed from the tubular fluid involves its combination with secreted protons to form carbonic acid. This encourages the equilibrium towards liberation of carbon dioxide, which is readily reabsorbed in to the tubular cell. Here, the carbon dioxide reacts with water, catalysed by carbonic anhydrase, to reform carbonic acid, which dissociates into bicarbonate and a proton. The proton is re-secreted to repeat the cycle while the bicarbonate ion is returned the blood via an antiport which exchanges it for a chloride ion.

Thus the reabsorption of bicarbonate involves the cycling of protons from tubular fluid to inside the cell and back again, with no net loss of protons. In circumstances where there is a proton excess (e.g. acidosis) the bicarbonate must be returned to the blood while the protons remain in the tubular fluid to be excreted in the urine. This is achieved by the excess protons combining with monohydrogen phosphate to form dihydrogen phosphate, which is not reabsorbed, thus 'locking' the protons in the tubular fluid and resulting in the passage of acidic (pH 4.5) urine. This is the so-called titratable acidity of urine.

Power I, Kam P. *Principles of Physiology for the Anaesthetist*. London: Arnold, 2001; pp. 221–34.

MTF Question 14: Congenital heart disease

The following congenital heart defects may progress to Eisenmenger's syndrome if left untreated:

a) Atrial septal defect (ASD)
b) Ventricular septal defect (VSD)
c) Tetralogy of Fallot (TOF)
d) Ebstein's anomoly
e) Patent ductus arteriosus (PDA)

Answer: a, b, e

Short Explanation
Eisenmenger's syndrome occurs when a left-to-right shunt, caused by an ASD, VSD or PDA, is reversed. TOF is a cyanotic congenital heart disease and already features a right-to-left shunt. Ebstein's anomaly is the apical displacement of the opening of the tricuspid valve without shunting of blood between the right and left ventricles.

Long Explanation
Eisenmenger's syndrome occurs when a right-to-left shunt, due to an ASD, VSD or PDA, is reversed. Normally, the left side of the heart generates the higher pressures required to supply blood to the whole body, and the right side of the heart generates the lower pressure required to circulate blood solely through the lungs. A right-to-left shunt causes increased blood flow through the pulmonary vasculature, resulting in pulmonary hypertension and increased right heart pressures.

This progresses until the pressure within the right side of the heart equals and exceeds that within the left side of the heart, causing the shunt to reverse. This is one of the commonest causes of adult congenital cyanotic heart disease, and results in end-organ and tissue damage.

Greater blood flow and pressure through the lungs damages the capillaries, causing scar tissue to form, which decreases the volume of functional pulmonary vasculature and reduces tissue flexibility. To compensate for this, the heart contracts at a faster rate in order to perfuse the lungs. Lung damage and pulmonary hypertension progress, resulting in a reduction in oxygen transfer and oxygen saturation in the blood. Erythrocytosis is another compensatory mechanism whereby rate of red blood cell synthesis increases in an attempt to increase oxygen saturation. Hyperviscosity syndrome occurs as a result. Patients are at risk of both uncontrolled haemorrhage due to the high pressures generated in the presence of damaged vessels, and thromboembolism due to hyperviscosity and stasis of blood.

Signs and symptoms of Eisenmenger's syndrome reflect the systemic flow of desaturated blood. They include cyanosis, polycythaemia, clubbing of fingernails, syncopal episodes, heart failure, arrhythmias, bleeding disorders and haemoptysis, cerebrovascular events and renal damage.

Anderson RH, Weinberg PM. The clinical anatomy of tetralogy of Fallot. *Cardiol Young* 2005; **15**: 38–47.
Vongpatanasin W, Brickner ME, Hillis LD, Lange RA. The Eisenmenger syndrome in adults. *Ann Intern Med* 1998; **128**: 745–55.

Yacobi S, Ornoy A. Is lithium a real teratogen? What can we conclude from the prospective versus retrospective studies? A review. *Isr J Psychiatry Relat Sci* 2008; **45**: 95–106.

MTF Question 15: Skin care: prevention and management of pressure sores

With reference to the prevention and management of pressure ulcers:

a) Damage can be caused by pressure, shearing, moisture and/or friction
b) Risk factors include anaemia and/or the use of noradrenaline infusions
c) A positive microbiology wound swab from a pressure sore will require antibiotics
d) A grade 1 pressure ulcer, using the European Pressure Ulcer Advisory Panel (EPUAP) scoring system, frequently requires surgical intervention
e) Sheepskins are useful in preventing pressure ulcers

Answer: a, b

Short Explanation

EPUAP grade 1 pressure ulcers are non-blanchable erythematous areas of intact skin, and they rarely require surgical intervention. Positive wounds swabs may represent colonisation, and care should be taken in the interpretation of results. Sheepskins are of no use.

Long Explanation

Pressure ulcers are defined as an area of local tissue damage caused by pressure, shearing, moisture and friction, or combinations thereof. ICU patients are at risk from these forces as they are frequently immobile and require assistance with movement. Pressure occurs when the patient's weight compresses tissue between a support surface and bony prominences, causing hypoperfusion in that area. Shearing frequently occurs as a result of friction and movement, such as sliding a patient up a bed.

A study of ICU patients found that anaemia, noradrenaline infusions, faecal incontinence, admission APACHE II scores greater than 13 and staying on ICU for longer than 3 days increased the risk of pressure ulcer development. Patient factors can also exacerbate the condition, including poor dietary intake, steroids, general health, weight, age and diabetes.

Prevention is best achieved using specific mattresses (and beds) and frequent repositioning while addressing the patient's underlying condition, maintaining nutrition and achieving early mobilisation. Mattresses aim to provide a comfortable surface while redistributing pressure. This is often achieved by timed inflation and deflation of air cells within the mattress.

The EPUAP is a grading system designed to classify the extent of injury. Grade 1 pressure ulcers are non-blanchable erythematous areas of intact skin. Grade 2 indicates partial thickness skin loss while grade 3 indicates full thickness skin loss with damage to the underlying subcutaneous tissue. Grade 4 pressure ulcers have extensive damage to muscle, bone or supporting structures with full thickness skin loss.

Prevention is key and early recognition essential. If they do develop, there are multiple treatment options from wound cleaning and specific dressings to surgical debridement. Sheepskins are ineffective, however. Antibiotics should be used with caution as many pressure ulcers will become colonised with organisms and not necessarily infected. Microbiology input should be sought.

Wound healing progresses through a number of phases from inflammation to proliferation and finally to maturation and remodelling. It may take several years until the pressure ulcer is fully healed.

Waldmann C, Soni N, Rhodes A. Pressure sores. In: *Oxford Desk Reference: Critical Care*. Oxford: Oxford University Press, 2008; pp. 504–5.

MTF Question 16: Mannitol

Which of the following statements regarding mannitol are true?

a) Mannitol increases cerebral blood flow
b) Mannitol is freely filtered at the glomerulus
c) Mannitol reduces intraocular pressure
d) Mannitol must be used with caution in patients with heart failure
e) Mannitol cannot be given orally due to its osmotic action on the gut mucosa

Answer: a, b, c, d

Short Explanation
Mannitol initially increases plasma volume and therefore cerebral blood flow, and this expansion can trigger acute heart failure. It is not absorbed from the gut, and is filtered but not reabsorbed in the kidney, causing an osmotic diuresis. It has been used to reduce intraocular pressure in ophthalmic surgery.

Long Explanation
Mannitol is a polyhydric alcohol that acts as an osmotic diuretic. It is freely filtered at the glomerulus but not reabsorbed in the nephron, increasing the osmotic gradient across the renal tubule and producing a diuresis. It cannot cross the intact blood–brain barrier, and by a similar mechanism draws water out of the brain, reducing cerebral oedema. However, if the blood–brain barrier has been damaged (e.g. by trauma) and mannitol enters the brain it can have the opposite effect and worsen brain swelling, and this occurs even in the intact brain after repeated doses. It has also been used to reduce intraocular pressure through its osmotic activity.

Mannitol cannot be given orally because it is only minimally absorbed from the gut, and when given intravenously it initially causes an expansion in plasma volume. This causes an increase in cerebral blood flow, and a small transient rise in intracranial pressure may be seen. The increased plasma volume may be sufficient to trigger ventricular failure in susceptible patients. Mannitol does not undergo significant metabolism.

Peck T, Hill S, Williams M. *Pharmacology for Anaesthesia and Intensive Care*, 3rd edn. Cambridge: Cambridge University Press, 2008.
Yentis S, Hirsch N, Smith G. *Anaesthesia and Intensive Care A–Z: an Encyclopaedia of Principles and Practice*, 4th edn. Edinburgh: Butterworth-Heinemann, 2009.

MTF Question 17: Troponin and other cardiac enzymes

Regarding the use of troponins in diagnosing acute myocardial infarction:

a) Troponin levels rise after 1–2 hours
b) They peak at 12 hours
c) They can be raised for 5–10 days
d) They may be elevated in chronic renal failure, cardiac trauma and pulmonary embolus
e) CK-MB is more sensitive and more specific than troponin enzymes for myocardial infarction

Answer: b, c, d

Short Explanation

Troponin enzymes rise after 3–6 hours and peak at 12 hours. Troponin I may be raised for up to 5 days and troponin T for 7–10 days. Causes of troponin rise other than myocardial infarction include chronic kidney disease due to myocardial toxicity, cardiac trauma and pulmonary embolus due to myocardial strain. Creatine kinase (CK) and CK-MB is also released from skeletal muscle damage, so a rise in CK-MB is less specific and less sensitive for cardiac muscle damage.

Long Explanation

Cardiac markers are molecules released into the circulation as a consequence of cardiac injury. They are used in the diagnosis of myocardial infarction (MI), but elevations are not always synonymous with an ischaemic mechanism of injury and results should be interpreted in the context of clinical and ECG findings. It is important to note that cardiac markers such as creatine kinase (CK), aspartate aminotransferase (AST) and lactate dehydrogenase (LDH) are of variable specificity to cardiac muscle.

Cardiac markers include:

- CK – earliest to rise
- CK-MB – second to rise, more specific for cardiac muscle than CK
- Cardiac troponin T and I – second to rise, at similar time to CK-MB
- AST – third to rise
- LDH – latest to rise

Troponins are protein components of striated muscle. Troponin is released during MI from the cytosolic pool of the myocytes. Its subsequent release is prolonged with degradation of actin and myosin filaments. There are three different troponins: troponin C (TnC), troponin T (TnT) and troponin I (TnI). TnT and TnI are found only in cardiac muscle, and have 84–90% sensitivity for myocardial infarction 8 hours after onset of symptoms, and 81–95% specificity. CK and CK-MB (defined as CK-muscle and brain types) are found in skeletal muscle as well as cardiac muscle. Therefore, if there is damage to skeletal muscle, elevations of CK and CK-MB will occur, which can make the diagnosis of MI difficult. In such a situation levels of TnT and/or TnI will not rise unless MI has occurred, and therefore the troponin enzymes are more specific and sensitive for MI than CK and CK-MB. These markers are also more sensitive and more specific than AST or LDH.

Due to the fact that troponins remain raised in the blood for up to 10 days, if a patient presents with symptoms within 10 days of having a raised troponin, CK-MB may be used to assess whether the patient has suffered a further cardiac event.

Elevation of TnT or TnI is absolutely indicative of cardiac damage, but in addition to MI a rise can also occur as a result of myocarditis, coronary artery spasm from cocaine use, severe cardiac failure, cardiac trauma from surgery or blunt chest wall injury, and pulmonary embolus – all of which can cause cardiac damage. Both TnT and TnI may be elevated in patients with chronic renal failure due to myocardial toxicity.

Failure to show a rise in TnT or TnI does not exclude the diagnosis of ischaemic heart disease.

Ebell MH, Flewelling D, Flynn CA. A systematic review of troponin T and I for diagnosing acute myocardial infarction. *J Fam Pract* 2000; **49**: 550–6.

MTF Question 18: Thirst

Regarding thirst:

a) The thirst centre is located in the thalamus
b) The thirst centre is sensitive to angiotensin II
c) Low-pressure sensors in the right atrium send afferents to the thirst centre

d) The thirst centre has osmoreceptors that are sensitive to extracellular tonicity
e) The sensation of thirst is sated once normal osmolality is restored

Answer: b, c, d

Short Explanation
The thirst centre is in the hypothalamus and is sensitive to hypotension, hypovolaemia, hypertonicity (despite the receptors being called osmoreceptors) and angiotensin II. Fortunately, pharyngeal sensors satisfy the thirst centre that water has been consumed. Awaiting restoration of tonicity could result in over-consumption of water in the meantime.

Long Explanation
The thirst centre in the hypothalamus tightly regulates extracellular fluid tonicity, where balance of water and sodium are inextricably linked. Although they are termed osmoreceptors, they are not sensitive to changes in osmolality (directly) but can respond to a 2% change in tonicity at the plasma membrane. Efferent activity here exerts a sensation of thirst in the subject and affects a behavioural change (to seek hydration).

Two sets of baroreceptors work cooperatively to sense the blood volume status and transmit it to the thirst centre. High-pressure baroreceptors in the carotid sinus increase firing frequency as pressure rises, inferring hypervolaemia and inhibiting the thirst centre. Low-pressure baroreceptors in the right atrium and central veins decrease firing frequency as pressure drops (such as in hypovolaemia), which disinhibits the thirst centre, promoting ingestion of water.

Angiotensin II is a potent 'dipsogen' acting at specific receptors outside the blood–brain barrier to activate interneurones to the hypothalamus which activate the thirst centre.

Satiety from thirst is induced by activation of pharyngeal receptors sensitive to water consumption. Once water is consumed there will be an inevitable delay (while it is absorbed from the intestine) before a change in tonicity results. If the thirst centre was relying on correction of the tonicity, the subject could continue to drink water whilst this occurred, potentially ending in water toxicity or dangerous hyponatraemia.

MTF Question 19: Pulmonary oedema

A 78-year-old man is admitted to the emergency department with central, crushing chest pain and sudden, increasing shortness of breath. ECG shows ST depression and T-wave inversion in the anterior chest leads. Troponin level is significantly elevated. On examination, he is distressed and agitated. There is a loud systolic murmur and bibasal crepitations on auscultation. He is extremely dyspnoeic, hypoxic and tachycardic. Which of the following statements are correct regarding the acute management of this patient?

a) Non-invasive ventilation (NIV) is indicated in refractory hypoxia
b) Ultrafiltration plays no role
c) Glyceryl trinitrate (GTN) reduces in-hospital mortality rate
d) Primary percutaneous coronary intervention (PCI) should be considered
e) Use of inotropes carries prognostic benefits

Answer: a, c, d

Short Explanation
This man has acute cardiogenic pulmonary oedema (CPO) secondary to non-ST-elevation myocardial infarction (NSTEMI). A new murmur suggests papillary rupture and valve incompetence. Inotropes have no evidence-based benefits in CPO,

but thrombolysis or primary PCI is appropriate if CPO is secondary to myocardial infarction. Ultrafiltration is appropriate if fluid overload is refractory to intravenous furosemide therapy.

Long Explanation

Cardiogenic pulmonary oedema (CPO) is defined as pulmonary oedema due to increased capillary hydrostatic pressure secondary to elevated pulmonary venous pressure. Increased left atrial pressure increases pulmonary venous pressure and pressure in the lung microvasculature, resulting in pulmonary oedema. CPO reflects the transudation of low-protein fluid into the lung interstitium and alveoli.

CPO may result from many causes, including excessive intravascular volume administration, pulmonary venous outflow obstruction or left ventricular (LV) failure. Progressive deterioration of alveolar gas exchange causes respiratory failure and rapid deterioration. In this case, acute CPO has occurred as a result of acute LV failure secondary to a myocardial infarction (MI), with likely acute mitral valve incompetence.

Urgent management of the patient is essential to reduce mortality and morbidity and improve symptom control. The patient should be managed in an upright posture. Oxygen therapy should be given, at 60–100% but with caution if there is concern regarding carbon dioxide retention. Oxygen is indicated if there is hypoxia, or if proceeding to non-invasive ventilation (NIV). Persistent hypoxia is an indication for NIV in these patients. If there is hypercapnia, invasive ventilation may be considered.

Furosemide is widely used in acute pulmonary oedema. The absolute indication for this is where CPO is secondary to volume overload. There is an evidence base for the use of ultrafiltration if fluid overload is gross and refractory to intravenous furosemide therapy.

Morphine or diamorphine improve symptoms and reduce agitation and respiratory distress, but studies fail to show a reduction in mortality despite the theoretical benefit of vasodilation and reduction in myocardial oxygen demand. Sublingual or infused glyceryl trinitrate (GTN) therapy reduces preload and is prognostically beneficial in reducing in-hospital mortality for patients with CPO if given early, as long as systolic blood pressure is > 100 mmHg. Other vasodilator therapies have a weaker or negative evidence base. Nitrates are contraindicated in severe obstructive valve disease.

If there is a precipitating myocardial infarction, primary percutaneous coronary intervention (PCI) or thrombolysis should be considered. Precipitating arrhythmias should be treated as appropriate. Inotropes have no evidence-based benefits in CPO.

Gray AJ, Goodacre S, Newby DE, *et al.* A multicentre randomised controlled trial of the use of continuous positive airway pressure and non-invasive positive pressure ventilation in the early treatment of patients presenting to the emergency department with severe acute cardiogenic pulmonary oedema: the 3CPO trial. *Health Technol Assess* 2009; **13**: 1–106.

Hollenberg SM. Vasodilators in acute heart failure. *Heart Fail Rev* 2007; **12**: 143–7.

Peacock WF, Fonarow GC, Emerman CL, Mills RM, Wynne J. Impact of early initiation of intravenous therapy for acute decompensated heart failure on outcomes in ADHERE. *Cardiology* 2007; **107**: 44–51.

Sosnowski MA. Review article: lack of effect of opiates in the treatment of acute cardiogenic pulmonary oedema. *Emerg Med Australas* 2008; **20**: 384–90.

MTF Question 20: Pseudo-obstruction

Regarding intestinal pseudo-obstruction:

a) Bowel sounds are usually absent
b) A caecum dilated to 8 cm suggests likely perforation
c) Colonoscopy is contraindicated

d) Hyperkalaemia is a common cause
e) Neostigmine is contraindicated because of the risk of perforation

Answer: all false

Short Explanation
Bowel sounds are typically present. Caecal dilation above 10–12 cm risks perforation. Hypokalaemia is a potential cause. Both neostigmine and colonoscopy are common treatment options.

Long Explanation
Pseudo-obstruction is a syndrome of apparent large bowel obstruction in the absence of mechanical obstruction. It was first described in a series of patients with malignant infiltration of the caecal plexus causing autonomic dysfunction (Ogilvie syndrome).

There are many risk factors. Local causes include trauma, abdominal surgery, urological surgery and post spinal injury. Systemic causes include sepsis, hypothermia and electrolyte imbalance (hypocalcaemia, hypokalaemia and hypomagnesaemia). Triggering medications include opioids, tricyclic antidepressants, phenothiazines, antiparkinson drugs and anaesthetic agents. The condition is more prevalent with increasing age. The pathophysiology is thought to relate to either increased sympathetic or decreased parasympathetic activity in the colon.

Patients typically present with features of obstruction – constipation, abdominal distension and vomiting – but on investigation have no mechanical cause. Bowel sounds may be abnormal but are present in 80%. Pseudo-obstruction can result in renal impairment (dehydration, compartment syndrome) and respiratory compromise due to abdominal distension. Mortality is 15% if managed medically, increasing to 30% if surgery is required. Caecal perforation is a major concern, and the risk increases as the diameter exceeds 12 cm.

Medical treatment includes rehydration, correction of electrolyte abnormalities, nasogastric drainage and discontinuation of contributory medications. Specific treatments include neostigmine and colonoscopy. Gastrograffin enema may be useful both diagnostically and therapeutically. Surgical treatment includes tube caecostomy and laparotomy with potential bowel resection.

Cagir B. Intestinal pseudo-obstruction surgery. *Medscape Reference* 2011. Available online at emedicine.medscape.com/article/187979-overview (accessed 30 June 2012).

MTF Question 21: Consent

Regarding consent from adults to medical treatment:

a) Adults who lack capacity to consent for a procedure cannot consent but are able to refuse treatment
b) A medical practitioner can perform a procedure in an unconscious adult patient if it is in that patient's best interests, but the next of kin has refused to consent for the procedure
c) Artificial nutrition and hydration is not deemed medical treatment
d) A patient who can consent for a procedure but cannot read or write is legally obliged to mark the consent form or find someone to sign on his/her behalf
e) If, during an operation, another procedure is found to be necessary but has not been discussed with the patient, and therefore has not been consented for, the surgeon may still go ahead with the procedure

Answer: b, e

Short Explanation

Adults who lack capacity are unable to consent or refuse medical treatment. Artificial nutrition and hydration is deemed to be medical treatment. There is no legal obligation on patients who cannot read or write to mark the consent form or find someone to sign for them. If another procedure is necessary during an operation but has not been consented for, the surgeon may proceed, if the procedure is in the patient's best interests and cannot be delayed.

Long Explanation

Adults are deemed to have capacity if they are able to:

- Understand the information given to them which is relevant to a decision
- Retain the information long enough to make a decision
- Weigh up the information to come to a decision
- Communicate the decision by any means

An adult who lacks capacity is unable to consent for or refuse medical treatment, and so there should be discussion with all parties concerned about what is in the patient's best interests.

A medical practitioner can perform a procedure in an unconscious adult if it is in that patient's best interests, even if the next of kin has refused to consent. This is particularly the case in emergency situations. Artificial nutrition and hydration has recently been defined in the courts as constituting medical treatment, so has the same status as artificial ventilation and medications when being discussed in terms of prolonging patients' lives.

A patient who has capacity and is able to consent for a procedure but is not able to read or write is not legally obliged to mark the consent form or find someone to sign for them. In these cases, this should be well documented in the notes.

During operations, it is sometimes necessary to perform procedures that were unforeseen before the operation. In these instances, the surgeon may proceed with the procedure while the patient is still under the general anaesthetic, so long as it is in the patient's best interests and cannot be delayed. It is up to the discretion of the surgeon as to what procedures fulfil these criteria in these circumstances.

Department of Health. *Reference Guide to Consent for Treatment*, 2nd edn, 2009. Available online at www.dh.gov.uk/dr_consum_dh/groups/dh_digitalassets/documents/digitalasset/dh_103653.pdf (accessed 30 June 2012).

MTF Question 22: Pregnancy and grown-up congenital heart disease

With regard to grown-up congenital heart disease in pregnancy:

a) In women with right-to-left shunts the drop in systemic vascular resistance (SVR) caused by pregnancy improves the shunt and decreases hypoxia
b) Pregnant women with pre-existing aortic regurgitation should be started on β-blockers, and tachycardia in labour should be avoided
c) Asymptomatic patients with small septal defects can be managed at their local district general hospital in a 'normal' manner
d) Pregnant women with pulmonary hypertension have the highest mortality out of all the specific cardiac lesions
e) Pre-eclampsia can cause significant cardiovascular decompensation in women with aortic regurgitation

Answer: c, d, e

Short Explanation

In women with right-to-left shunts the drop in SVR caused by pregnancy worsens the shunt, causing increased hypoxia. Aortic regurgitation is relatively well tolerated in pregnant women because vasodilation and tachycardia reduce regurgitant flow across the valve. Tachycardia should be avoided in women with aortic stenosis.

Long Explanation

With increasing numbers of patients surviving with complex congenital heart disease into adulthood, so the incidence of pregnancy in this group increases. Over the last few triennial reports into maternal death, there have been a significant number that could have been avoided if care had been provided by a tertiary centre.

Ideally all women with grown-up congenital heart disease (GUCH) should be counselled by suitably experienced obstetricians and cardiologists prior to conceiving, but this rarely happens in reality. All of these women should have at least one echocardiogram in early pregnancy, and maybe more, depending on the lesion.

In general, septal defects have a low mortality associated with pregnancy, and the degree of shunt will depend on whether or not correction has been attempted. Left-to-right shunts are generally of less concern, because oxygenation is not usually compromised. Small septal defects generally do not require treatment, but large ventricular septal defects are often associated with congestive cardiac failure, arrhythmias and pulmonary hypertension. For all patients with septal defects air filters should be placed on intravenous lines to minimise the risk of paradoxical air embolism.

In women with right-to-left shunts caused by pulmonary hypertension diverting blood away from the lungs, the drop in systemic vascular resistance (SVR) caused by pregnancy worsens the shunt and hypoxia. The principles of management for a patient with this condition include avoidance of hypotension, maintenance of preload, adequate oxygenation, and avoidance of air embolism. Pulmonary hypertension is extremely risky in pregnancy (30–50% mortality), and ideally pregnancy should be discouraged.

Mitral stenosis is the riskiest valvular condition in pregnancy. South Asian immigrant women have a relatively high prevalence of undiagnosed mitral stenosis and so may present with severe cardiac failure at 24–28 weeks, when increases in cardiac output are usually maximal. The main risk is pulmonary oedema, which will be greatly exacerbated by 'auto-transfusion' in the third stage of delivery and if pre-eclampsia develops. Women with mitral stenosis and aortic stenosis should be considered for β-blockers, and both tachycardia and sudden drops in SVR should be minimised in labour. Regurgitant valvular conditions are generally well tolerated in pregnancy, because tachycardia and decreased SVR cause a reduction in the regurgitant flow across the valve. An increase in SVR caused by pre-eclampsia would not be well tolerated and may provoke rapid cardiac decompensation.

Burt CC, Durbridge J. Management of cardiac disease in pregnancy. *Contin Educ Anaesth Crit Care Pain* 2009; 9: 44–47. Available online at ceaccp.oxfordjournals. org/content/9/2/44 (accessed 30 June 2012).

Centre for Maternal and Child Enquiries (CMACE). Saving Mothers' Lives: reviewing maternal deaths to make motherhood safer: 2006–08. The Eighth Report on Confidential Enquiries into Maternal Deaths in the United Kingdom. *BJOG* 2011; 118 (Suppl. 1): 1–203. Available online at onlinelibrary.wiley.com/doi/10.1111/ j.1471–0528.2010.02847.x/pdf (accessed 30 June 2012).

MTF Question 23: Ligaments of the vertebral column

Which of the following statements regarding the ligaments of the vertebral column are correct?

a) The posterior longitudinal ligament is found within the vertebral foramen
b) The ligamentum flavum connects adjacent laminae
c) The interspinous ligaments are continuous from the cervical vertebrae to the lumbar vertebrae
d) The supraspinous ligament connects the tips of the spinous processes and is continuous from the lower cervical vertebrae to the sacrum
e) The supraspinous ligament may become ossified

Answer: a, b, d, e

Short Explanation

The interspinous ligaments pass between adjacent spinous processes only; there is no connection between adjacent ligaments. The supraspinous ligaments may become ossified in the elderly.

Long Explanation

The primary means of connection between adjacent vertebrae is the intervertebral discs. The discs adhere to the hyaline cartilage covering the vertebral bodies. Each is composed of peripheral fibrous tissue, the annulus fibrosus, and a tough gel-like inner core, the nucleus pulposus.

The anterior longitudinal ligament is found running from C2 to the upper sacrum. It travels along the anterior aspect of the vertebral bodies. Along the posterior aspect of the vertebral bodies (and therefore at the anterior aspect of the vertebral foramen) is the posterior longitudinal ligament. The ligamenta flava are elastic ligaments which unite adjacent laminae. They provide much of the natural recoil of the spine (aiding standing from the stooped position) and become thicker in the inferior regions of the spine. The increase in thickness is notable clinically when siting an epidural: the ligamentum flavum is more easily 'felt' through a Tuohy needle in the lumbar than in the thoracic spine.

The interspinous ligaments connect adjacent spinous processes. There is no continuity from one to the next. In comparison, the supraspinous ligament is a tough fibrous ligament running along the tips of the spinous processes from C7 down to the sacrum. It is frequently ossified in the elderly, making centroaxial anaesthesia more difficult when performed from the midline approach.

Ellis H, Feldman S, Harrop-Griffiths W. The vertebrae and sacrum. In: *Anatomy for Anaesthetists*, 8th edn. Oxford: Blackwell, 2003; pp. 97–118.

MTF Question 24: Parkinson's disease

Regarding Parkinson's disease:

a) It consists of a tremor most marked on movement and absent when at rest
b) The cause is due to reduced activity of dopamine-secreting cells in the substantia nigra
c) Lewy bodies are seen at postmortem examination
d) Fatigability associated with blepharoptosis is a hallmark feature, but reflexes are normal
e) Surgery involving electrical stimulation of the sub-thalamic nucleus, thalamus or globus pallidus can be undertaken in those who become resistant to medication

Answer: b, c, e

Short Explanation

The tremor is most prominent at rest – a coarse, 'pill rolling'-type tremor. Fatigability associated with ptosis with sparing of reflexes is recognisable as the early presentation of myasthenia gravis. The intracytoplasmic inclusions are Lewy bodies.

Long Explanation

Parkinson's disease (PD) presentation consists of:

- Tremor – coarse, worse at rest, 4–6 Hz, 'pill-rolling'
- Rigidity – resistance to passive muscle stretch – 'lead piping', broken up by tremor – 'cogwheel rigidity'
- Bradykinesis – slowness of initiating movement and decreasing amplitude and speed of repeated actions
- Expressionless 'mask-like' face
- 'Festinant gait' – short shuffling steps and stoop, as if feet are frozen to the floor
- Micrographia
- There is also loss of postural reflexes

PD is one cause of this parkinsonism, caused by death of dopaminergic neurones in the pars compacta region of the substantia nigra in the midbrain. On postmortem examination Lewy bodies – eosinophilic, intracytoplasmic inclusions – are hallmark features. Later, cognitive decline may occur, and there is overlap between PD and Lewy body dementia. There is known to be increased risk of PD in those exposed to pesticides, and a curiously reduced risk in smokers. It is rare under the age of 50.

Treatments of early motor symptoms are mainly with levodopa (L-dopa) and dopamine agonists. A balance must be achieved between avoiding side effects (nausea and writhing movements) and improved mobility. As disease progresses, more dopaminergic neurones die and treatment becomes ineffective. Dyskinesia, exaggerated involuntary movements, then develop over years – leading to 'on/off' switching between such dyskinesia and immobility. For those suitable patients who become resistant to medication there is a surgical option that is growing in popularity. Called deep brain stimulation, it involves the placement of electrode(s) into the sub-thalamic nucleus, thalamus or globus pallidus. These areas of the brain are all involved in movement modification and interact with the substantia nigra. The electrodes are connected to a generator that fires a pulsed electrical signal, thus altering neuronal output from these areas. The effects in some patients can be dramatic.

Myasthenia gravis (MG), an autoimmune neuromuscular disease with antibodies to nicotinic acetylcholine receptors, often presents late with ptosis and ease of fatigability with repetitive actions – e.g. speaking, hence hypophonia on counting to 50; limb girdle weakness leading to head droop; facial muscle weakness leading to 'myasthenic snarl' on smiling. Such swallowing and speech difficulties in MG, as well as gait disturbance and poverty of facial expression, can overlap with or be mistaken for features of PD. In MG, however, there is sparing of reflexes, while postural reflexes are lost in PD.

For the patient with PD, rehabilitation and a multidisciplinary approach to coping with the disease is vital from the outset. This should involve general practitioner, physiotherapist, specialist nurse and neurologist.

Levin N, Karussis D, Abramsky O. Parkinson's disease associated with myasthenia gravis: a report of 4 cases. *J Neurol* 2003; **450**: 766–7.

Longmore M, Wilkinson I, Turmezei T, Cheung CK. *Oxford Handbook of Clinical Medicine*, 7th edn. Oxford: Oxford University Press, 2007; pp. 478–504.

MTF Question 25: Cephalosporins

Regarding cephalosporins:

a) Ceftazidime is more active than cefuroxime against Gram-positive bacteria
b) Cephalosporins were so named because they were good at crossing the blood–brain barrier and stopping bacterial proliferation
c) Cephalosporins are classified into one of four generations according to international consensus
d) Cephalosporins, in combination with probenecid, are effective against *Clostridium difficile*
e) In the absence of acquired bacterial resistance, first-generation cephalosporins can be used to treat any infection that is sensitive to penicillins

Answer: all false

Short Explanation
Cephalosporins are named after *Cephalosporium* fungi. There is no international consensus on cephalosporin classification, with some countries recognising five or six generations. Cefuroxime is more active than ceftazidime against Gram-positive bacteria. Cephalosporins are a major cause of *Clostridium difficile* infection. *Listeria* is sensitive to penicillins but not first-generation cephalosporins.

Long Explanation
Cephalosporins were first isolated from *Cephalosporium* fungi found in an Italian sewer in 1949. It is true that cephalosporins do cross the blood–brain barrier to varying degrees and have been used to treat meningitis, but that is not why they were so named.

Cephalosporins have been classed in generations, with major steps in development producing the announcement of further new generations. A fourth generation is well established and some are claiming ceftobiprole to be a fifth-generation agent. There are at least 15 cephalosporins that have not been assigned a generation. No international consensus exists, and some countries have different opinions as to which generation particular drugs should lie in.

For the first three generations, each new generation brought improved Gram-negative cover with decreased Gram-positive cover. So the third-generation cephalosporin ceftazadime has extended activity over Gram-negative bacteria compared to the second-generation cephalosporin cefuroxime, but is less active against Gram-positive bacteria. The fourth generation have a genuinely broad spectrum.

The first-generation cephalosporins have been shown to be able to treat almost all infections that are sensitive to penicillins apart from *Listeria monocytogenes*. Probenecid has been used to increase and prolong serum levels of cephalosporins and has been used to treat infections such as *Neisseria gonorrhoeae*. However, cephalosporins along with clindamycin and fluoroquinolones are the antibiotics most commonly implicated in the outbreaks of *Clostridum difficile* infections that have been a major problem in UK hospitals in recent years.

MTF Question 26: HME filter components

Which of the following are true regarding the use of heat and moisture exchange (HME) filters in anaesthetic practice?

a) As well as bacterial and viral particles, HME filters also filter latex particles
b) An HME filter that has no bacterial or viral filtration properties should be green in colour
c) According to the manufacturer's instructions, insertion of an HME filter between a patient and a breathing circuit allows that breathing circuit to be used for more than one patient

d) In general, hydrophobic filters are better than electrostatic ones in the prevention of fluid contamination of anaesthetic breathing circuits

e) In general, hydrophobic filters are better than electrostatic ones in the prevention of particulate contamination of anaesthetic breathing circuits

Answer: a, d, e

Short Explanation

Colour coding of HME filters: HME only = blue; HME + filtration = green; filtration only = yellow. Manufacturer's instructions remain that anaesthetic breathing circuits are single-use only, even if HME filters are used.

Long Explanation

HME filters usually have two functions, one as a heat and moisture exchange and the other as a filter for bacterial and viral particles. Some filters may only have one of these functions, but their use is rare in standard anaesthetic practice. Internationally recognised colour coding for filters is as follows: HME only = blue; HME + filtration = green; filtration only = yellow.

This question concentrates on the filtration of bacterial and viral particles component. The filtration component is made up of either a wad of electrostatically charged material or a pleated layer of hydrophobic material. The latter also has a role in HME, as a temperature gradient that builds up between the pleats acts allows condensation and evaporation to take place.

The manufacturers of all HME filters are expected to adhere to voluntary standard ISO 9360 *Anaesthetic and respiratory equipment – heat and moisture exchangers for use in humidifying respired gases in humans*. This standard provides advice concerning the construction of the filter housing, connections suitable for anaesthetic circuits, labelling and packaging. It also provides a framework for standardised testing of HME filters, thus allowing comparison.

In everyday UK anaesthetic practice, an HME filter is placed between the breathing circuit and the patient. This allows the breathing circuit to be reused, and most hospitals have a policy of routinely changing breathing circuits on a weekly basis unless they have been used in a patient with a known resistant infection or there is visible contamination of the circuit. Interestingly, this widespread practice goes against the manufacturer's recommendations for breathing circuit use, as they are produced to be single-use only.

Studies suggest that not all filters are equally effective. In general, hydrophobic filters are better than electrostatic ones in the prevention of both fluid and particulate contamination of anaesthetic breathing circuits, although manufacturers of both types claim prevention of transmission of all viral and bacterial particles of > 99.95%.

Lawes E. Hidden hazards and dangers associated with the use of HME/filters in breathing circuits: their effect on toxic metabolite production, pulse oximetry and airway resistance. *Br J Anaesth* 2003; **91**: 249–64.

MTF Question 27: Tocolytics

Regarding the use of drugs as tocolytics:

a) The β-adrenoreceptor agonist ritodrine is a good first-line agent

b) Nifedipine produces more cardiovascular instability than terbutaline

c) Indomethacin is effective but may cause premature closure of the ductus arteriosus

d) Atosiban works as an oxytocin receptor antagonist

e) Atosiban is the agent of choice if comorbidities such as pre-eclampsia or placental abruption are present because of favourable cardiovascular stability

Answer: c, d

Short Explanation

Ritodrine is no longer recommended as a first-line agent because of maternal cardiovascular instability. Nifedipine is preferred over the β-adrenoreceptor agonists for precisely these reasons. Atosiban is effective but is contraindicated in pre-eclampsia and abruption.

Long Explanation

Tocolytics are given to pregnant mothers experiencing premature contractions in which there is felt to be a benefit in delaying labour and delivery. This is usually for labour starting between 24 and 34 weeks into a pregnancy, and it allows the administration of corticosteroids to promote lung maturation in the fetus and also the transfer of the mother to a centre with neonatal intensive care. The Royal College of Obstetricians and Gynaecologists (RCOG) recommends at least 24 hours treatment with steroids, and delivery within 7 days of commencing therapy.

β-Adrenoreceptor agonists such as terbutaline or ritodrine are effective but may produce tachyarrhythmias, palpitations, chest tightness or hypokalaemia. In addition to the tachycardia they cause directly, they may also cause vasodilation and hypotension. This, when treated with excessive intravenous fluids, has produced a number of cases of pulmonary oedema. The calcium channel blocker nifedipine has been used but again has produced cardiovascular instability, although less than the β-adrenoreceptor agonists. Glyceryl trinitrate (GTN) has been administered intravenously or in patch form and is effective but may cause hypotension and headaches. Internationally, magnesium is used, but this practice is rarely used in the UK. The cyclooxygenase inhibitor indometacin reduces prostaglandin synthesis and may be used in situations where cardiovascular instability is particularly undesirable but may cause premature closure of the ductus arteriosus in the fetus after 32 weeks gestation. Atosiban is an oxytocin receptor antagonist with fewer adverse effects than β-adrenoreceptor agonists but is expensive and requires a complicated intravenous dosing regimen. It is also contraindicated in most of the major complications of obstetric practice (pre-eclampsia, placenta praevia, abruption, premature rupture of membranes) and so is only suitable in uncomplicated pregnancy with premature labour.

The current RCOG guidelines no longer recommend the β-adrenoreceptor agonists and favour atosiban or nifedipine.

British National Formulary. Available online at www.bnf.org (accessed 30 June 2012).

RCOG guidelines are available online at www.rcog.org.uk/files/rcogcorp/GT1BTocolyticDrug2002revised.pdf and www.rcog.org.uk/files/rcogcorp/GT7Antenata1Corticosterodsamended.pdf (accessed 30 June 2012).

MTF Question 28: Pathophysiology, diagnosis and management of asthma

Which of the following statements regarding severe acute asthma in adults are correct?

a) Asthmatic patients should be fluid resuscitated prior to intubation
b) Ketamine should be avoided as it causes bronchospasm and bronchorrhoea
c) Nitric oxide has been shown to be beneficial as an adjunct in ventilation of near-fatal asthma

d) Heliox has been shown to be beneficial as an adjunct in ventilation of near-fatal asthma

e) Initial ventilator settings should use no PEEP, low respiratory rates and long expiratory times

Answer: a, e

Short Explanation
Heliox has theoretical benefits as an adjunctive treatment, but has not been proven to be beneficial. Nitric oxide is a therapeutic manoeuvre for severe refractory hypoxaemia, which is not the primary problem in asthma. Ketamine is a bronchodilator.

Long Explanation
The patient with life-threatening asthma usually has high levels of circulating catecholamines with a high systemic vascular resistance. The combination of relative hypovolaemia secondary to dehydration and high intrathoracic pressures caused by gas trapping secondary to bronchospasm means that the patient has a reduced venous return, and upon induction of anaesthesia there is a chance of cardiovascular collapse and arrest.

It is prudent to fluid load the patient prior to induction and use a cardiovascularly stable induction agent. Ketamine is especially useful, as it acts as a bronchodilator in addition to its cardiovascular stability. Hypersecretion is a side effect of ketamine, but this is outweighed by its benefits in these patients.

Helium is a lightweight inert gas which decreases airways turbulence and facilitates diffusion due to its viscosity. When mixed with oxygen, helium can theoretically decrease airways resistance, reduce hyperinflation and improve CO_2 clearance. However, a Cochrane review found no benefit for the use of heliox in non-intubated patients with acute asthma, but did accept the possibility of benefit in patients with more severe obstruction.

The bronchospasm can lead to gas trapping and breath stacking if the expiratory phase of ventilation is not long enough. This acts as an 'auto PEEP', and if not corrected it will slowly increase with each breath, and the ensuing hyperinflation can compromise cardiac output. A slow respiratory rate and long expiratory time with zero PEEP reduces this risk, but the patient may still require periodic disconnection from the ventilator and manual decompression of the chest.

Brenner B, Corbridge T, Kazzi A. Intubation and mechanical ventilation of the asthmatic patient in respiratory failure. *Proc Am Thorac Soc* 2009; **6**: 371–9. Available online at pats.atsjournals.org/cgi/content/full/6/4/371 (accessed 30 June 2012).

Rodrigo GJ, Pollack CV, Rodrigo C, Rowe BH. Heliox for non-intubated acute asthma patients. *Cochrane Database Syst Rev* 2010; **(1)**: CD002884. Available online at onlinelibrary.wiley.com/doi/10.1002/14651858.CD002884.pub2/abstract (accessed 30 June 2012).

MTF Question 29: Wolff–Parkinson–White syndrome

A 10-year-old patient is admitted from the emergency department with palpitations. On examination his heart rate is 250 beats per minute. He is diagnosed with Wolff–Parkinson–White syndrome. Which of the following are features of this syndrome?

a) Delta wave on the ECG
b) Narrow QRS complex on the ECG
c) Prolonged PR interval on the ECG
d) Pre-excitation of the ventricles by the bundle of Kent
e) Most people remain asymptomatic throughout their lives

Answer: a, b, d, e

Short Explanation

Wolff–Parkinson–White (WPW) syndrome occurs due to pre-excitation of the ventricles by an accessory pathway called the bundle of Kent, which bypasses the atrioventricular (AV) node and bundle of His. ECG findings include shortened PR interval, a slurred upstroke of the QRS complex known as the delta wave and broad QRS complexes. Most people with a bundle of Kent remain asymptomatic.

Long Explanation

Wolff–Parkinson–White (WPW) syndrome is caused by pre-excitation of the ventricles by an accessory pathway called the bundle of Kent, an abnormal electrical communication from the atria to the ventricles. WPW is an atrioventricular re-entrant tachycardia. The prevalence is 0.1–0.3% of the general population.

In individuals with WPW syndrome, electrical activity travels down the accessory pathway as well as through the AV node, and therefore the ventricles are activated by both pathways. The bundle of Kent does not possess the rate-controlling properties of the AV node, so the electrical impulse first activating the ventricles originates from the accessory pathway, followed by electrical activity from the AV node. This gives the short PR interval and delta wave, representing the premature stimulation of the ventricles.

Most people with a bundle of Kent remain asymptomatic lifelong. However, there is a risk of sudden death due to the effect of the accessory pathway on tachyarrhythmias in these individuals. During a tachycardic episode, symptoms include palpitations, dizziness, dyspnoea and syncope.

WPW syndrome is diagnosed on ECG findings in an asymptomatic individual. The characteristic delta wave, a slurred upstroke in the QRS complex and a short PR interval are the most common findings. The QRS complex is also widened.

The definitive treatment of WPW syndrome is radiofrequency catheter ablation of the bundle of Kent.

Rosner MH, Brady WJ, Kefer MP, Martin ML. Electrocardiography in the patient with the Wolff–Parkinson–White syndrome: diagnostic and initial therapeutic issues. *Am J Emerg Med* 1999; **17**: 705–14.

Wolff L, Parkinson J, White PD. Bundle-branch block with short P-R interval in healthy young people prone to paroxysmal tachycardia. *Am Heart J* 1930; **5**: 685–70.

MTF Question 30: Calcium channel antagonists

Regarding calcium channel antagonists:

a) They cause vasodilation of the arterioles and venous capacitance vessels
b) All produce clinically effective lowering of the blood pressure
c) Nimodipine improves outcome after subarachnoid haemorrhage
d) Sublingual nifedipine is commonly used as a first-line antihypertensive agent
e) The effects of calcium channel antagonists in overdose can be reversed by magnesium

Answer: c

Short Explanation

Calcium channel antagonists cause selective arteriolar vasodilation with minimal effect on venous capacitance vessels. The phenylalkylamine verapamil has minimal antihypertensive action. Sublingual nifedipine can cause precipitous drops in blood pressure and is no longer recommended. CCA overdose is treated with intravenous calcium. Magnesium is the physiological antagonist of calcium and would exacerbate the vasodilation.

Long Explanation

Calcium channel antagonists block the inward movement of calcium by binding to L-type calcium channels in the heart and smooth muscle of the peripheral vasculature. In cardiac muscle, calcium antagonism reduces myocardial contractility and cardiac output in a dose-dependent fashion. Dilation of the coronary arteries increases myocardial oxygen supply. Automaticity at the SA node and conduction at the AV node are also calcium-dependent, and blockade decreases SA-node pacemaker rate and AV-node conduction velocity. In the peripheral vasculature arteriolar vasodilation occurs.

There are three major groups of calcium antagonists, which have variable affinity for L-type channels in myocardium, nodal tissue and vascular smooth muscle:

- Dihydropyridines – nifedipine, amlodipine, nimodipine
- Phenylalkylamines – verapamil
- Benzothiazepines – diltiazem

Dihydropiridines have minimal effect on cardiac conduction or heart rate, but cause potent arteriolar vasodilation. They are used predominantly as antihypertensive and antianginal agents. This class of drugs can cause reflex tachycardia and profound hypotension in patients with ventricular dysfunction, aortic stenosis and/or concomitant β-blockade. For this reason the use of sublingual nifedipine as a treatment of hypertensive emergencies is no longer recommended. Amlodipine has a similar pharmacodynamic profile to nifedipine but is thought to have additional anti-inflammatory and favourable lipid-modulating effects useful in patients with ischaemic heart disease. Nimodipine is a highly lipid-soluble analogue of nifedipine, which facilitates entry to the central nervous system, exerting selective cerebral vasodilatory effects. It is indicated in the prevention and treatment of vasospasm and ischaemic neurological deficit following subarachnoid haemorrhage.

Verapamil and diltiazem slow AV conduction, decrease SA node automaticity, and decrease heart rate. Verapamil is used predominantly as an antiarrhythmic and has limited vasodilatory actions. Diltiazem has vasodilatory effects that are intermediate between nifedipine and verapamil. It exerts minimal cardiodepressant effects and is used in the treatment of variant angina because of its coronary antispasmodic properties.

MTF Question 31: Cryoanalgesia

Regarding cryoanalgesia:

a) Cryoanalgesia results in an area of sensory loss
b) The probe uses the Joule–Thomson effect
c) Cryoanalgesia has a higher incidence of neuroma formation than phenol ablation
d) Cryoanalgesia is painful and therefore often requires sedation
e) A larger lesion is created by continuous rather than pulsed cooling

Answer: a, b

Short Explanation

Cryoanalgesia is used to disrupt sensory nerves without destruction of the endoneurium, minimising the chance of neuroma formation. The patient must be awake to locate the nerve, and local anaesthesia is generally adequate. Prolonged freezing is less effective than freeze–thaw as the ice ball insulates the probe and reduces its effect with time.

Long Explanation

Cryoanalgesia is effective for pain which is perpetrated by a peripheral sensory nerve. It is an alternative to surgical or alcohol ablation, which both have high incidences of neuroma formation. The neuronal vasculature is frozen, causing neuronal oedema which in turn disrupts the nerve structure. The effect is prolonged, but the nerve will grow back in time in the same location, as the endoneurium is left intact.

The probe is introduced via a sheath, to insulate and protect the surrounding tissues from damage. The probe incorporates a nerve stimulator for isolation of the specific nerve. Stimulation prior to cryoablation should produce discomfort in the painful area to ensure the correct nerve is treated. Cooling is achieved by passing carbon dioxide or nitrogen down a narrow tube at high pressure, which then cools the tube (to approximately −70 °C) as the gas expands and exits via an outer larger tube (the Joule–Thomson effect). Cycles of up to 3 minutes of cooling and 30–40 seconds of resting are repeated approximately three times.

Cryoablation has been used in the treatment of postoperative neuromas, trigeminal neuralgia, chest wall pain and abdominal and pelvic pain. It is not included in National Institute for Health and Clinical Excellence (NICE) guidelines for neuropathic pain, as these are for non-specialists. If successful, it may enable a reduction or discontinuation of systemic neuropathic pain medication. Contraindications include bleeding diathesis (relative) and overlying infection. Complications are mainly risk of damage to neighbouring structures, but overall the procedure is quite safe and well tolerated.

Trescot AM. Cryoanalgesia in interventional pain management. *Pain Physician* 2003; **6**: 345–60. Available online at www.painphysicianjournal.com/2003/july/ 2003;6;345-360.pdf (accessed 30 June 2012).

MTF Question 32: Drugs and the elderly

With regard to anaesthesia and the elderly, which of the following are true?

a) In the face of normal renal function vecuronium is preferable to atracurium due to the more predictable offset of action of the former drug
b) Gas induction occurs more slowly as the cardiac output is reduced
c) Spinal anaesthetic lasts longer than in a 30-year-old
d) By the age of 80 years, MAC values have reduced by 30% from the value in a 30-year-old
e) Confused patients with pain receive one-quarter the amount of morphine compared to patients with a mini mental state score of 10/10

Answer: d, e

Short Explanation
Vecuronium has an increased duration of action due to decreased hepatic enzyme activity whereas atracurium is unaffected. The decreased cardiac output should speed up a gas induction. It is the decreased alveolar ventilation that primarily slows induction. Spinal duration is relatively unaffected as you age.

Long Explanation
Many physiological changes occur that affect the way a person responds to drugs as he or she ages. For example, increased ventilation/perfusion mismatch and an overall reduced alveolar ventilation significantly delay a gas induction. This is not compensated for by the decreased cardiac output that is seen in the elderly, which would help to speed up a gas induction by increasing the partial pressure of the volatile agent at the alveolus.

The duration of action of spinal or epidural anaesthesia is relatively unaffected by age. Whereas the plasma protein binding and decreased hepatic microsomal enzymes would increase the effect and duration of an intravenous dose of amide anaesthetic, the offset of central neuraxial block is principally via a slow local redistribution that is relatively unimpaired as a person ages.

Atracurium is relatively unaffected by the age of the patient and is a particularly suitable drug if renal function is impaired. The aminosteroid neuromuscular blocking drugs require significant metabolism in the liver prior to excretion, and this is impaired with increasing age. Even in the face of normal renal function, atracurium usually has a superior offset of action in the elderly.

As working anaesthetists we are all aware that MAC drops with age. Different books quote a range of different percentages for the drop-off in MAC by the age of 80. If you have read in a book that MAC drops by 25%, it is unlikely that the examination board will have set a value of 30% as a false answer in the knowledge that 25% is true. For this sort of question, the true percentage would have to be substantially different from 30% for this answer to be false. You have a range from approximately 15% to 50% within which, if the value you believe to be true falls, the answer is likely to be true.

There is no evidence to support the belief that demented patients have an altered perception of pain, yet in audit data it has been shown that elderly patients with a mini mental state (MMS) score of 0/10 receive twice as much co-codamol, but only one-quarter the amount of parenteral morphine and 1/75th the amount of oral morphine compared to similar patients with a MMS score of 10/10.

MTF Question 33: Pulmonary thromboembolism

Regarding acute pulmonary thromboembolism (PTE):

a) Patients with proven pulmonary thromboembolism (PE) have a coexisting deep vein thrombosis in approximately 60% of cases
b) Acute PTE occurring within 6 weeks of surgery has a negligible recurrence rate
c) A patient suspected of having a massive PE should have urgent computed tomographic pulmonary angiography (CTPA) to confirm the diagnosis
d) The D-dimer assay is a useful diagnostic test in patients with a high probability of PE
e) Westermark's sign or Hampton's hump are signs on a chest radiograph suggestive of an acute PTE.

Answer: b, e

Short Explanation

Approximately 30% of patients with a proven PE have a coexisting deep vein thrombosis. A patient suspected of having a massive PE is unstable by definition, and the main diagnostic test is bedside echocardiography. A D-dimer assay maybe useful in excluding PE in patients with low to intermediate risk. High-risk patients should go straight for radiological investigation for PE.

Long Explanation

Approximately 30% of patients with a proven pulmonary embolus (PE) have coexisting deep vein thrombosis (DVT). Patients with proven DVT have (often silent) PE in 50% of cases. Acute pulmonary thromboembolism (PTE) occurring within 6 weeks of surgery has a negligible recurrence rate, and patients therefore do not require prolonged anticoagulation, whereas idiopathic PE has a recurrence rate of approximately 30% over 5 years, and long-term anticoagulation should be considered.

Massive PTE is characterised by haemodynamic instability, marked hypotension, or frank cardiopulmonary arrest. These unstable patients need urgent aggressive treatment if they are to survive. They should not be sent off for computed tomographic pulmonary angiography (CTPA), but should rather undergo bedside echocardiography to look for right ventricular dysfunction, with urgent consideration for thrombolytic therapy. These patients may be followed up after successful therapy with CTPA a week later to determine residual clot burden.

A negative D-dimer result is useful in helping to exclude a PE in patients with a low to intermediate risk of PE in an outpatient setting. However, patients with a high clinical suspicion of PE should go straight for radiological investigation, and a D-dimer should not be sent.

The chest radiograph in pulmonary embolism may demonstrate oligaemia distal to the pulmonary embolus (Westermark's sign) or an area of peripheral wedge-shaped pleural based consolidation suggesting infarction (Hampton's hump).

Torbicki A, Perrier A, Konstantinides S, *et al.*; ESC Task Force for the Diagnosis and Management of Acute Pulmonary Embolism. Guidelines on the diagnosis and management of acute pulmonary embolism. *Eur Heart J* 2008; **29**: 2276–315.

Van Beek EJR, Elliot CA, Kiely DG. Diagnosis and initial treatment of patients with suspected pulmonary embolism. *Contin Educ Anaesth Crit Care Pain* 2009; **9**: 119–24. Available online at ceaccp.oxfordjournals.org/content/9/4/119 (accessed 30 June 2012).

MTF Question 34: Malaria

Regarding treatments for malaria:

a) ECG monitoring is essential for administration of quinine, but not for quinidine
b) Artemisinins should not be given to a woman in the second or third trimester of pregnancy
c) Chloroquine can be used alone as prophylaxis and gives full protection
d) Benign malarias should be treated with chloroquine
e) Mefloquine should be avoided if there is a past medical or family medical history of epilepsy

Answer: d, e

Short Explanation

ECG monitoring is essential while administering quinidine, but not for quinine. Quinidine is an alternative to quinine and is not first line – it can cause torsade de pointes in toxicity. Artemisinin drug combinations are first line in children and women in second- and third-trimester of pregnancies. Chloroquine should never be relied upon as sole malaria prophylaxis and does not provide full protection, risks varying greatly with locality.

Long Explanation

It is important to get expert help when presented with a patient who has, within recent months, travelled abroad (to an approximately equatorial region), who is feverish with flu-like history and reduced conscious level.

Plasmodium falciparum malaria is a fulminating disease with an incubation of up to 10 days, whereas *P. ovale*, *P. malariae* and *P. vivax* are all benign malarias with slightly longer incubation periods. If there is infection with mixed types, or if the species is not known, it is safest to treat as for *P. falciparum*. Falciparum malaria is now almost wholly resistant to chloroquine, so it is safest to also treat as if resistant as well. Due to such resistances, artemisinin combination therapies (ACTs) are the best treatment regimens and are first line in children and in second- and third-trimester pregnancies (given with clindamicin), second line being quinine if ACTs fail. In the first trimester of pregnancy, however, the reverse is true, with quinine and clindamicin being first line.

ACT pills include:

- artesunate + amodiaquine
- artemether + lumefantrine
- dihydroartemisinin + piperaquine
- artesunate + mefloquine

These are better than quinine. If severe, then intravenous artesunate or intramuscular artemether can be used. If there is severe anaemia then exchange transfusion may be needed. Quinidine infusion (not a first-line therapy) requires continuous ECG monitoring because it is a class I antiarrhythmic agent as well as an anti-malarial and can cause long QT, U waves, depressed ST and wide QRS. In toxicity it can cause torsade de pointes.

Complications such as shock, acute respiratory distress syndrome (ARDS), acute kidney injury (AKI), metabolic acidosis and hypoglycaemia must be carefully looked for and treated accordingly. Daily platelet and parasite counts are helpful.

Benign malarias should be treated with chloroquine and, in the case of *P. ovale*, with primaquine after chloroquine to treat the liver stage of the disease. Primaquine is contraindicated in pregnancy, as it is contraindicated in glucose-6-phosphate dehydrogenase (G6PD) deficiency because of the potential for a severe haemolytic anaemia reaction, and the G6PD status of the fetus would not be known.

Prophylaxis will not give full protection, and risks vary greatly. In parts of Southeast Asia there is no really good protection. DEET repellent and long-sleeved clothing to avoid bites are advisable. Prophylaxis includes chloroquine and proguanil (and mefloquine and doxycycline or Malarone in sub-Saharan Africa, South America, Southeast Asia and Oceania). Malarone should be started the day before travel and continued for 7 days after return from the malaria-prone region. Other prophylactic agents should be started 2–3 weeks before to show up any side effects, of which there can be many, and continued for 4 weeks after return.

Chloroquine can cause psychosis or headaches. Pirimethamine and sulfadoxine can cause Stevens–Johnson syndrome or erythema multiforme. Primaquine gives haemolysis if G6PD deficient. Malarone causes abdominal pain and nausea and dizziness. Mefloquine gives nausea, dizziness and neuropsychiatric problems and hence is contraindicated in people with past or family histories of psychosis or epilepsy. It is also ill-advised in people needing to do careful precise work and in women who may become pregnant within the 3 months after therapy cessation.

World Health Organization. *Guidelines for the Treatment of Malaria*, 2nd edn. Geneva: WHO, 2010.

MTF Question 35: Defibrillation

Regarding the technique of defibrillation during cardiac arrest:

a) No person should touch the patient once the defibrillator has started charging
b) Oxygen should be disconnected from the tracheal tube before the shock is delivered
c) If using the standard sterno-apical pad position, the apical pad should be placed in the V_6 position
d) After shock delivery, CPR should not resume until a pulse check has confirmed the absence of return of spontaneous circulation
e) The recommended initial biphasic shock energy is 150–200 J

Answer: c, e

Short Explanation
Chest compressions should continue while the defibrillator is charging, and only stop once the shock is ready for delivery. Chest compressions should resume immediately

after a shock, without a pulse check. If the patient is intubated, the ventilation circuit should not be disconnected before shock delivery.

Long Explanation

The focus during cardiac arrest management should be on optimal cardiopulmonary resuscitation (CPR) while providing effective defibrillation. For this reason, the actual practicalities of managing the arrest are important.

Every pause in chest compressions causes a significant reduction in coronary and cerebral blood flow. For this reason, pauses should be minimised in frequency and length. If adhesive pads are used, modern defibrillators are relatively safe for staff. For this reason, it is recommended that chest compressions continue while charging the defibrillator, and hands are only removed once the shock is ready for delivery.

After the shock, the recommendation is to resume chest compressions immediately, without a pulse check. Even if the defibrillation has been successful and a cardiac output has been restored, there is likely to be some myocardial stunning. CPR will improve coronary and cerebral perfusion while the stunned myocardium recovers. CPR should only be stopped if there are signs of life, or if a palpable pulse is present at the next pulse check after 2 minutes.

High-flow oxygen over the chest during defibrillation causes a fire hazard, particularly if paddles (which are more prone to arcing and sparks) are used rather than pads. For this reason, a facemask oxygen supply should be moved well clear of the patient (at least 1 m) before defibrillation. If the patient is intubated and oxygen is supplied directly to the tracheal tube via an airtight circuit, oxygen is not flowing over the chest. Disconnection may delay delivery of the shock, increasing the length of the pause in chest compressions, and increases the risk of the tracheal tube becoming displaced. For this reason, the circuit should normally not be disconnected before defibrillation.

During defibrillation of VF or VT during cardiac arrest, the recommended first position of the pads is sterno-apical. The sternal pad should be placed below the right clavicle, while the apical pad should be placed in the V_6 position – in the mid-axillary line. For biphasic defibrillators the recommended starting energy is 150–200 J, while with monophasic defibrillators the recommended initial energy setting is 360 J.

Resuscitation Council UK. Adult advanced life support. Resuscitation Guidelines 2010. Available online at www.resus.org.uk/pages/guide.htm (accessed 30 June 2012).

MTF Question 36: Hypocalcaemia

The following features are typical of a patient presenting with hypocalcaemia:

a) Carpal spasm when inflating a blood pressure cuff
b) Torsades de pointes
c) QT shortening
d) Constipation
e) Recurrent infections and short fifth metacarpal

Answer: a, b, e

Short Explanation

Trousseau's sign is characteristic of hypocalcaemia (eliciting carpal spasm by inflating the blood pressure). There is intermittent QT prolongation, leading to torsades de pointes. DiGeorge syndrome, due to micro-deletion at chromosome 22, is a cause of hypoparathyroidism, producing variable features including T-cell dysfunction and skeletal abnormalities. Constipation is a feature of hypercalcaemia.

Long Explanation

Hypocalcaemia manifests as a symptom of a parathyroid hormone (PTH) deficiency or malfunction, a vitamin D deficiency, or unusually high or low magnesium levels. Hypocalcaemia may be associated with low PTH levels, as seen in hereditary hypoparathyroidism, acquired hypoparathyroidism (surgical removal), and hypomagnesaemia. Hypocalcaemia may be associated with high PTH levels when the parathyroid hormone is ineffective. In chronic renal failure, calcium levels in the blood fall, and high PTH levels are produced in response to the low calcium, but fail to return calcium levels to normal.

Features of hypocalcaemia include petechiae, paraesthesias and tetany. In particular, Trousseau's sign is carpal spasm elicited by inflating the blood pressure cuff and maintaining the cuff pressure above systolic. Chvostek's sign is less specific for hypocalcaemia, with tapping of the inferior portion of the zygoma producing facial spasms. There may also be hyperreflexia, laryngospasm and life-threatening cardiac arrhythmias, specifically intermittent QT prolongation leading to torsades de pointes if untreated.

DiGeorge syndrome occurs as a result of a micro-deletion on chromosome 22. The features of this syndrome vary widely. Characteristic signs and symptoms may include birth defects such as congenital heart disease, defects in the palate, learning disabilities, mild differences in facial features, recurrent infections and skeletal abnormalities, in particular shortened fourth and fifth metacarpals. Infections are common in children because of problems with the immune system's T-cell-mediated response that are due to an absent or hypoplastic thymus. Convulsions may occur due to hypocalcaemia arising from malfunctioning parathyroid glands.

Constipation is a feature of hypercalcaemia.

DiGeorge AM. *Congenital absence of the thymus and its immunologic consequences: concurrence with congenital hypoparathyroidism.* IV(1). White Plains, NY: March of Dimes-Birth Defects Foundation, 1968: 116–21.

MTF Question 37: Steroids

Regarding the clinical use of steroids:

a) Steroids reduce mortality in acute respiratory distress syndrome (ARDS) but only if administered in the fibroproliferative phase of the disease process
b) Steroids are useful in symptomatic treatment of brain cancer
c) Low-dose hydrocortisone may be of use in the management of septic shock
d) Topical steroids may prevent the rash of chicken pox developing into shingles in later life
e) High-dose steroids are contraindicated for reducing swelling of the brain following head injury

Answer: a, b, c, e

Short Explanation

All steroids, including topical presentations, should be avoided in chicken pox as they may worsen the severity of the disease

Long Explanation

Many different steroids are used in many different doses for many different diseases. A large number of rashes are responsive to topical steroid cream. Steroids are contraindicated in the management of some viral infections. In chicken pox, even topical steroids may increase the severity of the disease.

Since Meduri's original paper in 1998 there has been a strong body of evidence that commencing methylprednisolone may be beneficial during the fibroproliferative phase of ARDS. This is a majority view, but not universally held. Concerns have been raised about steroids too early or late in the disease, and also about dose selection.

Patients with septic shock may develop relative adrenal insufficiency. These patients can be identified by looking for a reduced or absent response when administering adrenocorticotrophic hormone. A low dose of hydrocortisone given to susceptible individuals has been found to improve 28-day survival. Steroids are frequently administered in neurosurgery for short-term relief of symptoms caused by solid expanding brain lesions. With regard to steroid use in head injury, the CRASH study update published in *The Lancet* in 2005 indicated a higher mortality following head injury in patients receiving steroids.

Alderson P, Roberts I. Corticosteroids for acute traumatic brain injury. *Cochrane Database Syst Rev* 2005; (1): CD000196. Available online at mrw.interscience. wiley.com/cochrane/clsysrev/articles/CD000196/pdf_fs.html (accessed 30 June 2012).

MTF Question 38: Epiglottitis

Which of the following statements regarding epiglottitis are true?

a) It is caused by *Haemophilus infuenzae* type B infection in approximately 25% of adult cases
b) It is most common in children aged 8–12 years
c) It has an insidious onset
d) A lateral neck x-ray will be unremarkable
e) Pulmonary oedema is a recognised complication

Answer: a, e

Short Explanation

It is most common in children aged 2–5 years but can also occur in adults, typically aged 20–40 years. It has an acute onset, and a lateral x-ray may show epiglottic enlargement. It should be noted, however, that interventions such as performing an x-ray may provoke airway obstruction, and therefore clinical assessment is usually appropriate in severe cases.

Long Explanation

Epiglottitis is an acute inflammation in the supraglottic region of the oropharynx with inflammation of the epiglottis, arytenoids and aryepiglottic folds. It is most often caused by an infection. This may be bacterial, fungal or viral in origin. Non-infectious causes include burns, including thermal, inhalational and caustic, and after foreign body ingestion. It can also occur following head and neck chemotherapy.

It has historically been most common in children aged 2–5 years but can also occur in adults, particularly those aged 20–40 years. Incidence has fallen over recent years due to the uptake of the Hib vaccination. Epidemiological data from the Health Protection Agency confirms this, with cases of epiglottitis caused by *Haemophilus influenzae* in the UK falling from 1315 in 1990 to 546 in 2010

Clinical features are of acute onset with fever, marked systemic upset, stridor and drooling. There is an absence of cough. Patients often adopt a position where they sit forward with an open mouth and jaw thrust forward. It can progress to complete airway obstruction, and this can be precipitated by pharyngeal examination, cannulation and stress. A lateral x-ray may show epiglottic enlargement, although interventions such as performing an x-ray may provoke airway obstruction, and therefore clinical assessment is usually appropriate in severe cases. Pulmonary oedema can occur if the obstruction is severe.

Maloney E, Meakin G. Acute stridor in children. *Contin Educ Anaesth Crit Care Pain* 2007; **7**: 183–6. Available online at ceaccp.oxfordjournals.org/content/7/6/183 (accessed 30 June 2012).

MTF Question 39: Visceral pain wind-up

Regarding visceral pain:

a) Repetitive noxious stimulation of viscera increases spinal cord neurone excitability
b) Frequency-dependent changes in neuronal excitability cause the 'wind-up' phenomenon
c) Somatic and visceral afferents both induce 'wind-up' by the same mechanism
d) Postsynaptic neurotransmitter actions are central to the effect of 'wind-up'
e) Positive feedback loops acting on visceral neurones may result in autonomic symptoms

Answer: a, b, e

Short Explanation
Although both somatic and visceral afferents can induce the phenomenon of central pain pathway 'wind-up', there are different mechanisms behind this. The increased excitability of the supraspinal pathways following prolonged and repetitive stimulation is central to the effect of 'wind-up'. Postsynaptic neurotransmitters may have a contributory role.

Long Explanation
The phenomenon of 'wind-up' is the mechanism which explains how, if left untreated, pain gets worse.

The nociceptor afferents enter the spinal cord dorsal horn and at this point exert an influence on the supraspinal pathways and the central nervous system. As a result, therapies are often concentrated on this area. Repetitive noxious visceral stimulus results in increased spinal cord excitability in a highly selective manner, such that the changes result only from viscerosomatic afferents specifically arising from the stimulated visceral cells.

Although the repetition of stimulus is central to somatic and visceral 'wind-up', the mechanisms behind 'wind-up' differ. Increased excitability resulting in frequency-dependent changes in neurone firing is important mainly in somatic pain systems. However, in visceral pathways it is thought that repetitive firing results in certain neurotransmitter release and complex neuronal network connections causes central sensitisation to pain. The autonomic effects (e.g. nausea associated with increasing pain) are due to sensitisation via positive feedback loops between supraspinal and spinal neurones.

Cervero F, Laird J M. Visceral pain. *Lancet* 1999; **353**: 2145–8.

MTF Question 40: Cholangitis and cholecystitis

Regarding cholangitis and cholecystitis:

a) Charcot's triad is classically seen in acute cholecystitis

b) The most common causative pathogens in ascending cholangitis are *Enterococcus* species
c) Patients with primary sclerosing cholangitis have a 25% chance of developing cholangiocarcinoma
d) Acalculous cholecystitis has a higher mortality than cholecystitis secondary to gallstones
e) Overall mortality of ascending cholangitis in the UK is approximately 10%

Answer: d, e

Short Explanation
Charcot's triad of fever, right upper quadrant pain and obstructive jaundice is associated with ascending cholangitis. The most common causative organism in ascending cholangitis is *Escherichia coli*. Patients with primary sclerosing cholangitis have approximately a 5–10% chance of developing cholangiocarcinoma.

Long Explanation
Charcot's triad comprises fever, right upper quadrant pain and obstructive jaundice, and it is classically associated with ascending cholangitis. Many patients, however, will not present with all the features. Acute cholecystitis does not give jaundice, but may present with right upper quadrant pain, fever and nausea.

Ascending cholangitis is the presence of infection that is superimposed on a background of biliary obstruction, be it with gallstones or malignancy. Organisms that are associated with cholangitis are *Escherichia coli* (most common), followed by *Klebsiella* and then the enterococci. Overall mortality of ascending cholangitis in the UK is approximately 10%.

Primary sclerosing cholangitis (PSC) is an autoimmune disorder that is associated with ulcerative colitis. Patients with PSC are at increased risk of developing cholangiocarcinoma, which is in the region of 5–10%. Testing the Ca19-9 tumour marker in patients has been shown to be fairly sensitive in detecting PSC patients who have developed cholangiocarcinoma.

Acalculous cholecystitis is cholecystitis that develops in the absence of gallstones, and it is usually associated with critical illness. Other causes included burns, sepsis and parenteral nutrition. Mortality rates in acalculous cholecystitis are therefore much higher than in cholecystitis secondary to gallstones. Variable rates are quoted, but it can be as high as 50–60%, compared with approximately 10% for cholecystitis secondary to gallstones. In acute cholecystitis, roughly 1 in 5 patients will require emergency surgery, for a gallbladder that has become gangrenous or has perforated. Delay in cholecystectomy for these patients increases mortality.

Burak K, Angulo P, Pasha TM, *et al*. Incidence and risk factors for cholangiocarcinoma in primary sclerosing cholangitis. *Am J Gastroenterol* 2004; **99**: 523–6.
Indar AA, Beckingham IJ. Acute cholecystitis. *BMJ* 2002; **325**: 639–43.

MTF Question 41: Medical diseases complicating pregnancy

With regard to pre-existing medical diseases complicating pregnancy:

a) Approximately 50% of women with asthma will experience worsened symptoms during pregnancy
b) Carboprost should be avoided in the management of post-partum haemorrhage (PPH) in an asthmatic woman

c) Misoprostolol should be avoided in the management of post-partum haemorrhage (PPH) in an asthmatic woman
d) Obstetric cholestasis is an indication for delivery by 37–39 weeks
e) Carbimazole is the preferred anti-thyroid drug in pregnancy

Answer: b, d

Short Explanation
Approximately 25% of women with asthma experience worsened symptoms during pregnancy. Misoprostolol is safe to give to asthmatic women because it does not cause bronchoconstriction. Propylthiouracil is the preferred drug because it prevents thyroxine release, blocks peripheral T4 to T3 conversion, and is not teratogenic, unlike carbimazole.

Long Explanation
Many women have pre-existing medical conditions prior to becoming pregnant, and most can be managed without much change to their current treatment regimens.

Asthma in pregnancy usually improves in about 25% of patients because of progesterone-mediated smooth muscle relaxation, 50% are unchanged, and the remaining 25% experience worsened asthma. Women who have moderate to severe asthma are at more risk of deterioration as pregnancy progresses. It is quite safe to continue taking inhaled β_2-agonists and corticosteroids. Additional oral steroids are not contraindicated for an acute exacerbation. The main treatment dilemma for asthmatic women is post-partum haemorrhage (PPH) management. Most bronchodilators such as salbutamol, terbutaline, volatile agents (the non-irritant ones!) cause uterine relaxation and promote haemorrhage. Incidentally ketamine increases uterine tone. Uterotonic agents such as Syntocinon (synthetic oxytocin) and ergometrine are not contraindicated in asthma. Misoprostolol is a synthetic prostaglandin E1 analogue used in labour induction and can be safely used as an uterotonic agent (usually given rectally). Carboprost is a synthetic analogue of prostaglandin F2α but can cause severe bronchoconstriction and is therefore contraindicated in asthmatic women.

Intrahepatic cholestasis of pregnancy affects approximately 0.7% of pregnancies but has a higher prevalence amongst women of South Asian origin. It commonly presents after 30 weeks gestation, possibly because there is a genetic predisposition to the cholestatic effect of oestrogens. The most common presenting feature is pruritus. Serum bile acids are elevated in addition to serum transaminases and bilirubin (usually stays below 100 μmol/L). The bile acids are the best marker for this condition. The main problem with obstetric cholestasis is the risk of pre-term labour, fetal distress (possible increased risk of meconium) and stillbirth. Although clotting is not usually deranged, there is an increased risk of PPH. Although a full evidence-based consensus on timing of delivery has not been reached, delivery by 39 weeks is reasonable to balance the risks of stillbirth versus neonatal prematurity problems.

The preferred drug treatment for hyperthyroidism during pregnancy is propylthiouracil, because it prevents thyroxine release and blocks peripheral T4 to T3 conversion. Thyroid-stimulating hormone (TSH) should be measured every 4–6 weeks and treatment should be adjusted accordingly. Use of radioactive iodine is absolutely contraindicated, and surgery is only indicated if medical treatment fails. Carbimazole is teratogenic and is associated with aplasia cutis congenita (a group of disorders characterised by loss of skin, either localised or widespread).

Norwitz E, Schorge J. *Obstetrics and Gynaecology at a Glance*, 3rd edn. Chichester: Wiley-Blackwell, 2010; pp. 100–3.

Royal College of Obstetricians and Gynaecologists. *Obstetric Cholestasis*. RCOG Green-top guideline 43, May 2011. Available online at www.rcog.org.uk/guidelines (accessed 30 June 2012).

Royal College of Obstetricians and Gynaecologists. *Postpartum Haemorrhage, Prevention and Management*. RCOG Green-top guideline 52, May 2009. Available online at www.rcog.org.uk/guidelines (accessed 30 June 2012).

MTF Question 42: Measures of tissue oxygenation: lactate

Regarding the use of the serum lactate concentration in critical illness:

a) Serum lactate concentration is a reliable indicator of tissue hypoxia
b) Elevated lactate is associated with worse outcomes in severe sepsis
c) In severe sepsis, lactate rise does not correlate well with blood pressure
d) Venous lactate will significantly overestimate arterial lactate concentration
e) The administration of exogenous lactate (e.g. by infusion of Hartmann's solution) significantly reduces the value of the serum lactate concentration as a measure of tissue oxygenation

Answer: b, c

Short Explanation

Assuming appropriate collection, venous and arterial lactate are normally very similar. Lactate is normally rapidly metabolised, and administration of small amounts in resuscitation fluids should not significantly alter levels. Lactate can be raised by several means, and does not reliably indicate tissue hypoxia.

Long Explanation

Serum lactate concentrations have recently been used as a marker of tissue hypoxia in critical illness, after a variety of publications demonstrated a worse outcome associated with lactaemia. This is true in severe sepsis, as well as in trauma and other causes of critical illness. As long as a tourniquet has not been applied for excessive periods (causing tissue hypoxia), the venous lactate concentration will be similar enough to the arterial concentration for clinical use.

Although useful for prognostication, single measurements of lactate are not reliable indicators of tissue hypoxia, as lactaemia can occur through several aerobic processes in critical illness, including deactivation of pyruvate dehydrogenase by severe sepsis. However, trends in the lactate level can be useful in judging adequacy of resuscitative efforts. Normal plasma lactate level is 0.3–1.3 mmol/L. A level of 5 mmol/L or higher in association with a metabolic acidosis would indicate a high likelihood of a poor outcome from an acute illness.

Under normal circumstances, exogenous lactate is rapidly broken down and should not influence serum concentrations. Lactate is metabolised in the liver to bicarbonate. This process may not occur during liver failure, so the administration of exogenous lactate such as in Hartmann's solution or lactate-containing dialysate may raise the lactate level and should be avoided.

In severe sepsis, profound lactaemia can occur despite normal haemodynamic state. This is because despite normal pressures, microvascular shunting can occur, resulting in ongoing tissue hypoxia despite adequate macrovascular resuscitation. In addition, as described above, lactate production in severe sepsis can be elevated by non-hypoxic processes. Adrenaline may raise lactate significantly by a perfusion unrelated mechanism.

MTF Question 43: Scoring systems in pancreatitis

Regarding the modified Glasgow score for pancreatitis:

a) The modification from the original Glasgow score results in a score out of 9
b) A point is scored for a serum amylase > 1000 units/L
c) The modified Glasgow score has been validated for pancreatitis caused by hyperlipidaemia
d) A point is scored if a criterion is met at any time during the 48 hours after onset of symptoms
e) An admission albumin concentration of 30 g/L would score a point

Answer: d, e

Short Explanation
The modified Glasgow score has eight criteria, resulting in a total score of 8. A raised amylase is virtually a precondition for assessing the Glasgow score, and so is not scored. It is only validated for gallstone/alcoholic pancreatitis.

Long Explanation
Pancreatitis is a common, often minor illness, which can become life-threatening. Considerable effort has therefore been devoted to developing scoring systems to high-light patients at high risk of developing severe pancreatitis, so that they can be cared for in a high-dependency environment.

Scoring systems in use include the Ranson, Imrie and Glasgow scores. The Glasgow score was originally out of 9, including transaminase levels, but this was dropped from the modified Glasgow score, resulting in a score out of 8. This modified Glasgow score has been validated for severity assessment in pancreatitis caused by gallstones or alcohol.

The criteria are (mnemonic P.A.N.C.R.E.A.S.):

- $PaO_2 < 60$ mmHg / 7.9 kPa
- Age > 55
- Neutrophils (WBC > $15 \times 10^9/mm^3$)
- Calcium < 2 mmol/L
- Renal (urea > 16 mmol/L)
- Enzymes (LDH > 600 units/L)
- Albumin < 32 g/L
- Sugar (blood sugar level > 10 mmol/L)

A point is scored if the criterion is met at any point in the first 48 hours after onset, even if the level subsequently drops back below the threshold. A score of 3 or more indicates severe disease.

Young SP, Thompson JP. Severe acute pancreatitis. *Contin Educ Anaesth Crit Care Pain* 2008; **8**: 125–8. Available online at ceaccp.oxfordjournals.org/content/8/4/125 (accessed 30 June 2012).

MTF Question 44: Phantom limb pain

After amputation of a limb:

a) Virtually all amputees will experience phantom limb pain
b) Phantom sensations occur almost immediately after amputation
c) Phantom pain can be precipitated by spinal anaesthetic

d) Stump revision is a useful treatment for intractable phantom limb pain
e) Pre-emptive epidural analgesia will reduce the risk of phantom limb pain

Answer: b, c

Short Explanation

Virtually all amputees will experience phantom sensations, not phantom pain, which is a separate entity. Stump revision is not a treatment for phantom limb pain, and is only useful for persistent stump pain (which is a distinct phenomenon) in specific circumstances. There is no strong evidence to suggest that pre-emptive analgesic techniques prior to limb amputation reduce the incidence of phantom pain.

Long Explanation

Following amputation of a body part, either due to trauma or as an elective intervention, three separate phenomena can occur: phantom painless sensation, phantom pain and stump pain.

Virtually all amputees will experience phantom sensations, which may consist of a perception of the missing limb or paraesthesia, and, over time, some upper limb amputees have a sensation of the missing forearm receding back into the stump, which is known as 'telescoping'.

The precise incidence of phantom limb pain is not known. Reports have estimated that up to 80% of amputees will experience phantom limb pain. Such pain normally occurs within a week after amputation, but may occur months or years afterwards. Lower limb phantom pain can present after a spinal anaesthetic for another procedure, or pre-existing pain may be exacerbated by spinal or epidural anaesthetic. This type of induced phantom limb pain is poorly understood, but it is possibly due to brainstem descending inhibition being 'overridden' by the sudden loss of input by spinal segmental afferents.

Stump pain occurs acutely after amputation and resolves with wound healing. However, the pain can persist beyond the healing period in up to 71% of cases, due to an ongoing pathological process, e.g. bone spurs, infection, or a neuropathic problem such as diabetic neuropathy. Surgery is best avoided and can make stump pain far worse unless there is a clearly defined, localised pathology. Stump resection is not a recommended treatment for phantom limb pain – which is a separate phenomenon, albeit part of the same pathophysiological process of central nervous system reorganisation.

Investigations into the use of pre-emptive analgesia (such as epidural and perineural blocks, and intravenous ketamine) in the 12–36 hours prior to a limb amputation have resulted in inadequate data to justify its use in routine practice. The theory is that such techniques can reduce the peripheral to central sensory input from a painful limb due to be amputated and start the process of undoing the central nervous system reorganisation that has resulted in increased sensitivity to such input. But it is considered unrealistic that reversing such reorganisation could be achieved in the days before surgery, given that it has taken a considerably longer period of time to develop. Such techniques are helpful, however, in the immediate postoperative period for acute pain relief.

Jackson MA, Simpson KH. Pain after amputation. *Contin Educ Anaesth Crit Care Pain* 2004; 4: 20–3. Available online at ceaccp.oxfordjournals.org/content/4/1/20 (accessed 30 June 2012).

MTF Question 45: Hypertension

A 34-year-old African businessman attends his general practitioner for an annual health check-up. He has been well over the past year but has been under some stress at work recently. He is a non-smoker, takes regular exercise and eats a healthy, balanced diet. His blood pressure was 165/89 mmHg. His cardiovascular risk is estimated at 10–20%. Regarding his management:

a) His blood pressure is an indication for immediate pharmacological intervention on this occasion
b) Amlodipine would be an appropriate first-choice antihypertensive
c) Ramipril would be an appropriate first-choice antihypertensive
d) Investigations should include plasma free metadrenaline and renal artery arteriogram
e) This gentleman has a healthy lifestyle, so lifestyle advice would not be indicated here

Answer: b, d

Short Explanation
This man has hypertension (BP > 140/90). Hypertension should be confirmed with ambulatory or home blood pressure monitoring prior to starting antihypertensive medication. Calcium channel blockers are first-line medical management for any hypertensive patient of African or Caribbean origin. Young hypertensive patients should be investigated for secondary causes, including phaeochromocytoma with plasma metadrenaline, and renal artery stenosis with an arteriogram. This patient may benefit from advice regarding stress management.

Long Explanation
According to the revised NICE guidelines issued in 2011, hypertension is defined as raised blood pressure above 140/90 mmHg in patients aged under 80 years, or 150/90 in those aged over 80 years, which should be confirmed with ambulatory, or home, blood pressure monitoring. If hypertension is confirmed, formal cardiovascular risk should be assessed, using tests to identify diabetes, cardiac or renal damage, and secondary causes of hypertension. Young patients in particular should be investigated for secondary causes of hypertension such as phaeochromocytoma, and early specialist input should be sought.

Ambulatory blood pressure monitoring (ABPM) is a new addition to the 2011 guidelines on blood pressure monitoring. It is used as a method for confirming hypertension, and should be offered to any patient with BP > 140/90. At least two blood pressure measurements should be taken each hour during the day, with hypertension diagnosed if average BP > 135/85 in patients aged under 80 years, or > 145/85 in patients aged over 80 years. If ABPM is not tolerated, home blood pressure monitoring (HBPM) may be used as an alternative method.

Drug therapy reduces cardiovascular risk, and should be offered to patients with stage 2 hypertension (BP > 150/95 on ABPM/HBPM), or stage 1 hypertension (BP > 135/85 on ABPM/HBPM) who also have target organ damage, diabetes, renal disease, established cardiovascular disease (CVD), or a 10-year risk of CVD 20%. A clinic blood pressure measurement of 180/110 is an indication for immediate medical management along with an urgent specialist referral. Hospital admission is indicated in accelerated hypertension (papilloedema or retinal haemorrhages seen on fundoscopy).

In hypertensive patients aged 55 or older, or black patients (African or Caribbean descent) of any age, first choice for initial therapy should be a calcium channel blocker (CCB). Thiazide-like diuretics such as indapamide may be considered as an alternative if CCBs are not tolerated or contraindicated due to oedema or heart failure. If a second drug is to be added, this should be an angiotensin-converting enzyme (ACE) inhibitor, or an angiontensin-II receptor blocker (ARB) if ACE inhibitor is not tolerated. In hypertensive patients younger than 55, the first choice for initial therapy should be an ACE inhibitor (or ARB if ACE inhibitor not tolerated). If a second drug is to be added, this should be a CCB.

If treatment with three drugs is required, combination of an ACE inhibitor, CCB and thiazide-like diuretic is advised. If hypertension is still uncontrolled, specialist help should be requested. Fourth drug choices include a higher thiazide-like diuretic dose, a second diuretic such as spironolactone, a β-blocker or a selective α-blocker.

If a diuretic is to be instigated, thiazide-like diuretics such as indapamide or chlortalidone are preferable to conventional thiazides such as bendroflumethiazide or hydrochlorothiazide. For hypertensive patients well controlled on conventional thiazide treatment, this should be continued.

NICE guidelines also advise clinicians to ascertain patients' diet and exercise patterns, because a healthy diet and regular exercise can reduce blood pressure. Appropriate guidance and written or audiovisual materials should be offered to promote lifestyle changes. Relaxation therapies can reduce blood pressure, and individual patients may wish to pursue these as part of their treatment – for example stress management, meditation, cognitive therapies, muscle relaxation and biofeedback. These are not currently provided by the NHS, however.

National Institute for Health and Clinical Excellence. *Hypertension: Management of Hypertension in Adults in Primary Care.* NICE Clinical Guideline 127, August 2011. Available online at guidance.nice.org.uk/CG127 (accessed 30 June 2012).

MTF Question 46: Administration of 100% oxygen therapy

Administration of 100% oxygen must be used with caution in the following patients:

a) An 18-month-old baby presenting for removal of an inhaled foreign body
b) A 22-year-old male presenting for elective surgery who has received chemotherapy in the past for testicular cancer
c) A 60-year-old male presenting with an acute exacerbation of chronic obstructive pulmonary disease (COPD)
d) A 50-year-old female presenting with a pulmonary embolus
e) A 70-year-old male with ischaemic heart disease presenting with carbon monoxide poisoning

Answer: b, c

Short Explanation

For a previously healthy baby presenting with an inhaled foreign body, pre-oxygenation with 100% oxygen for induction of anaesthesia would be appropriate. High-concentration oxygen is the appropriate treatment for acute carbon monoxide poisoning. Administration of 100% oxygen would be appropriate for pulmonary embolus but it should be titrated down.

Long Explanation

Basic physiology states that oxygen is good for us! However, too much oxygen for too long can lead to potentially serious and detrimental complications, especially in a few groups of patients.

The basic indications for oxygen as stated by the American College of Chest Physicians and National Heart, Lung, and Blood Institute are: cardiac and respiratory arrest; hypoxaemia ($PaO_2 < 7.8$ kPa, $SaO_2 < 90\%$); hypotension (systolic blood pressure < 100 mmHg, although this should be taken in context); low cardiac output and metabolic acidosis; respiratory distress (respiratory rate > 24/min); postoperatively, especially after general anaesthesia. On most occasions it is intuitive to commence oxygen therapy for a patient who is acutely unwell or to give 100% oxygen as part of induction of anaesthesia.

Patients who have received chemotherapy for testicular cancer will more than likely have received bleomycin. Bleomycin can cause pulmonary fibrosis, and this can be accelerated by administration of 100% oxygen. The high concentration of oxygen ultimately increases the alveolar and arterial oxygen tensions, and free-radical formation is promoted. It is the free-radical formation that is damaging. These patients should be managed with lower concentrations of oxygen and lower arterial oxygen saturation should be targeted (90–95%).

For a small group of COPD patients who chronically retain CO_2, high-concentration oxygen should be administered with caution. These patients depend on their hypoxic drive to maintain ventilation.

This can be blunted by administering too much oxygen, which will cause respiratory depression. Oxygen therapy should be administered using Venturi masks so that a known concentration of oxygen can be delivered. Serial arterial blood gases should be done to check that the arterial CO_2 tension is not rapidly rising.

Premature babies are at risk of retrolental fibroplasia when 100% oxygen is administered for too long a period. Premature infants are at risk up to 44 weeks post-conceptual age, and it would be prudent to avoid extended periods of 100% oxygen in healthy neonates. However, hypoxic infants should be given the appropriate amount of oxygen required.

A page on oxygen therapy and the physiology of oxygen delivery is available online at www.nda.ox.ac.uk/wfsa/html/u12/u1203_03.htm (accessed 30 June 2012).
Jackson RM. Pulmonary oxygen toxicity. *Chest* 1985; **88**: 900–5. Available online at chestjournal.chestpubs.org/content/88/6/900.long (accessed 30 June 2012).

MTF Question 47: Radiation sickness

Which of the following statements regarding radiation sickness are correct?

a) The earliest symptoms of acute radiation sickness are nausea, vomiting and fever
b) Frequent exposure to low-dose radiation does not cause radiation sickness
c) The absorbed dose of radiation is measured in a unit called the gray
d) There is higher incidence of cancer amongst survivors of radiation sickness
e) Decontamination by removing clothes and washing the skin can remove up to 50% of radioactive particles

Answer: a, b, c, d

Short Explanation
Nausea, vomiting and fever occur early in acute radiation sickness. It is usually caused by a very large amount of radiation being absorbed by the body over a short period of time. The gray (Gy) is the unit of measurement. Prussian blue can be used to treat some types of radiation sickness. Decontamination by removing clothes and washing the skin can remove more than 90% of radioactive particles

Long Explanation
Radiation sickness is still relatively rarely seen in the UK, but it does happen and therefore it is worth knowing a little about the signs, symptoms and treatment options. Radiation sickness is also known as acute radiation sickness, acute radiation syndrome (ARS) or acute radiation poisoning. It is basically damage to the body caused by a very large dose of radiation, often received over a short period of time. The amount of radiation absorbed by the body, which determines the severity of the illness, depends

on the strength of the radiated energy and the distance between the source and the patient.

The absorbed dose of radiation is measured in a unit called a gray (Gy). An x-ray can produce about 0.1 Gy of radiation and this is generally focused on a small area of tissue. Signs and symptoms of radiation sickness usually appear when the entire body receives an absorbed dose of at least 1 Gy. Doses greater than 6 Gy to the whole body are generally not treatable and usually lead to death within 2 days to 2 weeks, depending on the dose and duration of the exposure.

The early signs and symptoms include nausea, vomiting, diarrhoea and fever. In general, the greater the radiation exposure, the more rapid the onset of symptoms. The initial symptoms may come and go and last for varying amounts of time. Later problems include skin damage and hair loss. Most people who do not recover from radiation poisoning will die within several months of exposure. Bone marrow failure is responsible for death in the majority of cases of radiation poisoning.

Radiation sickness treatment is aimed at preventing further radioactive contamination. Decontamination by removing clothes and washing the skin can remove more than 90% of radioactive particles, which is important in reducing further contamination. The other treatments available are mainly supportive and treating organ failure. There are some specific treatments available for specific types of radiation exposure, for example potassium iodide and Prussian blue.

Centers for Disease Control and Prevention. Acute radiation syndrome (ARS): a fact sheet for the public. Available online at emergency.cdc.gov/radiation/ars.asp (accessed 30 June 2012).

MTF Question 48: Sickle cell disease

The clinical features of sickle cell anaemia include:

a) Pulmonary artery hypertension
b) Obstructive sleep apnoea
c) Cholesterol gallstones
d) Functional asplenism
e) Haemorrhagic stroke

Answer: a, b, d, e

Short Explanation

Haemolysis in sickle cell anaemia leads to pigment gallstone formation. Splenic auto-infarction results in functional asplenism and hypertrophy of other lymphoid tissue, including tonsils and adenoids. Repeated pulmonary infarction may culminate in pulmonary artery hypertension, and both thrombotic and haemorrhagic neurological events are seen.

Long Explanation

Sickle cell anaemia is due to a mutation on chromosome 11 resulting in an abnormality in the β-globin subunit of haemoglobin A, leading to the formation of haemoglobin S. The greater the proportion of haemoglobin S in the cell, the more likely it is to sickle. Sickle cell trait patients (heterozygous) commonly have a 30–40% haemoglobin S concentration, and the cells only sickle in exceptional circumstances or when the oxygenation saturation is below 40%. Homozygous sickle cell anaemia patients have almost 100% haemoglobin S and sickling of cells is common, starting when the oxygen saturation is below 85%.

Sickling results in small vessel occlusion (in any organ) and ongoing haemolytic anaemia, as the abnormal cells have a reduced life span. The clinical picture of sickle cell trait is benign with only a mild anaemia. Sickle cell anaemia patients have a chronic severe anaemia and present with chronic multisystem organ damage and acute vaso-occlusive crises. Recurrent pulmonary infarction and 'acute chest syndrome' results in dyspnoea, haemoptysis and pleuritic chest pain. It may also lead to pulmonary hypertension in the long term. Cardiomegaly is caused by anaemia and can lead to congestive cardiac failure.

There may be skeletal abnormalities from marrow hyperplasia and from avascular necrosis. Retinopathy is often seen, resembling that seen in diabetes, and renal impairment is also common. Acute splenomegaly with sequestration of red cells and platelets may be life-threatening, although in the long term the spleen tends to undergo auto-infarction with subsequent immunocompromise. Hypertrophy of other lymphoid tissue, including tonsils and adenoids, then occurs and may cause obstructive sleep apnoea. Haemolysis results in an increased formation of pigment gallstones. There is also an increase in both thrombotic and haemorrhagic neurological events.

Diagnosis of sickle cell disease is by haemoglobin electrophoresis. The Sickledex test is a screening tool used to detect haemoglobin S levels greater than 10%, but it will not differentiate between sickle cell trait and sickle cell anaemia.

Wilson M, Forsyth P, Whiteside J. Haemoglobinopathy and sickle cell disease. *Contin Educ Anaesth Crit Care Pain* 2010; **10**: 24–8. Available online at ceaccp.oxfordjournals. org/content/10/1/24 (accessed 30 June 2012).

MTF Question 49: Degradation products

Which of the following substances have degradation products with significant clinical pharmacological effects?

a) Paracetamol
b) Morphine
c) Atracurium
d) Rocuronium
e) Enalapril

Answer: a, b, e

Short Explanation
Paracetamol has a toxic metabolite that accumulates in overdose. Morphine has two active metabolites which can accumulate in renal failure. Enalapril is a prodrug which must be metabolised to become active. Atracurium is metabolised to laudanosine but not in sufficient quantities to have clinical relevance. Rocuronium is excreted largely (> 95%) unchanged.

Long Explanation
Drug metabolism tends to produce compounds with greater water solubility and less activity than the parent substance. This allows greater rates of elimination of the drug in the bile and urine. Two phases of metabolism may occur: phase I involves redox reactions and phase II involves conjugation with organic residues.

Sometimes the metabolites of a drug have activity equal to or even greater than the original substance: prodrugs such as enalapril have no activity until they have been metabolised (to enalaprilat in this case). Morphine is an example of a drug with active metabolites, being conjugated in the liver and kidney to produce two compounds. Morphine-3-glucuronide has arousal effects and is an opioid antagonist, while morphine-6-glucuronide is 13 times as potent as morphine itself with a similar duration of action: both compounds accumulate in renal failure and contribute to the toxicity of morphine in renal patients.

Atracurium is metabolised through two processes, non-specific ester hydrolysis in the plasma (60%) and Hofmann degradation (a pH- and temperature-dependent spontaneous breakdown). Both processes produce laudanosine, a glycine antagonist which has been shown to have pro-convulsant activity but which is not produced in sufficient quantities to have relevance to clinical practice.

The toxicity of drug degradation products is often less than that of the parent drug, but this is not always true. Alcohol is metabolised rapidly to acetaldehyde but its subsequent metabolism to acetic acid proceeds at a slower rate, leading to toxicity in hepatocytes where acetaldehyde accumulates.

A similar process occurs with paracetamol, where small amounts of the toxic metabolite N-acetyl-p-amino-benzoquinone-imine are produced in the liver and normally rapidly conjugated with glutathione. In overdose liver glutathione stores are rapidly exhausted, leading to build-up of the toxic product and acute hepatocyte necrosis.

Rocuronium is an example of a drug which undergoes only minimal metabolism and is largely excreted unchanged in the bile and (to a lesser extent) the urine.

Peck T, Hill S, Williams M. *Pharmacology for Anaesthesia and Intensive Care*, 3rd edn. Cambridge: Cambridge University Press, 2008.

MTF Question 50: Laser classification

Concerning the classification of lasers:

a) All lasers used in operative surgery are class 4
b) The blink reflex will fully protect the eye from potential damage caused by a class 3 laser
c) It is safe to view class 1 lasers with the naked eye
d) Class 3 lasers can set fire to materials upon which they are projected
e) For a laser to be classified as a class 2 laser it must be in the visible spectrum

Answer: a, c, e

Short Explanation
The blink reflex will protect the eye from class 1 and class 2 lasers. Class 4 lasers can set fire to materials upon which they are projected.

Long Explanation
LASER is an acronym that stands for light amplification by stimulated emission of radiation. There are strict safety guidelines that must be adhered to when laser is used in theatre, not least because all lasers used in surgery are in class 4 (potentially the most hazardous class).

All lasers are classified by the manufacturer and should be labelled with the appropriate warning labels. Lasers are classified according to a number of criteria that depend on whether the laser is a continuous-wave laser or a pulsed one. For both types, wavelength is important. For continuous-wave lasers, the average power output and any modifications to the laser design that may limit exposure time are considered. For pulsed lasers the total energy per pulse, pulse duration, pulse repetition frequency and emergent beam radiant exposure must all be considered. All lasers are then classified into one of four classes:

Class 1: all lasers in this class are eye-safe under all operating conditions, although those in subclass 1M may be hazardous to view if magnifying optical instruments are used. Lasers in this class can be visible, invisible or both.

Class 2: all lasers in this class are visible and are potentially hazardous if the natural aversion reflex to a bright light is overcome.

Class 3: radiation from lasers in this class is likely to be hazardous to the eyes or skin, but viewing any reflected light from the laser is not.

Class 4: radiation from lasers in this class is dangerous, as is any reflected light. Class 4 laser beams are capable of setting fire to materials onto which they are projected.

MTF Question 51: Heart murmurs

A 78-year-old lady with a childhood history of rheumatic fever is being investigated for a murmur, found incidentally during a preoperative assessment visit. The murmur is ejection systolic in nature. There are no signs of right or left heart failure and the apex is not displaced. Which of the following valvular abnormalities are associated with an ejection systolic murmur?

a) Aortic stenosis
b) Tricuspid regurgitation
c) Pulmonary regurgitation
d) Pulmonary stenosis
e) Mitral regurgitation

Answer: a, d

Short Explanation

Differential diagnoses for an ejection systolic murmur are aortic stenosis and pulmonary stenosis. Tricuspid regurgitation and mitral regurgitation present with a pansystolic murmur. Pulmonary regurgitation presents with a decrescendo diastolic murmur (Graham Steell murmur), similar to that heard in aortic regurgitation.

Long Explanation

Differential diagnoses for an ejection systolic murmur are aortic stenosis and pulmonary stenosis.

In aortic stenosis, the murmur is heard loudest in the right second intercostal space and may radiate to the carotid arteries. In addition, there is a reversed split S2 due to a delayed A2 heart sound, and there is an additional S4 heart sound. The pulse is slow rising and of small volume, the apex is not displaced but is heaving in nature, there is a left ventricular heave and systolic thrill. Aortic stenosis is asymptomatic until disease is moderate or severe, and symptoms include syncope, angina and dyspnoea on exertion. Hypertrophic obstructive cardiomyopathy (HOCM) presents in a similar way, but the pulse is described as 'jerky' in nature and symptoms present earlier in life. Bifid P waves (P mitrale) and left ventricular strain may be seen on electrocardiogram.

Pulmonary stenosis has an ejection systolic murmur heard loudest at the left second intercostal space, and it may radiate to the left shoulder. Heart sound S2 is split and there is an additional S4 heart sound. There is a right ventricular heave and palpable thrill. Signs include dyspnoea, fatigue, and right heart failure with right atrial and ventricular hypertrophy, peripheral oedema and ascites. A prominent 'a' wave is visible in the jugular venous pulse. Tall P waves (P pulmonale) are seen on electrocardiogram.

Tricuspid regurgitation presents with a pansystolic murmur, heard loudest at the left lower sternal edge. As severity progresses, signs of right heart failure and raised right atrial and venous pressure result, with raised jugular venous pressure and prominent 'v' waves and 'y' descent, peripheral oedema and ascites and pulsatile, painful hepatomegaly with jaundice.

Mitral regurgitation also presents with a pansystolic murmur, heard loudest in the left lateral position, radiating into the axilla. There is a right ventricular heave and palpable systolic thrill. S2 heart sound is split with an additional S3 heart sound. The apex is thrusting and displaced, and is complicated by left heart failure and, when severe, congestive cardiac failure. Bifid P waves (P mitrale) and left ventricular hypertrophy may be seen on electrocardiogram.

Pulmonary regurgitation is the commonest acquired abnormality of the pulmonary valve, caused by dilation of the pulmonary valve ring in pulmonary hypertension. There is a decrescendo diastolic murmur beginning at P2 heart sound, heard loudest at the lower sterna edge, which is known as a Graham Steell murmur. Pulmonary regurgitation is rarely symptomatic and rarely needs medical or surgical intervention. This murmur is similar to the early diastolic murmur heard in aortic regurgitation, also at the lower sternal edge. However, there are many other coexisting features in aortic regurgitation to help differentiate from pulmonary regurgitation.

Agabegi SS, Agabegi ED. Valvular heart disease. In: *Step-Up to Medicine*, 2nd edn. Hagerstown, MD: Lippincott Williams & Wilkins, 2008; pp. 36–43.

MTF Question 52: Valvular heart disease

Which of the following associations with aortic valvular heart disease are correct?

a) Aortic regurgitation and Quincke's sign (nail-bed capillary pulsations)
b) Aortic regurgitation and early diastolic murmur
c) Aortic stenosis and narrow pulse pressure
d) Aortic stenosis and Austin Flint murmur
e) Aortic stenosis and large-volume, 'collapsing' pulse

Answer: a, b, c

Short Explanation
Austin Flint murmur and a large-volume, 'collapsing' pulse are signs of aortic regurgitation, not stenosis.

Long Explanation
Aortic regurgitation (AR) is due to disease of the valve cusps or dilation of the aortic root. The left ventricle dilates and hypertrophies to compensate for the regurgitation. AR may be congenital, such as bicuspid valve, or may be acquired, such as in rheumatic disease, infective endocarditis, trauma and aortic dilation from Marfan's syndrome, aneurysm, dissection, syphilis or ankylosing spondylitis. Mild to moderate AR may be asymptomatic, or the patient may experience palpitations. If severe, there will be dyspnoea and angina. The pulses are bounding, large-volume, 'collapsing' pulses with a wide pulse pressure. Classical reported signs include Quincke's sign (nail-bed capillary pulsations), Duroziez's sign (femoral 'pistol shot' bruit) and de Musset's sign (head nodding with pulse). The murmurs heard on auscultation are an early diastolic murmur from the regurgitation, and a soft mid-diastolic 'Austin Flint' murmur due to fluttering of the anterior mitral cusp caused by the regurgitant stream. Increased stroke volume may also cause a systolic murmur to be heard. Other signs include a displaced, heaving apex beat due to volume overload and left ventricular dilation, a fourth heart sound and signs of pulmonary venous congestion.

The causes of aortic stenosis (AS) are dependent on age of onset. In infants and children, the commonest cause is congenital aortic stenosis, which presents early in life. Congenital bicuspid aortic valve presents in young to middle-aged adults as calcification and fibrosis develops over time.

Middle-aged to elderly patients present with senile degenerative aortic stenosis, and rheumatic aortic stenosis and calcification of a bicuspid valve. Mild and moderate AS is usually asymptomatic, but when severe, symptoms progress rapidly and prognosis is 3–5 years from onset of symptoms if untreated. Symptoms include exertional dyspnoea and syncope as the increased cardiac output required during exertion cannot be met. Other symptoms are angina, episodes of acute pulmonary oedema and, in severe cases, sudden death. Signs include an ejection systolic murmur that is heard loudest in the right second intercostal region and may radiate to the carotid arteries. Carotid pulse is slow-rising and the pulse pressure is narrow. The apex beat is thrusting due to left ventricular hypertrophy, but is not typically displaced, and there may be signs of venous congestion.

Investigation of valvular disease depends on a combination of the signs and symptoms the patient presents with and also any comorbidities that may influence whether valve replacement is appropriate in individual cases. All patients with valvular disease in which valve replacement is being seriously considered should receive an electrocardiogram, chest x-ray, echocardiogram with Doppler and cardiac catheterisation. Cardiac catheterisation is necessary to diagnose any occult coronary artery disease that may require bypass grafting at the same time.

MTF Question 53: Brown-Séquard syndrome

Which of the following are components of Brown-Séquard syndrome?

a) Flaccid paralysis at the level of the lesion on the ipsilateral side
b) Ipsilateral loss of temperature sensation
c) Ipsilateral spinocerebellar tract involvement
d) Ipsilateral extensor plantar response
e) No plantar reflex on the ipsilateral side

Answer: a, c, d

Short Explanation

Brown-Séquard syndrome is hemisection of the spinal cord. The plantar reflex is a painful stimulus and therefore is transmitted by the spinothalamic tract on the contralateral side. Temperature sensation is also transmitted via the spinothalamic tract. All other tracts lie on the ipsilateral side within the spinal cord.

Long Explanation

Brown-Séquard syndrome is hemisection of the spinal cord, involving the contralateral spinothalamic tract and all other tracts on the ipsilateral side. This is a rare syndrome resulting in ipsilateral hemiplegia with contralateral pain and temperature sensation deficits due to the spinothalamic tract crossing the midline within the spinal cord.

The plantar reflex is a painful stimulus, and absence of a response means the stimulus has not been transmitted. The plantar reflex itself is used to determine spinal or cranial pathology. Extensor plantar response means the stimulus has been transmitted by an intact spinothalamic tracts but it is abnormal due to pyramidal tract damage on the ipsilateral side.

Vibration sensation and proprioception are transmitted via the dorsal column, and therefore loss of these sensors would be on the ipsilateral side. This would also cause spastic paraparesis and brisk reflexes below the lesion on the same side. At the level of the lesion on the ipsilateral side there is loss of pain and temperature due to the

189

spinothalamic tract entering the cord and travelling ipsilaterally for a few segments before crossing the midline and travelling on the contralateral side.

There are many causes of Brown-Séquard syndrome, including tumour, trauma, ischaemia, infection, multiple sclerosis. Penetrating injury such as stabbing or gunshot wound is the most common cause. MRI is the investigation of choice to confirm clinical findings. Treatment depends on what is causing the Brown-Séquard syndrome.

Beeson MS. Brown-Séquard syndrome in emergency medicine. *Medscape Reference* 2011. Available online at emedicine.medscape.com/article/791539 (accessed 30 June 2012).

Börm W, Bohnstedt T. Intradural cervical disc herniation: case report and review of the literature. *J Neurosurg* 2000; **92**: 221–4.

MTF Question 54: Splenic rupture

Regarding traumatic splenic injury:

a) Vaccination against pneumococcus is recommended at 3 months post injury
b) Lifelong antibiotics are no longer recommended, because of the risk of multiresistance
c) The splenic artery supplies the stomach as well as the spleen
d) Fluid above the left kidney at ultrasound suggests a splenic injury
e) Hypotension at presentation is an indication for urgent laparotomy

Answer: c, d

Short Explanation

Vaccinations should be given at 14 days. Antibiotics are still recommended. A laparotomy can often be avoided in patients (even if hypotensive at presentation) who respond to fluids.

Long Explanation

Trauma to the spleen is common in blunt abdominal trauma. In adults it is frequently associated with rib fractures, but in children the spleen is lower and the ribs softer and it often occurs without fractures. The spleen is supplied by the splenic artery (off the coeliac trunk) which then also supplies part of the stomach. It takes approximately 5% of the cardiac output, and isolated splenic injury can be fatal and needs appropriate management.

Treatment options include conservative, radiographic and surgical. Ultrasonography (FAST scan) cannot identify the source of abdominal bleeding, but detection of fluid between the left kidney and spleen is suggestive of splenic injury. Initial hypotension is not in itself an indication for laparotomy, as a significant proportion of patients will respond to initial fluids. Where expertise is available, radiographic embolisation can often be used to avoid laparotomy.

If patients do require splenectomy they then become partially immunocompromised. They are at risk from encapsulated bacteria (e.g. pneumococcus, *Haemophilus influenzae*, meningococcus). Vaccination is recommended against these organisms, at 14 days post injury (delayed because the immune response may be damped immediately post injury). Three months post injury may be too late. Antibiotics are recommended post splenectomy, and the benefits outweigh the risk of multiresistance. Lifelong daily penicillin is a suitable choice, although compliance is often poor. Yearly influenza vaccination is also advocated, to reduce the risk of secondary bacterial infections.

Bjerke HS. Splenic rupture. *Medscape Reference* 2009. Available online at emedicine. medscape.com/article/432823-overview (accessed 30 June 2012).

MTF Question 55: Gender and pain

Regarding the differences between the sexes in chronic pain conditions:

a) Women of reproductive age have higher opioid binding than men of a similar age
b) Men are at greater risk of chronic pain than women as they complain about pain less
c) Women have greater pain tolerance than men
d) Chronic pelvic pain is a female-specific pain syndrome
e) Amitriptyline has an increased volume of distribution in women compared to men

Answer: a, e

Short Explanation
Women of reproductive age are more sensitive to opioids. Men self-report pain less than women, but this does not necessarily mean their risk of developing chronic pain is different. Women have demonstrable lower tolerance to pain than men. Chronic pelvic pain affects both sexes. Amitriptyline is highly lipid-soluble, and therefore has a higher volume of distribution (V_D) in women, who have a larger percentage of fat than men.

Long Explanation
Both gender and age influence μ-opioid (MOP) receptor agonist binding, as can be measured by positron emission tomography (PET). Women have higher opioid binding during their reproductive years and are more sensitive to opioids during this time. There are also differences in central nervous system MOP receptor binding in men and women. Women metabolise morphine differently to men, and exhibit greater opioid analgesia.

Social and cultural expectation affects pain reporting and seeking help from healthcare services. Men are less likely to complain of pain than women, and the pain history must be sensitive to this; a man is less likely to be as detailed as a woman, and disclosure needs to be encouraged. There is good evidence to suggest that females exhibit greater sensitivity to noxious stimuli and lower tolerance than males, while other studies suggest that women are better at coping with discomfort in the long term.

Chronic pelvic pain relating to the reproductive tract can affect both sexes. Women are more likely to present to gynaecology services before chronic pain services, with menstrual uterine cyclical problems or muscular pelvic pain after childbirth, whereas men are more likely to present with trauma-induced pain.

Tricyclic antidepressants such as amitriptyline are highly lipid-soluble. Women have a greater percentage of body fat than men, and lipid-soluble drugs will therefore have a higher volume of distribution (V_D) in females.

Baranowski A, Holdcroft A. Gender and pain. In: Holdcroft A, Jaggar S, eds., *Core Topics in Pain*. Cambridge: Cambridge University Press, 2005; pp. 195–200.

MTF Question 56: Invasive blood-pressure monitoring

Regarding invasive blood-pressure monitoring, which of the following statements are true?

a) A smaller cannula will lead to increased resonance
b) The transducer must be zeroed at the site of the catheter
c) The presence of air bubbles in the system leads to a damping effect
d) A low dicrotic notch is seen in sepsis
e) A damping value of 0.8 will lead to an elevated diastolic blood pressure reading

Answer: c, d, e

Short Explanation

Smaller cannulas can lead to increased damping of the signal. The transducer is zeroed at the level of the patient's right atrium, regardless of catheter position. Overdamping leads to decreased systolic and increased diastolic pressures.

Long Explanation

Classically 20G cannulas are used in adults, 22G in children and 24G in neonates. Larger cannulas increase the risk of distal thrombosis, while smaller cannulas lead to damping of the signal as the natural frequency of the system is directly related to catheter diameter.

The other factors determining the natural frequency of the system include the system compliance, compliance and length of tubing, and the density of the fluid in the system. Normally a continuous column of saline pressurised to 300 mmHg is contained within the system and will fluctuate against a diaphragm in the transducer with the pressure-wave changes in the artery. The presence of air or clot within the system increases the system compliance and causes a damping effect.

The arterial waveform seen on the monitor is the result of the summation of a series of sine waves of different amplitudes and frequencies. The system is said to be optimally damped at a damping value of 0.64. Increased resonance leads to higher systolic and lower diastolic values, and the opposite is true in the case of increased damping. In both instances the mean arterial pressure remains accurate.

The system should be zeroed at the level of the patient's right atrium. Above or below this level, a relative error of 7.6 mmHg for every 10 cm will occur. Adjusting for level, there is usually less than 10 mmHg difference in blood pressure between the major arteries in the body. This difference can become greater in conditions such as severe arteriosclerosis or coarctation of the aorta.

The dicrotic notch on the waveform represents pressure changes due to closure of the aortic valve.

In the vasodilated patient (sympathetic blockade, sepsis) it lies in a low position on the downstroke of the wave; in the vasoconstricted patient (excessive catecholamines) it lies higher.

Al-Shaikh B, Stacey S. *Essentials of Anaesthetic Equipment*, 2nd edn. London. Churchill Livingstone, 2002; pp. 134–5

MTF Question 57: Sacral plexus anatomy

Regarding the sacral plexus:

a) The sciatic nerve exits the pelvis via the greater sciatic notch
b) The superior gluteal nerve supplies gluteus maximus
c) The lateral cutaneous nerve of the thigh arises from the sacral plexus
d) The sciatic nerve only innervates muscles distal to the popliteal fossa
e) The inferior gluteal nerve supplies semitendinosus and semimembranosus

Answer: a

Short Explanation

The superior gluteal nerve supplies gluteus medius, gluteus minimus and tensor fascia lata. The inferior gluteal nerve supplies gluteus maximus. Proximal to the popliteal fossa, the sciatic nerve innervates the hamstring muscles. The lateral cutaneous nerve of the thigh is a branch of the lumbar plexus, L2 and L3.

Long Explanation

The sacral plexus arises from the nerve roots of L4, L5 and S1–S3 and gives rise to five nerves.

The sciatic nerve is the major nerve, arising from these same five nerve roots. It exits the pelvis via the greater sciatic notch and passes into the posterior thigh midway between the greater trochanter of the femur and the ischial tuberosity. In the thigh, it gives off motor branches to the hamstring muscles: semimembranosus, semitendinosus, biceps femoris and adductor magnus. Distal to this it divides into the common peroneal and tibial nerves in the upper pole of the popliteal fossa, which go on to supply the lower leg.

Of the remaining four nerves of the sacral plexus, two supply motor innervations: the superior gluteal nerve (L4, L5 and S1) supplying gluteus medius, gluteus minimus and tensor fascia lata, and the inferior gluteal nerve (L5, S1 and S2) supplying gluteus maximus. The two remaining nerves supply sensory innervation to the skin of the posterior thigh, these being the posterior cutaneous nerve of the thigh (S1–S3) and the perforating cutaneous nerve of the thigh (S2 and S3). Note that the lateral cutaneous nerve of the thigh is a branch of the lumbar plexus and arises from L2 and L3.

Erdmann AG. *Concise Anatomy for Anaesthesia*. Cambridge: Cambridge University Press, 2009; pp. 56–67.
Leslie RA, Johnson EK, Thomas G, Goodwin APL. *Dr Podcast Scripts for the Final FRCA*. Cambridge: Cambridge University Press, 2011; pp. 449–51.

MTF Question 58: Lower limb blocks

Regarding the lumbar plexus block:

a) The block provides good analgesia for a fractured neck of femur
b) To perform the block, the patient lies in the prone position
c) The needle insertion point is where Tuffier's line crosses a line drawn parallel to the spinous processes passing through the posterior superior iliac spine
d) The standard needle depth to the lumbar plexus is 8–12 cm
e) If the hamstring muscles are stimulated, the needle is too medial

Answer: a, c, d, e

Short Explanation

The patient should be in the lateral position for the block to be performed, with the operative side uppermost.

Long Explanation

The lumbar plexus is formed from the anterior primary rami of L1–L4, with a significant proportion of the population having contributions from T12 or L5. It lies posterior and lateral to the psoas muscle and fascia and gives rise to six main nerves:

- The iliohypogastric nerve arises from L1 and supplies sensation to the suprapubic skin.
- The ilioinguinal nerve also arises from L1 and supplies sensation to the skin of the upper thigh, root of the penis or mons pubis and of the scrotum or labia.
- The genitofemoral nerve arises from L1 and L2 and has two branches, the genital branch, which supplies the cremaster muscle and sensation to the scrotal skin or mons pubis and labia, and the femoral branch, which supplies the skin over the upper femoral triangle.
- The lateral cutaneous nerve of the thigh arises from L2 and L3 and supplies sensation to the lateral thigh.

- The obturator nerve arises from L2–L4 and supplies sensation to the medial thigh, hip and knee joints as well as motor innervation to the adductors of the hip (adductor longus, brevis and magnus, gracilis and external obturator).
- The femoral nerve also arises from L2–L4 and supplies motor innervation to iliacus, pectineus, sartorius and the quadriceps muscles of the thigh. It also supplies sensation to the hip joint, anterior thigh and medial aspect of the lower leg.

To block the lumbar plexus directly, a lumbar plexus block (also known as a psoas compartment block) can be performed. With the patient in the lateral position, the side to be blocked uppermost, a line is drawn parallel to the spinous processes passing through the posterior superior iliac spine. Where this line is intersected by Tuffier's line (a line connecting the iliac crests) the needle is inserted perpendicular to the skin. If the transverse process of the vertebra is encountered, the needle is re-angled to pass above or below it.

The standard depth to the plexus is usually between 8 and 12 cm, where approximately 0.5 mL/kg (a maximum of 30 mL) of local anaesthetic is injected. Correct needle placement is when contraction of the quadriceps tendon (patella twitch) is seen. If the hamstrings are stimulated then the needle is too medial or caudad. Complications of this block include absorption toxicity due to the block being primarily an intramuscular injection, renal injury, retroperitoneal haematoma and accidental epidural spread leading to bilateral sympathetic, motor and sensory block.

Leslie RA, Johnson EK, Thomas G, Goodwin APL. *Dr Podcast Scripts for the Final FRCA*. Cambridge: Cambridge University Press, 2011; pp. 446–9.

Nicholls B, Conn D, Roberts A. *The Abbott Pocket Guide to Practical Peripheral Nerve Blockade*. Abbott Anaesthesia, 2007; pp. 68–9.

MTF Question 59: Fixed-performance oxygen therapy devices

Which of the following are true regarding the use of high air flow oxygen enrichment (HAFOE) devices to deliver a fixed fractional inspired concentration of oxygen (FiO_2)?

a) Air entrainment through mask side holes helps determine delivered FiO_2
b) Gas flow must exceed peak inspiratory flow rate
c) A predetermined oxygen flow rate is required to give the desired FiO_2
d) They have no contribution to dead space
e) Re-breathing does not occur

Answer: b, c, d, e

Short Explanation

HAFOE devices entrain a predetermined volume of air through the Venturi gas flow inlet. The side holes on the mask are to vent exhaled gases.

Long Explanation

Fixed-performance oxygen delivery systems act independently of the patient's inspiratory and respiratory rate to deliver a predetermined fixed fractional inspired concentration of oxygen (FiO_2). These devices can be low flow, such as the Hudson mask with reservoir, or high flow. High air-flow devices such as the Venturi mask act by delivering a flow that exceeds the patient's peak inspiratory flow, and therefore air entrainment does not occur through the side holes of the mask to dilute the FiO_2.

Therefore, the predetermined FiO_2 of the high-flow gas is not affected by the patient's respiratory pattern and this concentration is delivered to the airway. For this to work, the gas flow must exceed the patient's peak inspiratory flow rate, which can be as much as 40 L/min. As most oxygen supplies only deliver a maximum 15 L/min, the flow rate must be increased somehow. The Venturi mask utilises the Bernoulli principle whereby the air flows through a constriction in the tubing at the inlet to the mask. As the air flow (kinetic energy) increases to pass through the constriction, the pressure falls (potential energy) distal to the constriction as the total energy (kinetic plus potential energy) must stay the same. If the tubing is open distal to the constriction, entrainment of ambient air occurs into the gas flow.

The Venturi mask has colour-coded attachments to connect the oxygen tubing to the mask. The attachments have different-sized constrictions (to determine flow) and apertures (to determine air entrainment), which determine the final delivered concentration of oxygen. The attachment is colour-coded for a specific FiO_2 and is marked with the flow required to deliver that FiO_2. The high air flow flushes exhaled gases through the mask side holes and rapidly fills the mask, so no re-breathing occurs, and as a result there is no functional dead space in the mask.

Ely J, Clapham M. Delivering oxygen to patients. *Br J Anaesth CEPD Rev* 2003; **3**: 43–5. Available online at ceacep.oxfordjournals.org/content/3/2/43 (accessed 30 June 2012).

MTF Question 60: Hypnosis

Which of the following statements concerning the use of hypnosis and imagery-based psychological interventions in pain management are correct?

a) These interventions are contraindicated in personality disorder and psychosis
b) There is no evidence for their use in chronic pain management
c) They are relaxation techniques only and not associated with adverse effects
d) They are useful in the management of acute postoperative pain
e) They are not helpful in pain associated with malignancy

Answer: a, d

Short Explanation
Adverse events are infrequent but can occur when therapy is not guided by a skilled therapist. Trance-like states encourage introspective focus, which is best avoided in severe mental illness. Pre-treatment with hypnosis can reduce the experience of acute pain associated with elective orthopaedic, bowel and gynaecological surgery, and with malignant disease. Imagery has been shown to help in the management of complex regional pain syndrome and phantom limb pain.

Long Explanation
Hypnosis, which induces a state of focused concentration and suspended peripheral awareness, allows the patient to experience relaxation, suggestibility, disassociation and altered perception of time and space. A trained therapist can lead the patient verbally to a calm and peaceful state of awareness. The aim of this therapy to is focus the attention away from the source of distress, such as pain or disease, and facilitate a healing process or develop skills which help patients cope with worrying symptoms and fears.

Imagery is a less passive form of hypnosis. Patients are encouraged to divert their attention away from upsetting symptoms or unhelpful thought patterns which limit function due to fear of pain (fear-avoidance behaviour) and instead to associate themselves, or a particular body part, with an image of health, strength, safety and capability. These theories are often combined with acceptance-based cognitive behavioural therapy techniques. These are psychological interventions aiming to challenge negative thought patterns while accepting that the condition 'has no cure'. The aim is to provide patients with realistic goal-setting skills and re-establish lost values, which often occur with chronic disease and pain conditions.

Beneficial results utilising imagery have been shown in the management of complex regional pain syndrome and phantom limb pain. Cancer pain management and acute procedural pain (e.g. bone marrow biopsy) in adults and children are an important area for the potential impact of the hypnosis practitioner. Several good quality randomised controlled trials have shown that patients can reduce their experience of pain, anxiety and distress when pre-treated with hypnosis or guided image therapy.

Similarly, attention control techniques (also known as mindfulness) learned during guided hypnosis or imagery sessions have been shown to reduce pain experiences associated with elective colorectal, gynaecological and orthopaedic surgery, and in burns management, with lower consumption of analgesia postoperatively and during procedures such as dressing changes.

Adverse affects of hypnosis and imagery are infrequent when therapies are delivered by a skilled practitioner, but the introspective nature of these methods means that they are generally contraindicated for treating patients with severe mental illness, psychotic states and personality disorders. Reports of false memories generated in the trance state, and the revelation of repressed memories, can lead to considerable psychological distress and harm to the patient.

Ernst, E, Pittler M, Wider B, eds. *Complementary Therapies for Pain Management: an Evidence-Based Approach*. London: Mosby, 2007.

Keefe FJ, Somers TJ, Abernethy A.. Psychologic interventions for cancer pain. In: Stannard C, Kalso E, Ballantyne E, eds., *Evidence-Based Chronic Pain Management*. Oxford: Blackwell, 2010; pp. 337–47.

McCracken LM, Carson JW, Eccleston C, Keefe FJ. Acceptance and change in the context of chronic pain. *Pain* 2004; **109**: 4–7.

SBA Question 61: Neuromuscular monitoring

With regard to the use of a nerve stimulator for monitoring neuromuscular function following administration of a non-depolarising muscle relaxant, the following statements are true, EXCEPT for which one?

Answers
a) Satisfactory recovery from neuromuscular block has not occurred until the train-of-four (TOF) ratio is > 0.9
b) The train-of-four count should be at least 3 before administering a neuromuscular antagonist
c) The use of a nerve stimulator is contraindicated in a patient with myotonic dystrophy
d) It is preferable for a nerve stimulator to deliver a constant current, rather than a constant voltage
e) Double-burst stimulation allows detection of small degrees of residual neuromuscular block

Answer: c

Short Explanation
Myotonic dystrophy is characterised by difficulty with initiating muscular contraction and delayed relaxation. A nerve stimulator is not contraindicated in myotonia but the response to stimulation needs careful interpretation as muscle stimulation may trigger myotonic contraction. This might share the appearance of tetany and recovery from neuromuscular blockade might incorrectly be assumed to have occurred.

Long Explanation

Residual neuromuscular block is common and can adversely affect patient outcome. There are a number of methods available to the anaesthetist to monitor neuromuscular block and to assess the degree of recovery.

Using a nerve stimulator can help the anaesthetist detect optimal conditions for intubation at induction, monitor the degree of neuromuscular blockade during maintenance of anaesthesia, and assess the suitability for administration of a reversal agent at the end of an operation. Neuromuscular monitoring should be used routinely when a neuromuscular blocking drug is given.

A nerve stimulator works by applying a supramaximal stimulus to a peripheral nerve and then measuring the associated response. An electrical current is applied transcutaneously to stimulate the nerve, aiming to generate an action potential in all the nerve fibres within a motor nerve. The current applied is typically 25% above the stimulus needed to produce a maximal muscular contraction, hence the term supramaximal stimulus.

Ideally, the nerve stimulator should be able to deliver a constant current up to 80 mA. This is preferable to a nerve stimulator that can only deliver a constant voltage because it is current magnitude that determines whether a nerve depolarises or not. If a constant voltage is used, the current will vary depending on the resistance of the skin (Ohm's law, $V = IR$).

The negative electrode is placed directly over the most superficial part of the nerve, and the positive electrode is placed proximally along the course of the nerve. The nerve stimulator should then be capable of delivering a variety of patterns of stimulation, the response to which will vary depending on the pattern of stimulation used, the type of drug used to produce neuromuscular block, and the degree of neuromuscular blockade.

Myotonic dystrophy is characterised by difficulty with initiating muscular contraction and delayed relaxation. Suxamethonium should always be avoided in these patients, and if necessary neuromuscular blockade can be achieved with short-acting non-depolarising neuromuscular blockers. A reduced dose should be used, as there is increased sensitivity to these agents.

McGrath CD, Hunter JM. Monitoring of neuromuscular block. *Contin Educ Anaesth Crit Care Pain* 2006; **6**: 7–12. Available online at ceaccp.oxfordjournals.org/content/6/1/7 (accessed 30 June 2012).

SBA Question 62: Sugammadex

Which of the following doses of sugammadex should be used to reverse neuromuscular blockade in an 85 kg man who received 100 mg of rocuronium bromide 3 minutes ago?

a) 170 mg
b) 340 mg
c) 680 mg
d) 1360 mg
e) 2720 mg

Answer: d

Short Explanation

Administration of 16.0 mg/kg sugammadex 3 minutes following a bolus dose of 1.2 mg/kg rocuronium bromide provides a median time to recovery of the T4/T1 ratio to 0.9 of approximately 1.5 minutes.

Long Explanation

Sugammadex is a modified γ-cyclodextrin which binds with the steroidal neuromuscular blocking drugs. In binding in a 1:1 ratio with these drugs within the plasma, it establishes an effective concentration gradient, causing movement of the neuromuscular blocking agent away from the neuromuscular junction. It can be used to reverse partial or dense neuromuscular blockade in a dose-dependent fashion as follows:

Routine reversal

- 4.0 mg/kg sugammadex is recommended if recovery has reached 1–2 post-tetanic counts following rocuronium or vecuronium-induced blockade. Median time to recovery of the T4/T1 ratio to 0.9 is around 3 minutes.
- 2.0 mg/kg sugammadex is recommended if spontaneous recovery has occurred up to the appearance of T2 following rocuronium- or vecuronium-induced blockade. Median time to recovery of the T4/T1 ratio to 0.9 is around 2 minutes.

Immediate reversal

- If there is a clinical need for immediate reversal following administration of rocuronium, a dose of 16.0 mg/kg sugammadex is recommended. Administration of 16.0 mg/kg sugammadex 3 minutes following a bolus dose of 1.2 mg/kg rocuronium bromide provides a median time to recovery of the T4/T1 ratio to 0.9 of approximately 1.5 minutes.

Product information on sugammadex (Bridion) can be found online at www.medicines.org.uk/EMC/medicine/21299/SPC/Bridion (accessed 30 June 2012).
Naguib M. Sugammadex: another milestone in clinical neuromuscular pharmacology. *Anesth Analg* 2007; **104**: 575–81.

SBA Question 63: Fluid resuscitation

A previously healthy 64-year-old has presented with pneumonia and septic shock. He is hypotensive, with a serum lactate level of 6 mmol/L. He appears dehydrated. Which of the following statements is LEAST CORRECT regarding his fluid therapy?

a) Correct fluid therapy will reduce his mortality
b) Early fluid therapy should be limited to 4 L to reduce the risk of acute respiratory distress syndrome (ARDS) and pulmonary oedema
c) Central venous pressure (CVP) should be used to help guide fluid therapy
d) Serial lactate concentrations will help guide fluid therapy
e) There is a place for blood products during fluid resuscitation from septic shock

Answer: b

Short Explanation

Patients with severe sepsis may require considerable volumes for adequate early resuscitation, and predetermined limits on these are unlikely to be helpful. Correct fluid therapy can reduce mortality, and should be guided by physiological targets.

Long Explanation

In a classic paper from 2001, Rivers *et al.* demonstrated a significant reduction in the mortality of severe sepsis through implementation of a goal-directed early resuscitation protocol. Although the paper and exact protocol has been criticised, it has demonstrated that correct early fluid therapy can reduce the mortality of severe sepsis, and that using physiological goals to guide fluid therapy can be helpful.

The protocol specified use of central venous pressure (CVP) to determine response to boluses of crystalloid. Central venous oxygen saturations were measured, and used to further guide fluid and inotropic therapy, with low central venous saturations despite a lack of rise in CVP in response to a fluid bolus being an indication to start inotropes. In the presence of anaemia and failure to achieve physiological targets despite apparently adequate volume of fluid administration, red cell transfusion should be considered.

Lactate concentrations have a use in guiding fluid therapy. Once an adequate perfusion is restored, the lactate should start to fall. The problem with using this to guide therapy is that firstly serum lactate concentration may depend on more than just volume status (in sepsis, microvascular compromise may cause ongoing tissue hypoxia despite restoration of circulating volume), and secondly the lactate fall will be delayed, so relying on serial lactate measurements will tend to slow resuscitation.

Patients with severe sepsis may require significant volumes of fluid, as they may start dehydrated, and have ongoing fluid losses into the interstitium. It is therefore not helpful to set limits to the volume to be administered in advance. However, it is true that excessive fluid administration is associated with development of acute respiratory distress syndrome (ARDS), so volume resuscitation needs to be targeted rather than excessive.

Rivers E, Nguyen B, Havstad S, *et al.*; Early Goal-Directed Therapy Collaborative Group. Early goal-directed therapy in the treatment of severe sepsis and septic shock. *N Engl J Med* 2001; **345**: 1368–77.

SBA Question 64: Rhabdomyolysis

A 34-year-old man is admitted to the emergency department after being found trapped under a tractor for several hours. Both his legs have been crushed and are now very swollen. His urine is dark. Which one of the following is the most important step in his management?

a) He should have delayed fasciotomies to prevent the sudden release of myoglobin
b) He needs to have a bicarbonate infusion to alkalinise his urine and prevent myoglobin precipitation
c) He needs to have a mannitol infusion to induce a diuresis and prevent myoglobin deposition
d) He should have immediate angiography to determine which parts of his legs are viable
e) He should be given a 0.9% saline infusion sufficient to induce a diuresis

Answer: e

Short Explanation
The key priority is to resuscitate and achieve a diuresis with 0.9% saline. Fasciotomies may be required but should not be delayed, as muscle injury may increase. There are theoretical benefits to both bicarbonate (alkalinisation) and mannitol (diuresis), but neither has shown improved outcome compared to 0.9% saline. It is important to avoid other renal insults such as intravenous contrast.

Long Explanation
Rhabdomyolysis is the breakdown of striated muscle and the release of intracellular constituents into the circulation, including potassium, myoglobin and haem (pigment). The clinical picture includes hyperkaelemia (and associated arrhythmias), hepatic injury (due to protease release), acute kidney injury (acute tubular necrosis) and disseminated intravascular coagulation. There are a number of causes of

rhabdomyolysis including muscle trauma (crush, immobility), muscle ischaemia, excessive muscle activity (sport), drugs (amphetamine, chlorpromazine) and hyperthermia. Renal failure occurs in 20–50% of cases of rhabdomyolysis and is due to dehydration, haem toxicity and myoglobin causing tubular cast formation.

Rhabdomyolysis should be suspected if the history suggests possible muscle injury. Urine is typically discoloured, from pink to dark brown ('cola' coloured). Diagnosis is confirmed by elevated serum creatine kinase and urine myoglobin.

Management of rhabdomyolysis is largely supportive. Further muscle damage must be prevented by appropriate surgery as needed. There is no evidence that delaying surgery is protective, and it is likely to cause further injury. Additional renal insults should be avoided, and intravenous contrast is likely to worsen renal failure. Aggressive fluid resuscitation should be used both to prevent dehydration and to induce a diuresis. Bicarbonate has been advocated to induce an alkaline urine, which reduces cast formation. Mannitol induces a diuresis and its free-radical scavenging effect may be renal-protective. Although advocated by some, neither mannitol nor bicarbonate has been shown to improve outcome compared to aggressive 0.9% saline resuscitation.

Prognosis is variable (10–80% mortality, depending on series). Dialysis-dependent renal failure increases mortality to 20% and multi-organ failure to > 50%. Despite this, if the patient survives the prognosis for renal recovery is excellent.

Huerta-Aiardfn AL, Varon J, Marik PE. Bench-to-bedside review: rhabdomyolysis. An overview for clinicians. *Crit Care* 2005; **9**: 158–69. Available online at ccforum. com/content/9/2/158 (accessed 30 June 2012).

SBA Question 65: Preoperative fasting

Regarding fasting for elective surgery, which of the following patients is most appropriately starved for theatre?

a) A patient who has just drunk 500 mL of water 2 hours before surgery
b) A patient who is chewing gum 4 hours before surgery
c) A patient who has eaten a hamburger 6 hours before surgery
d) A patient eating a boiled sweet 4 hours before surgery
e) A patient who has drunk 500 mL of lemonade 2 hours before surgery

Answer: a

Short Explanation

Residual gastric volume and pH are unaffected by the volume of clear fluid ingested up to 2 hours prior to surgery. Patients should be fasted for 6 hours following a light meal, longer for fatty food. Sweets are considered to be food, and chewing gum should not be allowed on the day of surgery. Residual carbonated liquid may delay diagnosis of an oesophageal intubation.

Long Explanation

The purpose of preoperative fasting is to ensure minimal residual gastric volume at induction of anaesthesia. It is incorrect to think of the stomach as full or empty, because even starved patients have some residual gastric content. The risk of aspiration is dependent on the volume and pH of fluid aspirated. Studies on rhesus monkeys involving the direct instillation of gastric contents into the right main bronchus have led to the assertion that patients are at risk of aspiration with a residual gastric volume of 25 mL with a pH < 2.5.

Guidelines for preoperative fasting recommend the following periods for adult patients: 6 hours for a light meal and 2 hours for clear liquids. The mantra 'nil by mouth from midnight' has no place in modern anaesthetic practice. There is no evidence that unrestricted fluid intake up to 2 hours prior to surgery increases gastric volume, lowers gastric pH or affects lower oesophageal sphincter tone. In fact there is evidence that shorter fast times reduce gastric volume and increase gastric pH. Gastric emptying for fluid is an exponential process, and the half-time for water is approximately 10 minutes. Gastric emptying for solids is constant, and starts 1 hour after a meal. Fatty or fried foods prolong gastric emptying, and fasting is recommended for 8 hours or more.

Chewing gum should not be permitted on the day of surgery, based on a small but statistically significant increase in gastric volume in patients included in a meta-analysis. Sweets and lollipops are considered to be solid food in published guidelines. The American Society of Anesthesiologists considers carbonated drinks to be acceptable as clear fluids, but the potential for late detection of oesophageal intubation because of the presence in the stomach of carbon dioxide from the lemonade means that the first of the five options is the best.

American Society of Anesthesiologists. Practice guidelines for preoperative fasting and the use of pharmacologic agents to reduce the risk of pulmonary aspiration: application to healthy patients undergoing elective procedures. *Anesthesiology* 2011; **114**: 495–511.

Levy DM. Preoperative fasting: 60 years on from Mendelson. *Contin Educ Anaesth Crit Care Pain* 2009; **9**: 10–13. Available online at ceaccp.oxfordjournals.org/content/6/6/215 (accessed 30 June 2012).

Royal College of Nursing. Perioperative fasting in adults and children. An RCN guideline for the multidisciplinary team, November 2005. Available online at www.rcn.org.uk/_data/assets/pdf_file/0009/78678/002800.pdf (accessed 30 June 2012).

SBA Question 66: Gastro-oesophageal reflux

A man presents for elective knee arthroscopy with a history of regular acid indigestion for which he uses over-the-counter antacid remedies. During your preoperative assessment he describes waterbrash on bending forward, and tells you that he sleeps propped up in bed due to reflux symptoms. What would be the most appropriate premedication to administer?

a) Metoclopramide 10 mg orally 2 hours prior to induction
b) Ranitidine 150 mg orally 2 hours prior to induction
c) Rabeprazole 20 mg orally 2 hours prior to induction
d) Sodium citrate 0.3 M 30 mL orally prior to induction
e) Omeprazole 20 mg orally the night before and the morning of surgery

Answer: b

Short Explanation

Both H$_2$ antagonists and proton-pump inhibitors (PPIs) reduce gastric volume and increase pH, but a meta-analysis has shown that ranitidine is more effective. PPIs work best given in two doses, but that would require cancellation of the operation. Sodium citrate would increase gastric volume. Metoclopramide has not been studied in patients with gastro-oesophageal reflux.

Long Explanation

Acid aspiration syndrome (AAS) is a rare but potentially serious complication of anaesthesia. The risk of an episode of aspiration depends on the volume aspirated, the presence of particulate matter and the pH of the aspirate. The top factors predisposing to aspiration in the Australian Anaesthetic Incident Monitoring Study were non-elective surgery, inadequate depth of anaesthesia, acute or chronic gastrointestinal pathology, obesity, neurological disease, impaired conscious level, sedation, opioid medication, lithotomy position, difficult intubation or airway, gastro-oesophageal reflux and hiatus hernia.

Prevention of AAS involves preoperative fasting, use of rapid sequence induction and administering agents that increase gastric pH and reduce gastric volume. Acid aspiration is a rare event, and routine use of pharmacological agents is not recommended; treatment should be reserved for at-risk patients. No comparison studies exist on the effect of agents in patients with gastro-oesophageal reflux, so the data are extrapolated from studies of gastric contents in healthy patients and obstetrics. Practice recommendations have been made by the Royal College of Nursing and the American Society of Anesthesiologists.

Metoclopramide is effective in reducing gastric volume and increasing pH in pregnant patients studied prior to caesarean section; no studies exist in patients with gastro-oesophageal reflux. Sodium citrate is effective in raising gastric pH but will increase gastric volume and have no effect on lower oesophageal sphincter (LOS) tone.

Compared head to head, ranitidine (an H_2 antagonist) is more effective than proton-pump inhibitors (PPIs) in increasing gastric pH and reducing gastric volume. PPIs are most effective given in two doses (the night before and the morning of surgery). However, a single dose of an H_2 antagonist is as effective as two doses of any of the PPIs included in the meta-analysis (omeprazole, lansoprazole and rabeprazole).

Clark K, Lam LT, Gibson S, Currow D. The effect of ranitidine versus proton pump inhibitors on gastric secretions: a meta-analysis of randomised controlled trials. *Anaesthesia* 2009; **64**: 652–7.

Ng A, Smith G. Gastroesophageal reflux and aspiration of gastric contents in anesthetic practice. *Anesth Analg* 2001; **93**: 494–513.

SBA Question 67: Bacterial translocation

Which ONE of the following measures to improve gastrointestinal integrity in critically ill polytrauma patients has been shown to reduce both septic complications and mortality?

a) Early enteral nutrition with glutamine supplementation
b) Arginine
c) Oropharyngeal decontamination
d) Probiotics
e) Dopexamine

Answer: a

Short Explanation
While all of the above measures have been shown to have a beneficial effect on gut barrier function and/or reduction in septic complications, only early enteral nutrition with glutamine supplementation has been shown to reduce mortality.

Long Explanation
Breakdown of gastrointestinal (GI) barrier function has been associated with bacterial translocation, whereby viable bacteria and their antigens access mesenteric lymph nodes and portal and systemic circulations. The pathogenesis of bacterial translocation in critical illness involves splanchnic hypoperfusion, ischaemia–reperfusion injury and pro-inflammatory responses in the GI tract.

Many therapeutic measures to reduce bacterial translocation and septic complications in critical care patients have been tried and tested, and while many have beneficial effects few have been demonstrated to improve outcome. But early enteral nutrition started within 24–72 hours of ICU admission is widely accepted to reduce mortality. Adequate nutritional intake should be maintained by whatever means. However, the enteral route is cheaper, easier, safer and more physiological, maintaining GI function.

Glutamine is a conditionally essential amino acid, important in the catabolic state of critical illness. An essential fuel for rapidly dividing cells including gut epithelium and gut-associated lymphoid tissue, it also has trophic effect on enterocytes and helps maintain gut integrity under conditions of stress. Both enteral and parenteral nutritional supplementation with glutamine have been associated with improved outcomes and reduced length of stay in select groups, particularly trauma and burns patients. Other immunomodulatory enteral feed supplements have been studied. Most have failed to show benefit, and in fact arginine has been associated with increased mortality in severe sepsis, which may reflect its mechanism of action as a precursor of nitric oxide synthase.

The administration of topical oral antimicrobial agents (selective orophayrngeal decontamination, or SOD) with or without the administration of short-term systemic preparations (selective decontamination of the digestive tract, or SDD) has been trialled as a means of reducing sepsis from enteric bacteria. These regimes aim to 'selectively' reduce pathogenic Gram-negative microbes in preference to commensal organisms. Current evidence suggests that only SDD reduces mortality (OR 0.75, NNT 17). SOD impacts on the incidence of respiratory infections without an effect on survival.

Probiotics have been shown to improve gut transit and microbial balance, reducing the prevalence of potentially pathogenic bacteria in the upper GI tract. However, there are no clinical data to suggest improved outcome.

Attenuating the ischaemia–reperfusion injury by maintaining adequate gut perfusion and oxygen delivery seems intuitive. In addition to early resuscitation, avoidance of hypovolaemia and maintenance of an adequate cardiac output, various inotropic agents have been investigated for their selective vasodilatory properties. Dopexamine has been found to increase splanchnic blood flow and increase intramucosal pH in sepsis and critical illness, but no mortality benefit has been demonstrated.

Gatt M, Reddy BS, Macfie J. Bacterial translocation in the critically ill: evidence and methods of prevention. *Aliment Pharmacol Ther* 2007; **25**: 741–57.
Liberati A, D'Amico R, Pifferi S, *et al.* (2009) Antibiotic prophylaxis to reduce respiratory tract infections and mortality in adults receiving intensive care. *Cochrane Database Syst Rev* 2009; (4): CD000022.
Guidelines available at www.criticalcarenutrition.com (accessed).

SBA Question 68: Transfusion triggers

Which of the following is NOT an evidence-based transfusion trigger?

a) Hb 10 g/dL in a patient with active bleeding
b) Hb 7 g/dL in a haemodynamically stable resuscitated trauma patient
c) Hct > 30% in the early resuscitation phase of severe sepsis
d) Hb 12 g/dL in a patient with evidence of myocardial ischaemia
e) Hb 7 g/dL in a long-term ventilated patient with a history of stable cardiac disease

Answer: d

Short Explanation

The current recommended haemoglobin (Hb) target for a patient with an acute coronary syndrome is 8 g/dL. While the decision to transfuse a patient should be based on individual assessment, there is no evidence of benefit from red blood cell transfusion in the stable critically ill above an Hb of 7 g/dL. More liberal transfusion may cause harm.

Long Explanation

Current clinical practice guidelines suggest that the only well-established recommendation for red blood cell (RBC) transfusion is acute haemorrhage with haemodynamic instability or inadequate oxygen delivery. In the absence of major bleeding a restrictive transfusion strategy (maintaining Hb > 7 g/dL) is suggested to be as effective as a liberal strategy (Hb > 10 g/dL) in critically ill patients with haemodynamically stable anaemia, including resuscitated trauma patients, those requiring mechanical ventilation and those with stable cardiac disease.

Possible exceptions to restrictive RBC transfusion practice are the early phases of local or global tissue ischaemia, as seen in acute coronary syndromes (ACS) and severe sepsis/shock. In ACS the data are somewhat conflicting, although available evidence supports transfusion at a slightly higher haemoglobin (8 g/dL). Similarly in severe sepsis, optimal transfusion triggers are unclear. The Surviving Sepsis guidelines suggest a liberal transfusion practice in the early phase of resuscitation (haematocrit > 30% as needed to achieve $ScvO_2$ 70%). However, there is no clear evidence that blood transfusion increases tissue oxygenation, and these recommendations are based on a single-centre study not specifically designed to assess transfusion practice.

It is hoped that the implementation of evidence-based transfusion practices in the ICU will reduce inappropriate transfusion. Current evidence suggests that the use of RBC transfusion is widespread in the critically ill, with 40% of patients receiving a transfusion and an average pre-transfusion Hb of 8.5 g/dL. The vast majority of transfusions are used in the treatment of anaemia. The efficacy of RBC transfusion in this setting has not been demonstrated, with adverse microcirculatory effects of stored RBCs potentially failing to improve end-organ oxygen delivery. There is also a heightened awareness of the risks associated with allogenic RBC transfusion, including infection, pulmonary complications such as transfusion-related acute lung injury (TRALI) and transfusion-associated circulatory overload (TACO), transfusion-related immune modulation (TRIM), multi-organ failure and an increase in risk-adjusted mortality.

Napolitano LM, Kurek S, Luchette FA, *et al.* Clinical practice guideline: red blood cell transfusion in adult trauma and critical care. *Crit Care Med* 2009; **37**: 3124–57.

Surviving Sepsis Campaign Guidelines. Available online at www.survivingsepsis.org/Guidelines (accessed 30 June 2012).

SBA Question 69: Anaesthesia and endovascular aneurysm repair

A 76-year-old is listed for endovascular aneurysm repair (EVAR) of an extensive infrarenal abdominal aortic aneurysm. The surgeon wishes to use a fenestrated trouser graft, as the neck below the renal arteries is short. Which of the following is the LEAST suitable method of providing anaesthesia?

a) Lumbar epidural with sedation
b) Combined spinal–epidural
c) Local anaesthesia with sedation
d) Spinal
e) General anaesthesia

Answer: d

Short Explanation
All of the above methods have been used successfully in the endovascular repair of abdominal aortic aneurysms. However, a fenestrated trouser graft is complicated to insert and there is a significant risk that the spinal anaesthetic would wear off prior to the end of the procedure.

Long Explanation
The repair of abdominal aortic aneurysm via the endovascular route is becoming increasingly popular. Advantages include a less invasive procedure, shorter duration of operation, reduced haemodynamic and metabolic stress response, early postoperative ambulation and a 50% decrease in length of stay, as well as reducing the need for blood products.

The aim when providing anaesthesia for endovascular aneurysm repair (EVAR) is similar to that for any vascular anaesthetic. Invasive arterial monitoring and urinary catheterisation are considered essential, although central venous catheter placement is rarely required.

All of the anaesthetic techniques listed in the question have been used successfully in the provision of anaesthesia. However, consideration must be given to the suitability of each technique, taking into account both the pathology and surgical complexity of the procedure and the individual patient and his or her comorbidities. Where the procedure is anticipated to exceed 2 hours a spinal is not the method of choice because of the risk that it might wear off before the end of the procedure.

The potential advantages of both local and regional anaesthesia are that they provide peri- and postoperative analgesia and cardiovascular stability. Sedated patients must be able to cooperate with breath-holding during the contrast runs imaging the proximal end of the aneurysm. Local infiltration anaesthesia of the groins has been shown to provide adequate anaesthesia, as deployment of the stent graft within the aorta is usually pain-free.

SBA Question 70: Pleural effusion in the critically ill

A 45-year-old man was admitted to the ICU 5 days ago with a right-sided community-acquired pneumonia and acute respiratory distress syndrome (ARDS). He remains ventilated and has developed a right-sided pleural effusion. A pleural aspiration was performed this morning and 30 mL of sero-sanguinous fluid was aspirated and sent for analysis. You have been asked to review the results: pH 7.1, LDH 1200 IU/L, protein 35 g/L, no organisms on Gram staining. Which one of the following would constitute the most appropriate management plan?

a) No immediate action is required; observe the patient clinically and radiologically
b) Insertion of a large-bore chest drain
c) Urgent CT chest
d) Insertion of a small-bore chest drain under ultrasound guidance
e) Thoracocentesis under ultrasound guidance to drain the remaining fluid

Answer: d

Short Explanation
The results indicate an exudative effusion. The low pH, high lactate dehydrogenase (LDH) and protein levels are suggestive of an infected parapneumonic effusion/empyema. Although a CT chest may well be indicated at some point, the first clinical priority is to drain the infected fluid. Current BTS guidelines recommend initial drainage under ultrasound guidance, although the bore of the chest drain tube remains controversial.

Long Explanation

An empyema develops when fluid in the pleural space becomes infected. It progresses from an acute exudative stage through a transitional fibrinolyic phase where fluid becomes increasingly viscous to a final organising stage where loculations and adhesions develop. Empyemas may be associated with infected parapneumonic effusions, lung abscess rupture, oesophageal rupture and mediastinitis, or they may complicate thoracic trauma, surgery and chest drains. Common organisms implicated include streptococci, *Staphylococcus aureus* (especially in nosocomial and postoperative infections), *Escherichia coli*, *Pseudomonas* species, *Haemophilus influenzae* and *Klebsiella* species. Occasionally anaerobic or mixed growth can be found.

The cornerstones of empyema management are drainage, appropriate antibiotics (which should include anaerobic cover), good supportive care (including nutritional supplementation), venous thromboembolism prophylaxis, and early surgical intervention should these measures fail.

Indications for drainage are frank pus or turbid fluid on aspiration, organisms on Gram stain or culture, pleural fluid pH < 7.2, LDH > 1000 IU/L, loculated effusion or poor clinical progress during treatment with antibiotics alone. In the early stages most effusions can be managed with antibiotics and closed drains. British Thoracic Society guidelines strongly recommend the use of ultrasound for all procedures with pleural fluid, although there is little experimental evidence to support this. Small-bore 12–16F Seldinger-type chest drains are suggested initially as they are often effective and are better tolerated. However, they can block easily and should be flushed regularly. Large-bore drains may be indicated if fluid is particularly viscous. There is little evidence to support one bore of tube over the other, and some clinicians in this setting would look to initially insert a larger tube. CT imaging and multiple drains may be required for loculated effusions. Routine administration of intrapleural fibrinolytics is not recommended, and surgical intervention should be considered in organised effusions and those not responding to treatment. Options include video-assisted thoracic surgery or open thoracotomy with decortication.

British Thoracic Society. Pleural Disease Guidelines, 2010. Available online at www.brit-thoracic.org.uk/guidelines/pleural-disease-guidelines-2010.aspx (accessed 30 June 2012).

SBA Question 71: Phaeochromocytoma: preoperative preparation

Which of the following is INCORRECT regarding the preoperative preparation of a patient with phaeochromocytoma?

a) Labetolol provides optimal preoperative preparation, as it is both an α-adreno- and β-adrenoreceptor blocker
b) Phenoxybenzamine provides irreversible α-adrenoreceptor blockade but may contribute to postoperative hypotension
c) Selective α-adrenoreceptor blockade does not necessitate β-adrenoreceptor blockade
d) Preoperative blockade is not essential in patients with normotensive phaeochromocytoma
e) Echocardiography should be performed in patients with persistent hypertension

Answer: a

Short Explanation

Labetolol is a non-selective adrenoreceptor blocker with α- and β-receptor antagonist properties in a ratio of 1 to 7. Therefore, paradoxical hypertension may occur. In normotensive patients with an incidental finding of phaeochromocytoma, tumour may be safely excised without preoperative hypotensive drugs. All other statements are correct.

Long Explanation

Phaeochromocytomas are functionally active tumours usually found in the adrenal medulla. The symptoms associated with these tumours are due to the uncontrolled release of catecholamines. Preoperative preparation has predominantly focused on adrenoreceptor blockade, with the aim of minimising haemodynamic instability during surgery as well as managing symptoms preoperatively.

Traditionally, sympathetic blockade commences with an α-receptor blocker. Phenoxybenzamine irreversibly inhibits α_1- and α_2-adrenoreceptors. This results in arteriolar dilation but leads to an increased release of noradrenaline due to the blockade of prejunctional α_2-receptors. Common side effects include significant postural hypotension and reflex tachycardia. Therefore, β-blockade is often required (although β-blockade must never be initiated prior to established α-blockade).

Oral phenoxybenzamine has a long half-life of 24 hours and may, therefore, contribute to postoperative hypotension (and is usually stopped a couple of days before surgery to minimise this). Doxazosin, terazosin and prazosin are selective α_1-receptor blockers that are shorter-acting due to their competitive inhibition. They do not inhibit prejunctional α_2-receptors and thus avoid tachycardia. These agents are still associated with significant postural hypotension. They provide comparable preoperative blood pressure control but are less effective intraoperatively, where large catecholamine surges may displace the agent from the α_1-receptor.

Small studies have demonstrated that patients with normotensive phaeochromocytoma may undergo surgery without preoperative hypotensive drugs. In fact, results have shown that those treated with such drugs required more intraoperative vasoactive drugs and colloid infusions.

The most commonly observed cardiovascular pathology is severe hypertension, which may be sustained or paroxysmal, and palpitations. Less commonly, patients may present with symptoms of myocardial ischaemia or heart failure associated with catecholamine cardiomyopathy. Improvement or reversal of cardiomyopathy weeks after tumour excision is well documented.

Leissner K, Mahmood F, Aragam, J, Amouzgar A, Ortega R. Catecholamine-induced cardiomyopathy and pheochromocytoma. *Anesth Analg* 2008; **107**: 410–12.

Lentschener C, Gaujoux S, Tesniere A, Dousset B. Point of controversy: perioperative care of patients undergoing pheochromocytoma removal – time for a reappraisal? *Eur J Endocrinol* 2011; **165**: 365–73.

Pace N, Buttigieg M. Phaeochromocytoma. *Br J Anaesth CEPD Rev* 2003 3; 20–3. Available online at ceaccp.oxfordjournals.org/content/3/1/20 (accessed 30 June 2012).

SBA Question 72: Laser safety

You are anaesthetising a patient who is having laser surgery to his upper airway. You have placed a specific laser endotracheal tube and are ventilating with 40% oxygen and 2% sevoflurane in air. Suddenly, the surgeon tells you there is a fire in the airway. What is the most appropriate course of action after switching off the laser and flooding the site with saline?

a) As you are using a laser-specific endotracheal tube, continue to ventilate the patient through the tube with 40% oxygen and 2% sevoflurane in air

b) As you are using a laser-specific endotracheal tube, continue to ventilate the patient through the tube but with 2% sevoflurane in air

c) Disconnect the anaesthetic circuit, remove the endotracheal tube and ventilate the patient on air using a bag-valve-mask circuit

d) Disconnect the anaesthetic circuit, remove the endotracheal tube and ventilate the patient on 50% oxygen using a bag-valve-mask circuit

e) Disconnect the anaesthetic circuit, remove the endotracheal tube and ventilate the patient on 100% oxygen using a bag-valve-mask circuit

Answer: c

Short Explanation

Management of an airway fire requires promptly switching off the laser (removing the energy source), flooding the site with saline, removing the endotracheal tube (removing the fuel) and using air to ventilate the patient (reducing the oxygen concentration). Even laser-specific tubes can ignite.

Long Explanation

The use of lasers in surgery has increased in recent decades, as they allow the precision cutting of tissues with almost perfect haemostasis. With their increased use it is important to have a good grasp of laser safety, particularly with laser surgery to the airway. In such cases, a variety of anaesthetic techniques have been described. Some centres intubate and ventilate patients with a laser endotracheal tube, others use a jet ventilator attached to a rigid laryngoscope, while others use a spontaneously ventilating technique via a laser endotracheal tube or nasopharyngeal airway.

Whichever method is used, it is important to appreciate that an airway fire is a real possibility, and you should be prepared to manage such a case. When considering a fire it is helpful to recall the three ingredients required to cause a fire: energy, oxygen and a fuel. In the case of an airway fire, these are the laser (energy), the endotracheal tube/circuit (fuel) and oxygen from the ventilator gases.

Managing an airway fire requires all three elements to be dealt with. Firstly, the laser should be switched off and the site flooded with saline. Secondly, the ventilator should be temporarily disconnected and, if feasible, the endotracheal tube removed. It is important to note that even laser endotracheal tubes can become ignited. Finally, the patient should be ventilated with air using a bag-valve-mask circuit. Once the fire is extinguished, the surgeon should inspect the airway via a rigid bronchoscope to assess the extent of the burn.

Airway fires can result in significant lung injury, with worsening hypoxaemia developing over the subsequent 48 hours. It is therefore prudent to transfer the patient (re-intubated) to ICU postoperatively for a period of ventilation and a course of dexamethasone (to reduce airway oedema), so that any deterioration in respiratory function can be closely monitored.

Kitching AJ, Edge CJ. Lasers and surgery. *Br J Anaesth CEPD Rev* 2003; **3**: 143–6. Available online at ceaccp.oxfordjournals.org/content/3/5/143 (accessed 30 June 2012).

SBA Question 73: Complex regional pain syndrome and neuromodulation

Which ONE of these interventions is recommended in the management of complex regional pain syndrome (CRPS) of the lower limb?

a) Surgical lumbar sympathectomy

b) Spinal cord stimulation

c) Intravenous regional sympathetic blockade with guanethidine

d) Acupuncture
e) Amputation of the affected limb

Answer: b

Short Explanation

Surgical sympathectomy may achieve long-standing results but risks recurrence of symptoms within 2 years. Sympathetic blockade with intravenous guanethidine lacks supporting evidence. Acupuncture is commonly used but its efficacy is disputed. Pain relief is rarely achieved with amputation, which can lead to intractable phantom limb pain. In 2008 NICE issued guidance recommending spinal cord stimulation to treat CRPS.

Long Explanation

Complex regional pain syndrome (CRPS) is described as a triad:

1. Pain, often excruciating, that can be evoked by touch or movement and is present at rest. The pain may be allodynia (pain due to a stimulus that does not normally provoke pain) and/or hyperalgesia (increased pain from a stimulus that normally provokes pain)
2. Trophic changes affecting the skin, hair and nails
3. Vasomotor disturbances, resulting in sweating and flushing, or pallor and cold extremities, and oedema.

Motor dysfunction may also occur. This may be the result of a direct motor nerve injury, or movement may be restricted by pain, resulting in disuse atrophy and joint stiffness. Involuntary movements such as dystonia and tremor may also occur.

The aim of treatment is pain reduction and restoration of function. Therapies remain controversial, and the evidence base for certain procedures is weak. Reports of benefit are anecdotal and possibly due to placebo. Intravenous regional guanethidine has been found to be no better than placebo in confirmed cases of sympathetically maintained pain (SMP). SMP can be established by local anaesthetic blockade of the lumbar sympathetic chain paravertebral ganglia or stellate ganglion, which is both diagnostic and can provide temporary relief for resumption of activity and physiotherapy. Surgical sympathectomy and radiofrequency ablative techniques have achieved more long-standing results, but with the risk of recurrence of symptoms and neuralgia at 6 months to 2 years.

Acupuncture is used widely but there is little supporting evidence for its efficacy.

Neuromodulation is gaining interest, and in 2008 the National Institute for Health and Clinical Excellence (NICE) recommended the use of spinal cord stimulation (SCS) in neuropathic pain conditions, including CRPS. SCS modifies the perception of neuropathic pain by stimulating the dorsal columns of the spinal cord. The neurostimulator generates an electrical pulse and is surgically implanted subcutaneously in the abdomen or in the buttock area. Electrodes connected to the stimulator are implanted near the spinal cord either surgically or percutaneously. The device can be controlled remotely and adjusted according to individual requirements. In combination with physiotherapy, SCS has been found to have a statistically significant, albeit modest, effect on pain.

Amputation of the affected limb is considered in the presence of ongoing disease such as infection or ischaemia. Pain relief is rarely achieved, however, and a significant proportion of patients go on to develop intractable phantom limb pain.

National Institute for Health and Clinical Excellence (NICE). *Spinal Cord Stimulation for Chronic Pain of Neuropathic or Ischaemic Origin.* NICE Technology Appraisal Guideline 159, October 2008. Available online at www.nice.org.uk/TA159 (accessed 30 June 2012).

Wilson J G, Serpell M G. Complex regional pain syndrome. *Contin Educ Anaesth Crit Care Pain* 2007; 7: 51–4. Available online at ceaccp.oxfordjournals.org/content/7/2/5 (accessed 30 June 2012).

SBA Question 74: Hypertensive response to laryngoscopy

Extra steps are often taken to obtund the hypertensive response to laryngoscopy. In which of the following situations are these extra steps LEAST likely to be required in order to avoid increased morbidity or mortality?

a) A 49-year-old female who is fit and well presenting for coiling of a berry aneurysm
b) A 79-year-old treated hypertensive with asymptomatic triple-vessel disease presenting for repair of an incarcerated inguinal hernia
c) A 29-year-old male with complete spinal cord transection at C6 who presents for appendicectomy
d) A 42-year-old pre-eclamptic woman presenting for a caesarean section under general anaesthesia
e) A 19-year-old fit scaffolder presenting for removal of a metal shard from his eye under general anaesthesia

Answer: c

Short Explanation
Cardiovascular responses to intubation vary in patients with spinal cord injuries. In patients with complete transection of the cord above C7, there is no hypertensive response to laryngoscopy and intubation, although tachycardia is still seen and there is elevation of plasma levels of catecholamines.

Long Explanation
Both laryngoscopy and intubation have been shown independently to cause a sympathetic response, which is of varying magnitude and has variable consequences depending upon the individual situation.

Patients with underlying hypertension (including pre-eclampsia) and cerebrovascular or cardiovascular disease demonstrate an exaggerated response. The degree to which this is important depends on the comorbidities of the patients. Severe perioperative hypertension is a major threat to hypertensive patients, especially increases of blood pressure in excess of about 20% of the preoperative value. Consequences of pressure surges include bleeding from vascular suture lines, cerebrovascular haemorrhage, and myocardial ischaemia/infarction. The mortality rate of such events may be as high as 50%.

Any patient with known risk of intracranial haemorrhage such as an unprotected aneurysm requires special measures to attenuate the hypertensive response.

In patients with penetrating eye injury, the resulting increase in intraocular pressure can cause expulsion of the contents of the globe.

Cardiovascular responses to intubation vary in patients with spinal cord injuries. In patients with complete transection of the cord above C7, there is a reduced hypertensive response to laryngoscopy and intubation, although tachycardia is still seen and there is elevation of plasma levels of catecholamines. In patients with cord transections below C7, the hypertensive response to laryngoscopy is similar to that of normal controls, although there is a disproportionate increase in heart rate in those with transections between T1 and T4.

Yoo KY, Lee JU, Kim HS, Im WM. Hemodynamic and catecholamine response to laryngoscopy and tracheal intubation in patients with complete spinal cord injury. *Anesthesiology* 2001; **95**: 647–51.

SBA Question 75: Lower limb blocks

You are anaesthetising a 67-year-old male for a transurethral resection of a bladder tumour under general anaesthetic. Midway through the operation, the surgeon complains that the patient's right leg is moving as he resects the right side of his bladder tumour. Which of the following blocks would have been most likely to prevent this occurring?

a) A spinal anaesthetic
b) A lumbar plexus block
c) A femoral nerve block
d) A sciatic nerve block
e) A caudal block

Answer: b

Short Explanation

Direct stimulation of the obturator nerve as it passes close to the lateral wall of the bladder can cause sudden, violent adductor muscle spasm. This reflex is not abolished by spinal anaesthesia and is suppressed only by a selective obturator nerve block, i.e. a lumbar plexus block. A femoral block is unlikely to spread to cover the obturator nerve. A sciatic nerve block or a caudal block would only reliably anaesthetise the lower levels of the spinal cord.

Long Explanation

The obturator nerve is a mixed motor and sensory nerve arising from L2–L4. It descends within the psoas muscle before emerging within the pelvis, where it is in close proximity to the ureter and subsequently the lateral wall of the bladder. From here it gives rise to branches which innervate the parietal peritoneum before exiting the pelvis via the obturator canal. Outside the pelvis, the nerve supplies sensation to a variable portion of skin over the medial aspect of the thigh, but more consistently it supplies sensation to the hip and knee joints as well as a small area of skin behind the knee. The nerve also provides motor innervation to the adductors of the hip, these being adductor longus, brevis and magnus, gracilis and the external obturator.

Since the nerve passes so close to the lateral wall of the bladder, during a transurethral resection of the lateral wall of the bladder the resector can directly stimulate the nerve causing sudden, violent adductor muscle spasm. This is potentially dangerous, as it will increase the risk of serious complications, including perforating the bladder wall. This reflex is not abolished by spinal anaesthesia and is suppressed only by a selective obturator nerve block.

There are multiple ways of blocking the obturator nerve, including a 3 in 1 and lumbar plexus block. It is also possible to selectively block the obturator nerve, the most common technique being the paravascular selective inguinal block, where the anterior and posterior branches are selectively blocked. This technique is more caudad than the original Labat's technique, which had a high level of discomfort for the patient. To perform the paravascular block, the needle insertion point is identified by a line drawn over the inguinal fold from the pulse of the femoral artery to the tendon of the adductor longus muscle. The needle is inserted at the mid-point of this line at an angle of 30 degrees cephalad. Stimulation of the nerve results in twitching seen in the adductor compartment of the thigh. On identifying the nerve, 5–7 mL of local anaesthetic is injected. Of note, performing an obturator nerve block at this site will miss blocking the articular branches to the hip joint.

New York School of Regional Anaesthesia. Obturator nerve block, March 2009. Available online at www.nysora.com/peripheral_nerve_blocks/nerve_stimulator_techniques/3095-obturator-nerve-block.html (accessed 30 June 2012).

SBA Question 76: Epidural anaesthesia

A 69-year-old lady undergoes an abdominoperineal (AP) resection for colonic cancer. She has a thoracic epidural sited for analgesia that works well. On postoperative day 3 she complains of left- sided weakness in her ankle joint and altered sensation on the outside of her left lower leg. You are asked to review her sensory loss. The most likely explanation to this neuropathy is:

a) Unilateral epidural blockade
b) Direct nerve injury during insertion of the epidural catheter
c) Spinal haematoma
d) Peripheral neuropraxia from leg supports
e) Residual paraesthesia from epidural infusion

Answer: d

Short Explanation

A unilateral block will have revealed itself during the immediate postoperative period. Direct nerve injury must be suspected if there is a history of paraesthesia or pain during insertion of the epidural or injection of local anaesthetic. A spinal haematoma is a serious complication that must be diagnosed early; it presents with back pain, usually bilateral altered motor and sensory function, urinary and faecal incontinence. Residual paraesthesia will be bilateral and improving such that the patient's motor and sensory function return with time.

Long Explanation

Abdominoperineal (AP) resection is a prolonged major colorectal procedure that involves the patient being in the Lloyd Davies position (legs in stirrups). One of the pitfalls of this position is direct pressure on the common peroneal nerve (CPN) at the fibula neck. This can cause direct nerve palsy.

The symptoms of CPN nerve palsy are:

- weakness in dorsiflexon and eversion of foot
- sensory deficit to anterolateral aspect of lower leg and dorsum of foot
- foot drop
- normal tendon reflexes
- pain and Tinel's sign over the fibula neck

When assessing a neurological deficit following insertion of an epidural, we must exclude immediate spinal-cord-threatening pathology. There are several red flag symptoms to identify:

- significant motor block with a thoracic epidural
- unexpectedly dense motor block, including unilateral block
- markedly increasing motor block during epidural infusion
- motor block that does not regress when an epidural is discontinued
- recurrent unexpected motor block after restarting an epidural infusion that was stopped because of motor block

If all significant central neuraxial block complications are excluded (from history and examination, looking for red flag symptoms), a direct nerve injury can be suspected.

Management of CPN palsy is conservative, with physiotherapy and ambulation. A significant foot drop may require orthotic treatment to limit damage to toes and falls.

Agrawal P. Peroneal mononeuropathy. *Medscape Reference* 2010. Available online at emedicine.medscape.com/article/1141734 (accessed 30 June 2012).

Royal College of Anaesthetists. *Major Complications of Central Neuraxial Block in The United Kingdom* (NAP3). London: RCA, 2009. Available online at www.rcoa.ac. uk/docs/NAP3_web-large.pdf (accessed 30 June 2012).

SBA Question 77: Risks of central neuraxial blockade

You are asked to see a woman on the maternity ward who is considering an epidural for pain relief. She is concerned as she has heard stories about nerve damage and has heard that this is 'quite common'. During your discussion, you quote an incidence of postdural puncture headache, transient nerve root damage and vertebral canal haematoma. The correct values for these, respectively, are:

a) 1 in 200, 1 in 15 000, 1 in 55 000
b) 1 in 1000, 1 in 50 000, 1 in 500 000
c) 1 in 100, 1 in 3000, 1 in 160 000
d) 1 in 10, 1 in 1000, 1 in 75 000
e) 1 in 20, 1 in 5000, 1 in 260 000

Answer: c

Short Explanation
Accidental dural puncture occurs in approximately 1%. Transient nerve root damage occurs in 1 in 3000, permanent neurology related to nerve root damage 1 in 15 000. A study of 1.37 million women in 2006 calculated the risks of serious complications as epidural haematoma 1 in 168 000, deep epidural infection 1 in 145 000, persistent neurological injury 1 in 240 000, transient neurological injury 1 in 6700.

Long Explanation
Regional analgesia in the pregnant and labouring population is long established and well researched. It provides very safe analgesia and anaesthesia for labour, instrumental deliveries, caesarean section and occasionally non-obstetric surgery. It is favoured over general anaesthesia because of the risks associated with general anaesthesia in the pregnant population. It is accepted, however, that one in ten women will require instrumental delivery as a result of the epidural.

Approximately 25% of labouring women undergo epidural analgesia in the UK, equating to around 140 000 women per year. The most commonly occurring complication is that of accidental dural puncture, which occurs in approximately 1400 women (1 in 100). The risk of transient nerve root damage is in the region of 1 in 3000, and permanent neurology as a result of root damage occurs in approximately 1 in 15 000. It is important to note, however, that the process of childbirth itself may also result in nerve damage. The femoral, peroneal, lateral cutaneous nerve of the thigh, the lumbosacral plexus and even the conus medullaris are potentially vulnerable to damage, either from maternal posture or from pressure of the fetal head on the nerves or blood vessels, resulting in hypoperfusion.

Infective complications of central neuraxial blockade are rare in the obstetric population. Figures have been quoted as 0.2–3.7 in 100 000 for epidural abscess formation and 1.5 in 100 000 for bacterial meningitis. Ruppen *et al.* (2006) reviewed 1.37 million women over 27 separate studies regarding the risk of serious complications including, epidural haematoma formation and deep epidural formation. Risks are quoted at 1 in 168 000 and 1 in 145 000, respectively.

It is important to recognise that any central neuraxial blockade can result in maternal hypotension and hypoperfusion of the utero-placental unit, and inadvertent intrathecal placement of epidural catheters risks a very high block or total spinal. Another rare and often forgotten complication is that of subdural haematoma formation, following accidental puncture of the dura with a large-bore epidural needle and subsequent traction on the meningeal blood vessels with precipitous drops in CSF pressure.

Maternal death is thankfully an extremely rare complication of central neuraxial blockade, but cases in the recent past have included respiratory failure secondary to a high spinal and maternal cardiac arrest as a result of 'wrong route' administration of local anaesthetic solution.

Royal College of Anaesthetists. *Major Complications of Central Neuraxial Block in the United Kingdom* (NAP3). London: RCA, 2009. Available online at www.rcoa.ac. uk/docs/NAP3_web-large.pdf (accessed 30 June 2012).

Royal College of Anaesthetists Faculty of Pain Medicine. *Best Practice in the Management of Epidural Analgesia in the Hospital Setting*, November 2010. Available online at www.aagbi.org/sites/default/files/epidural_analgesia_2011.pdf (accessed 30 June 2012).

Ruppen W, Derry S, McQuay H, Moore RA. Incidence of epidural hematoma, infection, and neurologic injury in obstetric patients with epidural analgesia/anesthesia. *Anesthesiology* 2006; **105**: 394–9.

SBA Question 78: Anti-embolic stockings

A 68-year-old is on your list for a paraumbilical hernia repair. He is a well-controlled insulin-dependent diabetic and otherwise had a myocardial infarction 5 years ago. Previous surgery includes a carpal tunnel release and a right aorto-femoral bypass graft. The surgeon asks you whether anti-embolic stockings are suitable for this gentleman. What is the best treatment option?

a) Anti-embolic stockings are not suitable in this patient
b) Left side only knee-length anti-embolic stockings
c) Bilateral knee-length anti-embolic stockings
d) Left side only thigh-length anti-embolic stockings
e) Bilateral thigh-length anti-embolic stockings

Answer: a

Short Explanation

This man is likely to have significant cardiovascular disease, being diabetic and having had a myocardial infarction and peripheral arterial bypass grafting in the past. 2010 NICE guidelines advise that patients who have had peripheral arterial bypass grafting or with suspected or proven peripheral arterial disease should not be offered anti-embolic stockings.

Long Explanation

Venous thromboembolism (VTE) is an important cause of morbidity in patients undergoing surgery. Because of its importance, the National Institute for Health and Clinical Excellence (NICE) updated its guidelines in 2010 with the aim of reducing the risk of VTE in all patients admitted to hospital. The guideline provides a list of all persons who have an increased risk of developing a VTE during their admission.

The patient in the case presented here has at least two of these risk factors, having significant cardiac disease and being over the age of 60. For patients undergoing surgery such as this, those with at least one risk factor for developing VTE should be offered a mechanical method of thromboprophylaxis from the time of their admission. Mechanical methods available are anti-embolic stockings, foot pump devices or intermittent pneumatic compression devices.

Patients for whom anti-embolic stockings are not suitable include those with suspected or proven peripheral arterial disease, peripheral arterial bypass grafting, peripheral neuropathy, local skin conditions that may be aggravated by the stockings, known allergy to the material of the stockings, cardiac failure, severe leg oedema or pulmonary oedema from congestive heart failure, and patients with unusual leg size or shape. For any patients falling into this category who need mechanical thromboprophylaxis, one of the other two methods available should be offered.

The guideline also provides extensive advice on the appropriate methods of thromboprophylaxis for all different types of surgery, and it is important to have a good grasp of these.

Barker RC, Marval P. Venous thromboembolism: risks and prevention. *Contin Educ Anaesth Crit Care Pain* 2011; **11**: 18–23.

National Institute for Health and Clinical Excellence. *Venous Thromboembolism: Reducing the Risk.* NICE Clinical Guideline 92, February 2010. Available online at guidance.nice.org.uk/CG92 (accessed 30 June 2012).

SBA Question 79: Pain relief in labour: epidural analgesia

A primigravida who has been induced for labour is 2–3 cm dilated and is requesting an epidural. She is currently being treated for pre-eclamptic toxaemia (PET). Her blood pressure was 170/110 mmHg, and after commencing a labetalol and magnesium sulphate infusion this decreased to 140/85 mmHg. She has proteinuria of 7 g/24 hours and her most recent platelet count, taken 4 hours ago, was 100×10^9/L (6 hours before that it was 150×10^9/L). What is the best management of this parturient's labour analgesia?

a) Insert epidural as usual
b) Send repeat full blood count and clotting screen and await results. Only insert epidural if platelet count is $> 80 \times 10^9$/L and clotting screen is within acceptable limits
c) Advise remifentanil PCA
d) Give 50 mg intramuscular pethidine and send repeat full blood count and clotting screen and await results. Only insert epidural if platelet count is $> 80 \times 10^9$/L and clotting screen is within acceptable limits
e) Send repeat full blood count and clotting screen and await results. Only insert epidural if platelet count is $> 60 \times 10^9$/L and clotting screen is within acceptable limits

Answer: b

Short Explanation
In severe PET it would be prudent to wait for a repeat full blood count and clotting prior to epidural insertion. Intramuscular injections should be minimised in patients who are potentially coagulopathic. The platelet count should be above 80×10^9/L and the INR should be 1.4 or less.

Long Explanation
Contraindications to epidural analgesia include maternal refusal, local anaesthetic allergy, localised infection, coagulopathy and hypovolaemia. Cardiac diseases such as aortic stenosis and peripartum cardiomyopathy are considered relative contraindications.

Pre-eclamptic toxaemia (PET) is a multisystem disorder specific to pregnancy. Early on in the disease process PET enhances the normal hypercoagulable state of pregnancy. However, in severe PET there is the potential for rapid development of thrombocytopenia and coagulopathy. The drop in platelet count is caused by an increase in consumption, and fibrin activation may lead to the development of disseminated intravascular coagulation (DIC). Significant thrombocytopenia occurs in about 15% of parturients with severe PET and DIC in about 7% of cases.

HELLP (haemolysis, elevated liver enzymes, low platelets) syndrome is a recognised complication of severe PET and can develop in about 4% of cases. Epigastric pain is often one of the presenting symptoms, because of tension on the liver capsule. Full blood count analysis is recommended within the 4 hours prior to inserting an epidural. If the platelet count is $< 100 \times 10^9$/L, then a clotting screen should be sent. It is generally accepted that it is reasonably safe to perform regional techniques with a platelet count $> 80 \times 10^9$/L with INR < 1.4, but it is still an area of much debate. It would be prudent to have a multidisciplinary discussion with the obstetricians, midwives and consultant anaesthetist on call to ascertain the likelihood of the parturient having a successful induction of labour if haematological parameters are worsening.

Dalgleish DJ. Pre-eclampsia. *Anaesthesia UK* 2006. Available online at www.anaesthesiauk.com/article.aspx?articleid=100463 (accessed 30 June 2012).

McGrady E, Litchfield K. Epidural analgesia in labour. *Contin Educ Anaesth Crit Care Pain* 2004; 4: 114–17. Available online at ceaccp.oxfordjournals.org/content/4/4/114 (accessed 30 June 2012).

SBA Question 80: Orthopaedic cement

An 80-year-old patient with severe chronic obstructive pulmonary disease (COPD) is undergoing an elective total hip replacement under spinal anaesthesia and propofol target-controlled infusion (TCI) sedation (1.0–1.5 g/mL). As the hip is reduced following joint insertion there is a fall in SpO_2 associated with significant hypotension. What is the likely cause?

a) A combination of severe COPD, sedation and hypoventilation worsening pulmonary hypertension and cardiac output
b) Acute coronary syndrome
c) Reduced systemic vascular resistance secondary to spinal anaesthesia with associated reduced coronary perfusion and cardiac output
d) A 'high spinal' resulting in progressive loss of intercostal muscle function on the background of severe COPD, resulting in hypoxia and pulmonary hypertension
e) Bone cement implantation syndrome

Answer: e

Short Explanation
The placement of orthopaedic cement results in intramedullary hypertension causing the embolisation of cement, fat, marrow, air, bone and aggregated fibrin into the venous circulation. Reduction of the hip following joint replacement 'unkinks' veins, resulting in systemic release, pulmonary hypertension, hypoxia and hypotension. Complications associated with the spinal are more likely to occur earlier during the onset of block. An acute coronary syndrome is a possibility, though the temporal association with manipulation of the hip joint makes this a less likely cause than bone cement implantation syndrome.

Long Explanation
Bone cement implantation syndrome (BCIS) is still poorly understood but remains an important cause of intraoperative morbidity and mortality in those undergoing cemented hip joint replacement. Because of the wide spectrum of presentation and associated comorbidities in this patient group it is difficult to establish a true incidence. It is also difficult to classify but is known to be associated with hypoxia, hypotension, cardiac arrhythmias, increased pulmonary vascular resistance and cardiac arrest. It is

also considered to be part of a less severe postoperative syndrome of hypotension, hypoxia and postoperative confusion.

There are numerous theories as to its pathophysiology, and it is likely that this is multimodal. Initial theories focused on the release of methylmethacrylate (MMA) monomers during cementation. Studies have demonstrated that such monomers cause vasodilation in vitro but not in vivo. Much recent research has concentrated on embolisation in BCIS at the time of cementation but also as vessels are 'unkinked'. The embolic showers that result are thought to be due to a mechanical effect in pulmonary, coronary and cerebral circulations but also subsequent mediator release (thrombin, thromboplastin, prostaglandins) and complement activation. It is also important to note that histamine release may occur in BCIS, and that true anaphylaxis to bone cement can also present in a similar fashion.

Risk factors for BCIS can be broadly classified into patient and surgical. Patient risk factors include old age, multiple comorbidities, poor cardiopulmonary function and pre-existing pulmonary hypertension. Osteoporosis, bony metastases and pathological intertrochanteric fractures also significantly increase risk by providing abnormal vascular channels through which marrow contents can access the systemic circulation. Surgical risk factors include primary hip replacement and the use of long-stem femoral components.

BCIS can be anticipated with careful surgical and anaesthetic care including preoperative assessment and multidisciplinary approaches. Anaesthesia should be tailored on a case-by-case basis, and in high-risk patients appropriate invasive monitoring should be undertaken. The avoidance of nitrous oxide is recommended, as is increasing inspired oxygen concentrations prior to cementing while maintaining adequate circulating volume.

Donaldson AJ, Thomson HE, Harper NJ, Kenny NW. Bone cement implantation syndrome. *Br J Anaesth* 2009; **102**: 12–22. Available online at bja.oxfordjournals.org/content/102/1/12 (accessed 30 June 2012).

SBA Question 81: Paediatric anaesthesia: anatomy and physiology

You are asked to intubate a 2-year-old for a routine operative procedure. When considering this child's airway, which one of the following would you consider the LEAST likely to present a challenge?

a) This child is likely to have frequent upper respiratory tract infections, which can increase the risk of laryngospasm and other respiratory complications
b) The narrowest part of this child's airway is the cricoid ring. Your endotracheal tube may cause trauma at this level
c) The child may have loose teeth that can be dislodged and aspirated
d) The child will have a relatively large occiput compared to an adult patient, and excessive head extension may occlude the airway
e) The distance between cricoid and main bronchi is short, increasing the risk of endobronchial intubation

Answer: c

Short Explanation

All of these are relevant to the paediatric airway. The key point is the age of the child. At 2 years of age the large occiput, short trachea and cricoid diameter are always pertinent. Toddlers suffer on average from eight or more upper respiratory tract infections during winter months. Often parents report that their child is never without a runny nose. Age 2, however, is not an age when deciduous dentition or milk teeth are normally shed.

Long Explanation

The differences between the adult and the paediatric airway constitute core knowledge for anaesthetic exams. Of course the paediatric airway is a heterogeneous entity, varying considerably with age. As in the adult, it can be affected by disease processes. It is not uncommon to encounter congenital abnormalities, and children with these conditions can frequently present for surgery.

As a generalisation, the paediatric patient has a relatively larger occiput than the adult, a variable number of teeth, teeth that may be loose, a relatively large tongue compared to the adult, fragile mucosa that can be damaged by instrumentation, and soft compressible tissues in the neck and floor of the mouth. Infants are often described as obligate nasal breathers. This does not mean that they cannot breathe through their mouth but that the airway is designed to function while breastfeeding. This explains why infants with nasal blockage have difficulty feeding.

The larynx is high and anterior compared to the adult, and the epiglottis is floppy and U-shaped. The narrowest part of the airway is at the level of the cricoid, which of course is not visible. Care must be taken to avoid causing trauma with the endotracheal tube at this level. The cricoid itself is not fully formed, and in fact continues to ossify late into adult life. The distance between larynx and carina is short.

One of the most common findings on neonatal intensive care chest radiographs is endobronchial intubation. The physiological changes associated with laryngoscopy can be particularly damaging, especially in premature neonates, where inadequately sedated babies show an increase in intraventricular haemorrhage.

Frequent upper respiratory tract infections are common in the paediatric population, as any parent will attest to.

Eruption of deciduous dentition or milk teeth starts at around 6 months of age and continues until about 2.5 years. Decay and dental caries are not uncommon, especially in children over 12 months who take a bottle to bed. However, shedding or exfoliation of milk teeth does not occur until about 6 years of age.

SBA Question 82: Pulse oximetry

All of the following will potentially render the pulse oximeter reading inaccurate, EXCEPT which one?

a) A patient with cyanide poisoning
b) A patient with methaemoglobinaemia
c) A patient with methaemoglobinaemia treated with methylene blue
d) A patient with a LiMON global liver function monitor in use
e) A patient with carbon monoxide poisoning

Answer: a

Short Explanation

Methaemoglobinaemia causes pulse oximetry to trend towards 85%. Methylene blue and indocyanine green (used in the LiMON) both significantly affect readings. Carboxyhaemoglobin causes overestimation of oxygen saturation. Cyanide prevents tissue utilisation, but does not affect arterial oxygen saturation or pulse oximetry measurements.

Long Explanation

The pulse oximeter uses the different absorption spectra of oxygenated and deoxygenated haemoglobin (Hb) to calculate the ratio of the former to the latter, and thus the oxygen saturation of the haemoglobin in a sample. This is achieved using light-emitting diodes (LEDs) which emit light at two different wavelengths. These flash on and off at high frequency, and the light is received via sensors which also account for ambient light. The changes in absorbance occurring over time are therefore due to changes in the substance lying between the emitters and the sensors (i.e. the passage of arterial blood into tissue during systole).

However, numerous factors can interfere with the readings obtained:

- poor perfusion (decreased pulsatile proportion, as seen in vasoconstriction, or poor cardiac output, also seen with high and/or pulsatile venous pressure)
- interference (bright overhead lights, surgical diathermy, patient motion or shivering)
- nail varnish
- dyes (e.g. indocyanine green, methylene blue)
- haemoglobin forms (e.g. carboxyhaemoglobin, methaemoglobinaemia – treated by methylene blue – which, in excess, is a cause of methaemoglobinaemia)

Fetal haemoglobin and bilirubin have no clinically significant effect on readings.

Davis PD, Kenny GNC. *Basic Physics and Measurement in Anaesthesia*, 5th edn. Oxford: Butterworth-Heinemann, 2003; pp. 201–2.
Ralston AC, Webb RK, Runciman WB. Potential errors in pulse oximetry. III: Effects of interference, dyes, dyshaemoglobins and other pigments. *Anaesthesia* 1991; **46**: 291–5.

SBA Question 83: Awake craniotomy

A patient is scheduled to undergo an awake craniotomy. Which of the following would be most likely to prevent the surgery being done in this way?

a) The presence of a frontal lobe tumour
b) That the patient is registered blind
c) That the patient has a benign essential tremor
d) The presence of significant dural involvement of the tumour
e) That the patient is known to be epileptic

Answer: d

Short Explanation
A low occipital, not frontal, tumour would be a contraindication to awake craniotomy as the patient would need to be in the prone position. A common indication for this type of surgery is in the treatment of epilepsy. Verbal and not visual communication with the patient during the procedure is essential, and a tremor is not a contraindication as the head will be in pins for the surgery. Dural involvement of the tumour is likely to make surgery too painful to be done awake.

Long Explanation
Awake craniotomy is performed on carefully selected patients for neurosurgery for three main reasons:

(1) in eloquent areas of the brain, where the neurosurgeon can perform precise, controlled resection with real-time feedback from the patient that important tissue is not being infringed upon;
(2) where stimulation of deep brain nuclei is required together with monitoring of effects (e.g. Parkinson's disease);
(3) where anaesthetic agents must be kept to a minimum for the close monitoring of electrophysiology (e.g. epilepsy surgery).

Numerous techniques have been described in the literature, and their usage will vary from centre to centre. The key components are focused around the balance between safe, effective anaesthesia/analgesia and optimal operating conditions. The most stimulating parts of the procedure involve the opening and closure of the cranial vault (skin, periosteum and dura). Brain resection or electrode insertion is not considered to be painful. Asleep-awake-asleep techniques provide anaesthesia with safe airway management for stimulating parts of the procedure. A ProSeal laryngeal mask airway (LMA) offers a 'secure' airway, facilitates ventilation and management of $PaCO_2$ and can be easily inserted and removed as required. Awake craniotomies have been performed with patients spontaneously ventilating on an LMA during the 'awake' phase, but this has been associated with a higher incidence of complications.

Numerous drugs have been used for awake craniotomies, including propofol, opioids, benzodiazepines and α_2-receptor agonists. Effective anaesthesia is likely to be best provided by potent, short-acting and easily titratable agents. Remifentanil and propofol used as target-controlled infusions seem ideal. Effective local anaesthetic infiltration by the surgeon is also paramount for the 'awake' phase. The skin, scalp, periosteum and pericranium are innervated by cutaneous nerves arising from branches of the trigeminal nerve and can be blocked effectively by field blocks. The dura is innervated by all three divisions of the trigeminal nerve, by the recurrent meningeal branch of the vagus nerve and by branches of the upper cervical roots. Local anaesthetic infiltration around the nerve trunk running with the middle meningeal artery provides effective anaesthesia of these.

Jones H, Smith M. Awake craniotomy. *Contin Educ Anaesth Crit Care Pain* 2004; **4**: 189–92. Available online at ceaccp.oxfordjournals.org/content/4/6/189 (accessed 30 June 2012).

SBA Question 84: Cleft palate

A child presents for cleft palate repair and is known to have an associated syndrome. That syndrome is most likely to be:

a) Treacher Collins syndrome
b) Pierre Robin syndrome
c) Klippel–Fiel syndrome
d) Down's syndrome
e) DiGeorge syndrome

Answer: b

Short Explanation
Cleft lip and palate exists most frequently as an isolated defect. However, it is associated with many congenital conditions, and other associated underlying abnormalities must be investigated prior to surgery. Pierre Robin sequence describes a condition of micrognathia and glossoptosis where cleft palate occurs in 80%.

Long Explanation
Many patients presenting with cleft lip and palate are relatively straightforward, presenting minimal airway or intubation challenges to the anaesthetist. However, other associated abnormalities can cause profound upper airway obstruction in certain cases.

The most important group of cleft lip and palate patients with airway problems are those with Pierre Robin sequence. The primary deformity in these infants is micrognathia, resulting in a tongue position further back in the mouth. In utero the reduced pharyngeal space prevents palatal fusion, and after birth upper airway obstruction can present a real challenge. Conservative management consists of placing the infant prone, and this may be all that is required. If an artificial airway is required, a nasopharyngeal adjunct can be tried. Very rarely tracheostomy is necessary.

All the other conditions mentioned are known to be associated with cleft palate to varying degrees except DiGeorge syndrome.

Pierre Robin sequence can also be associated with other syndromes and abnormalities. Surgery is usually performed after 3 months for cleft lip and 6 months or more for cleft palate. This allows time for investigation of other underlying pathology. Some advocate the 10,10,10 rule for cleft palate (deferring surgery until the patient is 10 months, 10 kg and with a haemoglobin above 10 g/dL).

Somerville N, Fenlon S. Anaesthesia for cleft lip and palate surgery. *Contin Educ Anaesth Crit Care Pain* 2005; **5**: 76–9. Available online at ceaccp.oxfordjournals. org/content/5/3/76 (accessed 30 June 2012).

SBA Question 85: Cauda equina syndrome

A 65-year-old man presents to the emergency department. He has a history of prostate cancer and describes a 2-month history of worsening low back pain which is now severe and unresponsive to simple analgesia. Which one of the following symptoms/ signs points AGAINST a diagnosis of cauda equina syndrome?

a) Saddle anaesthesia
b) Hyperreflexia in the lower limbs
c) Difficulty urinating
d) Constipation
e) Unilateral radicular pain

Answer: b

Short Explanation

Cauda equina syndrome is a surgical emergency, and in a patient presenting in this way one would expect reduced or absent lower limb reflexes rather than hyperreflexia.

Long Explanation

'Red flags' are features in the back pain history that arouse suspicion of serious spinal pathology. They aim to detect malignancy, infection, fracture and inflammatory arthritides, as follows:

- Malignancy: age over 50, prior history of malignancy, unexplained weight loss, progressive symptoms unresponsive to simple treatments, failure of bed rest to relieve symptoms.
- Infection: systemically unwell, history of immunocompromise, history of tuberculosis, history of intravenous drug use, source suggesting infective metastasis (e.g. indwelling urinary catheter), skin infection.
- Fracture: history of trauma, history of osteoporosis, long-term steroid therapy.
- Inflammatory arthritides: family history, widespread persisting limitation of spinal movement, peripheral joint involvement, associated rheumatological phenomena (iritis, colitis, urethritis, rashes). High sensitivity and specificity if four positive answers to: Morning stiffness? Improvement with exercise? Onset before age 40? Slow onset? Pain persisting longer than 3 months?

Our patient is over 50 with a history of prior malignancy and worsening symptoms unresponsive to simple treatments, and therefore a malignant cause of his back pain should be suspected.

Cauda equina syndrome is a compression of the cauda equina. Symptoms include low back pain, unilateral or bilateral radicular pain, saddle and perineal hypoaesthesia/anaesthesia, bowel and bladder disturbance, motor and sensory deficits of the lower limb, reduced or absent lower limb reflexes. It is a neurosurgical emergency.

Urinary manifestations of cauda equina syndrome include urinary retention, difficulty initiating urination and decreased urethral sensation. The initial presentation of bladder dysfunction may be of difficulty initiating or terminating urination, and although urinary manifestations classically begin with urinary retention and are later followed by an overflow urinary incontinence, difficulty initiating urination is not reassuring.

Bowel disturbances of cauda equina syndrome include constipation, incontinence of stool and loss of anal tone and sensation. Therefore, although constipation classically progresses to overflow incontinence, constipation cannot be regarded as reassuring. His leg weakness remains subjective, and so his ventral roots are currently spared. Leg weakness develops as the ventral roots become compromised.

Dawodu ST. Cauda equina and conus medullaris syndromes. *Medscape Reference* 2011. Available online at emedicine.medscape.com/article/1148690 (accessed 30 June 2012).

Stannard C S, Booth S. *Pain*, 2nd edn, Edinburgh: Churchill Livingstone, 2004; p. 266.

SBA Question 86: Temperature loss in a patient under anaesthesia

When anaesthetising a patient for a laparotomy, which ONE of the following options is the most important implementation to reduce heat loss during surgery?

a) Using a heat and moisture exchange (HME) filter
b) Ensuring the patient is not in contact with any cold metallic objects
c) Avoiding the use of neuromuscular blocking agents, to allow thermogenesis via shivering
d) Use of total intravenous anaesthesia (TIVA), to prevent inactivation of the central thermoregulatory mechanisms
e) Use of a forced-air warming device

Answer: e

Short Explanation
Use of an HME filter will reduce heat loss via respiration and humidification, and avoiding contact with cold objects is sensible to reduce heat loss via conduction, but neither of these represents the main mechanism by which heat is lost from the body. Avoidance of neuromuscular blocking agents is not an appropriate or sensible implementation. TIVA still lowers the body's thermoregulatory thresholds, so the body's thermoregulatory mechanisms are not triggered until lower temperatures. A forced-air warming device helps to prevent heat loss by convection, which accounts for approximately 30% of total heat loss.

Long Explanation
Heat loss from the body is by five main mechanisms, which are given varying levels of importance depending on which text you read, but generally the contribution of each is as follows: radiation 40%, convection 30%, evaporation 15%, respiration 10%, conduction 5%.

Patients undergoing anaesthesia have their physical and behavioural responses to cold abolished, and so it is down to the theatre team to ensure that heat loss via these routes is minimal.

Of the options provided in the question, the use of a forced-air warming device would help to prevent heat loss via convection, which can contribute up to 30% of total heat loss. Convection refers to the movement of molecules away from a warm object as a consequence of their reduced density as they gain heat and expand. This creates convection currents, which transfer heat away from the object.

Conduction of heat occurs between two objects in direct contact where a temperature gradient exists between them. It is of course extremely important to prevent a patient coming into contact with any metal objects during any operation because of the risks associated with the flow of electricity and pressure areas, as well as heat loss. But this contributes very little towards heat loss unless the area exposed is large, for example if the patient were lying on a cold metal table.

Evaporation refers to latent heat losses – i.e. when a liquid converts to a gas it needs to gain energy to do so, and this energy in the form of heat is taken from the patient. Heat lost through respiration is in the form of evaporative heat loss.

Several studies have shown that hypothermic patients have potentially severe physiological disturbances. A temperature of 36 °C is the standard used in NICE guidance, below which is termed inadvertent perioperative hypothermia.

Sullivan G, Edmondson C. Heat and temperature. *Contin Educ Anaesth Crit Care Pain* 2008; 8: 104–7. Available online at ceaccp.oxfordjournals.org/content/8/3/104 (accessed 30 June 2012).

SBA Question 87: Anaesthesia in a patient with Parkinson's disease

A patient with Parkinson's disease has undergone general anaesthesia for an upper limb orthopaedic procedure. Postoperatively he feels nauseated, but is not vomiting. He is due his next dose of oral dopaminergic agent shortly. Which one of the following is the best first-line antiemetic therapy in this case?

a) Metoclopramide intravenously
b) Domperidone orally
c) Prochlorperazine intramuscularly
d) Droperidol intravenously
e) Olanzapine orally

Answer: b

Short Explanation
Metoclopramide, droperidol and prochlorperazine may all cause Parkinsonism. Olanzapine does have antiemetic action, but is not first line here. Domperidone is a dopamine antagonist that does not cross the blood–brain barrier, so it is suitable for use in Parkinson's disease

Long Explanation
Parkinson's disease is a syndrome characterised by the triad of bradykinesia, tremor and rigidity. Postural instability is also a common feature. It is increasingly common with advancing age, with up to 3% of the population over the age of 66 years affected. It is caused by a reduction in dopaminergic activity in the basal ganglia, and therefore treatment is aimed at increasing central dopamine activity, or reducing the activity of the associated antagonistic cholinergic pathways.

Parkinson's disease manifests itself as a multisystem disorder, with many implications for anaesthesia:

- Airway. Sialorrhoea results, probably from less swallowing/dysphagia, and in association with an increased risk of gastro-oesophageal reflux represents an increased risk of aspiration.
- Respiratory. Respiratory function may be compromised by bradykinesia and chest wall muscle rigidity.
- Cardiovascular. Dysautonomia and drug-induced hypotension mean that haemodynamic instability may be problematic. Commonly used drugs also increase the risk of arrhythmias.
- Renal. Urinary retention is a common problem.
- Neurological. High risk of postoperative cognitive dysfunction (dementia is common), hallucinations and speech impairment. Patients can be very reliant on medications, and it is vital to ensure that times of drug administration are adhered to as rigidly as possible. It may be necessary to insert a nasogastric tube to ensure that medications can be given.
- Drug interactions. Many drugs have central dopaminergic or cholinergic actions – it is important to avoid these to avoid worsening of symptoms.

In the case given here, the first-line drug of choice would be domperidone (only available as an oral preparation – the intravenous preparation was withdrawn following multiple case reports of cardiac arrest associated with its use). Domperidone is a peripherally acting dopamine antagonist which has minimal central activity. Suitable alternatives would include intravenous serotonin antagonists (e.g. ondansetron), or antihistamines (e.g. cyclizine). Olanzapine does have antiemetic properties, but it is not commonly used for this purpose outside of malignancy-related emesis.

Nicholson G, Pereira AC, Hall GM. Parkinson's disease and anaesthesia. Br J Anaesth 2002; **89**: 904–16. Available online at bja.oxfordjournals.org/content/89/6/904 (accessed 30 June 2012).

SBA Question 88: Headache and chronic facial pain

A 32-year-old woman complains of headaches associated with photophobia, phonophobia and visual disturbances. It has a throbbing, pulsating quality with moderate to severe intensity, and lasts between 4 and 6 hours. Which of the following best describes this condition?

a) Migraine
b) Tension-type headache
c) Cluster headache
d) Trigeminal neuralgia
e) Post-herpetic neuralgia

Answer: a

Short Explanation
Migraine is a primary headache disorder characterised by the features described above. Tension-type headaches are described as generalised pressure or tightness in the head. Cluster headaches occur in attacks and are associated with autonomic hyperactivity. Trigeminal neuralgia and post-herpetic neuralgia tend to affect the face.

Long Explanation
Migraine is characterised by various combinations of neurological, autonomic and gastrointestinal symptoms. It is divided into two types: migraine without aura (70%) and migraine with aura (30%). Migraine with aura, previously termed classic migraine, has a reversible preceding aura comprising one or more of the following visual

disturbances: homonymous hemianopsia, tunnel vision, scotoma, photopsia. Migraine headache can be unilateral (60%) or bilateral (40%), located anywhere about the head or neck, and it lasts for 4–72 hours. It has a throbbing, pulsating quality with moderate to severe intensity, and numerous accompanying features including nausea (90%), vomiting (33%), vertigo, fatigue, confusion, ataxia, drowsiness, photophobia, phono-phobia and nasal congestion. Migraine is aggravated by postural change, activity and raised intracranial pressure. Migraine attacks are triggered by stress, menses, preg-nancy, dietary habit (e.g. red wine, cheese, chocolate and nuts), odours, light and poor sleep.

Tension-type headache is the most common primary headache disorder. These headaches are characterised by generalised pressure or tightness in the head. The discomfort is mild to moderate and is unaffected by activity. Nausea, photophobia or phonophobia are not prominent features.

Cluster headache is included in the trigeminal autonomic cephalagias and com-prises headache with signs of cranial autonomic hyperactivity. Attacks occur for a period of several weeks or months, then remit, leaving the patient pain-free for several months or years, only for the attacks to recur. The pain is so intense that the sufferer becomes extremely agitated and restless. One symptom of localised autonomic hyper-activity occurring in about 20% of patients is a Horner's syndrome, affecting the ipsilateral side. Unlike in migraine, nausea and vomiting are uncommon.

The hallmark of trigeminal neuralgia is agonising, paroxysmal lancinations con-fined strictly to one or more branches of the trigeminal nerve. Non-noxious stimuli trigger the pain, typically around the perioral region. The pain is nearly always unilateral.

Post-herpetic neuralgia consists of pain persisting in the zoster-affected dermatome at 3 months. It typically affects the first division of the trigeminal nerve and may be associated with trophic changes such as scarring, loss of pigmentation and allodynia.

Farooq K, Williams P. Headache and chronic facial pain. *Contin Educ Anaesth Crit Care Pain* 2008; **8**: 138–42. Available online at ceaccp.oxfordjournals.org/content/8/4/138 (accessed 30 June 2012).

SBA Question 89: Sub-Tenon's block

A 79-year-old male presents for cataract surgery. He has a past medical history of hypertension which is well controlled with medication, a previous myocardial infarc-tion (5 years ago), type 2 diabetes (tablet-controlled) and atrial fibrillation for which he takes warfarin. His current INR is 2.8. What is the most suitable course of action?

a) Advise the patient that the surgery will have to be cancelled as his INR is too high to safely carry out a regional anaesthetic technique today
b) Give 1 mg of vitamin K by slow intravenous injection, repeat his INR in 4 hours and proceed with surgery if it is < 2
c) Providing the surgeon is happy, proceed with surgery under general anaesthesia
d) Providing the surgeon is happy, proceed with surgery, performing a peribulbar block
e) Providing the surgeon is happy, proceed with surgery, performing a sub-Tenon's block

Answer: e

Short Explanation

Current guidelines recommend that in patients on warfarin, the INR should be checked to ensure it is within the normal range for the condition it is being used to treat (which is the case here). If so, consideration should be given to using either sub-Tenon's or topical anaesthesia. There is no reason to delay the operation, and sharp needle techniques should be avoided as they increase the risk of bleeding.

Long Explanation

This is not an uncommon case presenting on an eye list – a patient with multiple medical problems on warfarin. The current guidelines for cataract surgery from the Royal College of Ophthalmologists advise that for patients on warfarin the INR should be checked to ensure it is within the desired therapeutic range. Providing the INR is within the recommended range, if local anaesthesia is opted for, sub-Tenon's or topical anaesthesia should be considered, as sharp needle techniques increase the risk of orbital haemorrhage. It is suggested that if needle local anaesthesia is performed, the risk of orbital haemorrhage is increased by 0.2–1.0% from the normal population.

For the prevention of thromoembolic events in patients with atrial fibrillation, the National Institute for Health and Clinical Excellence (NICE) has published guidelines recommending that the therapeutic range of warfarin is for an INR between 2.0 and 3.0. In this case, the INR is within the recommended therapeutic range and therefore there is no need to delay surgery. A peribulbar block can be ruled out as a sharp needle technique increases the risk of orbital haemorrhage above that of a sub-Tenon's block. It would not be incorrect to continue with a general anaesthetic, but this is not the most suitable course of action, because a general anaesthetic in a patient with multiple comorbidities has significant risks. Also, the patient is diabetic and a local anaesthetic will allow him to resume a normal diet earlier than if he had a general anaesthetic.

This leaves the sub-Tenon's block as the most suitable answer. To perform such a block, topical local anaesthetic drops are instilled into the eye. The patient is then asked to look up and out to expose the inferonasal quadrant. The conjunctiva is then raised with Moorfield's forceps and a small incision made in the conjunctiva using Westcott spring scissors. A blunt, curved sub-Tenon cannula is inserted backwards beyond the equator and 3–5 mL of local anaesthetic solution is injected.

National Institute for Health and Clinical Excellence. *Atrial Fibrillation*. Quick Reference Guide. London: NICE, June 2006. Available online at www.nice.org. uk/nicemedia/live/10982/30054/30054.pdf (accessed 30 June 2012).

Nicholls B, Conn D, Roberts A. *The Abbott Pocket Guide to Practical Peripheral Nerve Blockade*. Abbott Anaesthesia, 2007; pp. 12–13.

Royal College of Ophthalmologists. *Cataract Surgery Guidelines*. London: RCO, 2004.

SBA Question 90: Neonatal/infant physiology

A category 1 caesarean section delivers an apnoeic, pale, floppy, 40-week-gestation baby covered in thin meconium. Which of these signs would be most likely to suggest that this baby is in primary rather than terminal apnoea?

a) Meconium stains the vocal cords and is suctioned from the lungs
b) Heart rate is approximately 70 beats per minute
c) Colour and tone improve with inflation breaths and chest compressions
d) The baby starts to display shuddering gasps
e) Approximately 5 minutes has passed since delivery

Answer: d

Short Explanation

Shuddering whole-body gasps at a rate of approximately 12 per minute occur at the end of the primary apnoea period. If the airway is unobstructed these gasps ventilate the lungs and the baby will often recover spontaneously. The other signs are non-specific.

Long Explanation

Primary and terminal apnoea are the result of a hypoxic insult to the neonate. The physiology of the neonate has developed to help it survive the normal birth process, which inherently involves periods of hypoxia. The initial effect of hypoxia on the neonate is to stimulate breathing. If the hypoxia persists then the child will lose consciousness. As hypoxia progresses the central stimulation of respiration is impaired and respiratory effort ceases. Cardiac metabolism shifts from aerobic to the less efficient anaerobic state and heart rate falls. This is termed primary apnoea.

If hypoxia continues, then primitive spinal centres initiate a rescue mechanism in the form of gasps. These shuddering whole-body movements aim to aerate the lungs and restore oxygenation. In most cases with an unobstructed airway this is successful. However, if the airway is not clear or the baby is still in utero then the gasping movements will gradually fade away. This is secondary or terminal apnoea, so called because, from this point, the neonate will not be able to establish ventilation for itself and without support will die. The whole process from onset of anoxia may take approximately 20 minutes.

Resuscitation involves ensuring the neonate is dry and warm, opening the airway, inflating the lungs and establishing ventilation. If the heart rate is low the baby may require chest compressions to move oxygenated blood from the lungs to the heart, converting the myocardium from anaerobic to aerobic conditions. If drugs are required in neonatal resuscitation the outcome is likely to be poor.

There has been debate about the significance of meconium in resuscitation of the newborn. In theory the aspiration of meconium in utero is more likely if gasping has taken place. This suggests that if meconium is suctioned from the lungs then it may be that the baby has reached terminal apnoea. In practice this convoluted reasoning is not overly useful, and resuscitation guidelines stipulate when tracheal toilet should take place.

Resuscitation Council UK. Newborn life support. Resuscitation Guidelines 2010. Available at www.resus.org.uklpages/guide.htm (accessed 30 June 2012).

Index

Printed in the United States
by Baker & Taylor Publisher Services

Printed in the United States
By Bookmasters